Clinical Research Made Easy®
A Guide to Publishing in Medical Literature

Clinical Research Made Easy®

A Guide to Publishing in Medical Literature

Second Edition

Revised and Edited by

Mohit Bhandari
MD PhD FRCSC

Professor and Head
Division of Orthopaedic Surgery
McMaster University
Hamilton, Ontario, Canada

Parag Kantilal Sancheti
FRCS (Ed) MS (Ortho) DNB (Ortho) MCh (UK)

Professor and Chairman
Sancheti Institute for Orthopaedics and Rehabilitation
Pune, Maharashtra, India

Foreword
KH Sancheti

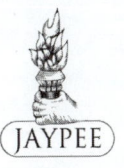

JAYPEE *The Health Sciences Publisher*
New Delhi | London | Panama

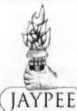

Jaypee Brothers Medical Publishers (P) Ltd

Headquarters

Jaypee Brothers Medical Publishers (P) Ltd
4838/24, Ansari Road, Daryaganj
New Delhi 110 002, India
Phone: +91-11-43574357
Fax: +91-11-43574314
Email: jaypee@jaypeebrothers.com

Overseas Offices

J.P. Medical Ltd
83 Victoria Street, London
SW1H 0HW (UK)
Phone: +44 20 3170 8910
Fax: +44 (0)20 3008 6180
Email: info@jpmedpub.com

Jaypee-Highlights Medical Publishers Inc
City of Knowledge, Bld. 235, 2nd Floor, Clayton
Panama City, Panama
Phone: +1 507-301-0496
Fax: +1 507-301-0499
Email: cservice@jphmedical.com

Jaypee Brothers Medical Publishers (P) Ltd
17/1-B Babar Road, Block-B, Shaymali
Mohammadpur, Dhaka-1207, Bangladesh
Mobile: +08801912003485
Email: jaypeedhaka@gmail.com

Jaypee Brothers Medical Publishers (P) Ltd
Bhotahity, Kathmandu, Nepal
Phone +977-9741283608
Email: kathmandu@jaypeebrothers.com

Website: www.jaypeebrothers.com
Website: www.jaypeedigital.com

© 2017, Jaypee Brothers Medical Publishers

The views and opinions expressed in this book are solely those of the original contributor(s)/author(s) and do not necessarily represent those of editor(s) of the book.

All rights reserved. No part of this publication may be reproduced, stored or transmitted in any form or by any means, electronic, mechanical, photocopying, recording or otherwise, without the prior permission in writing of the publishers.

All brand names and product names used in this book are trade names, service marks, trademarks or registered trademarks of their respective owners. The publisher is not associated with any product or vendor mentioned in this book.

Medical knowledge and practice change constantly. This book is designed to provide accurate, authoritative information about the subject matter in question. However, readers are advised to check the most current information available on procedures included and check information from the manufacturer of each product to be administered, to verify the recommended dose, formula, method and duration of administration, adverse effects and contraindications. It is the responsibility of the practitioner to take all appropriate safety precautions. Neither the publisher nor the author(s)/editor(s) assume any liability for any injury and/or damage to persons or property arising from or related to use of material in this book.

This book is sold on the understanding that the publisher is not engaged in providing professional medical services. If such advice or services are required, the services of a competent medical professional should be sought.

Every effort has been made where necessary to contact holders of copyright to obtain permission to reproduce copyright material. If any have been inadvertently overlooked, the publisher will be pleased to make the necessary arrangements at the first opportunity.

Inquiries for bulk sales may be solicited at: jaypee@jaypeebrothers.com

Clinical Research Made Easy®—A Guide to Publishing in Medical Literature

First Edition: 2010
Second Edition: **2017**
ISBN: 978-93-86056-09-2
Printed at Rajkamal Electric Press, Plot No. 2, Phase-IV, Kundli, Haryana.

Dedicated to

*our patients for whom the practice of evidence-based medicine informs
decisions to improve their lives and their futures*

Section Editors

Section 1: **Ilyas Aleem** MD FRCSC
University of Michigan
Ann Arbor, Michigan, USA

Section 2: **Moin Khan** MD MSc FRCSC
University of Michigan
Ann Arbor, Michigan, USA

Section 3: **Tahira Devji** PhD (Cand)
McMaster University
Hamilton, Ontario, Canada

Section 4: **Kim Madden** MSc
McMaster University
Hamilton, Ontario, Canada

Ydo V Kleinlugtenbelt MD
Deventer Hospital
Deventer, Overijssel, The Netherlands

Section 5: **Harman Chaudhry** MD MSc
McMaster University
Hamilton, Ontario, Canada

Raman Mundi MD MSc
McMaster University
Hamilton, Ontario, Canada

Section 6: **Nathan Evaniew** MD PhD
McMaster University
Hamilton, Ontario, Canada

Contributors

Akhila Rachakonda BMSc (Cand)
University of Western Ontario
London, Ontario, Canada

Alisha Garibaldi MSc
McMaster University
Hamilton, Ontario, Canada

Alonso Carrasco-Labra DDS PhD
McMaster University
Hamilton, Ontario, Canada

Andrew Duong MSc
McMaster University
Hamilton, Ontario, Canada

Anil Jain MS MAMS
Professor of Orthopaedics
University College of
Medical Sciences
University of Delhi, India

Arnav Agarwal BSc
McMaster University
Hamilton, Ontario, Canada

Ashok Rajgopalan MS MCh Ortho FRCS (Edinburgh)
Chairman, Bone and Joint Institute, Fortis Escorts
Okhla, Delhi, India and Fortis Memorial Research Institute
Gurgaon, Haryana, India

Ashok Shyam MS (Ortho)
Sancheti Institute for Orthopaedics and Rehabilitation
Pune, Maharashtra, India

Austin MacDonald MD
McMaster University
Hamilton, Ontario, Canada

Chloe Bedard BHSc
McMaster University
Hamilton, Ontario, Canada

Christopher Scott Smith MSc
OrthoEvidence
Burlington, Ontario, Canada

Chuan Silvia Li MSc (Cand)
McMaster University
Hamilton, Ontario, Canada

Colm McCarthy MDCM
McMaster University
Hamilton, Ontario, Canada

Enal Hindi BSc MHSc
Harvard University
Boston, Massachusetts, USA

Erika Arseneau MSc
McMaster University
Hamilton, Ontario, Canada

Feng Xie PhD
McMaster University
Hamilton, Ontario, Canada

Gurava Reddy MB D Ortho DNB Ortho MCh (Ortho) FRCS (Ed) FRCS (GI)
Managing Director and CEO
Chief of Division of Joint Replacement Surgery
Sunshine Hospitals
Secunderabad, Telangana
India

Hamza Jalal MD
University of Toronto
Toronto, Ontario, Canada

Hiba Mannan BSc MOptom
McMaster University
Hamilton, Ontario, Canada

Ilyas Aleem MD MSc FRCSC
University of Michigan
Ann Arbor, Michigan, USA

Jean-Eric Tarride PhD
McMaster University
Hamilton, Ontario, Canada

Kathleen G Dobson MSc
McMaster University
Hamilton, Ontario, Canada

Kerry Tai BSc
McMaster University
Hamilton, Ontario, Canada

Kim Madden MSc
McMaster University
Hamilton, Ontario, Canada

Lawrence Mbuagbaw MD PhD
McMaster University
Hamilton, Ontario, Canada

Lyubov Lytvyn MSc
McMaster University
Hamilton, Ontario, Canada
Oslo University Hospital
Oslo, Norway

Madhav Borate MS (Ortho)
Head of Academics
Sancheti Institute for Orthopaedics and Rehabilitation
Pune, Maharashtra, India

Mandeep Dhillon MS FRCS MAMS
Professor and Head
Department of Orthopaedics
PGIMER, Chandigarh, India

Manraj Kaur PT PhD (Cand)
McMaster University
Hamilton, Ontario, Canada

Mark Gichuru BSc CCRP
Global Research Solutions
Burlington, Ontario, Canada

Mark Phillips MSc (Cand)
McMaster University
Hamilton, Ontario, Canada

Mohit Bhandari MD PhD FRCSC
Professor and Head
Division of Orthopaedic Surgery
McMaster University
Hamilton, Ontario, Canada

Moin Khan MD MSc FRCSC
McMaster University
Hamilton, Ontario, Canada
University of Michigan
Ann Arbor, Michigan, USA

Nikhita Singhal BHSc MD (Cand)
McMaster University
Hamilton, Ontario, Canada

KH Sancheti MBBS FCPS D(Ortho) MS(Ortho) FICS FACS PhD FRCS
Founder-Sancheti Institute for Orthopaedics and Rehabilitation
Pune, Maharashtra, India

Parag Kantilal Sancheti FRCS (Ed) MS (Ortho) DNB (Ortho) MCh (UK)
Professor and Chairman
Sancheti Institute for Orthopaedics and Rehabilitation
Pune, Maharashtra, India

Patrick Thornley MD
McMaster University
Hamilton, Ontario, Canada

Rajeev Jetly BSc
McMaster University
Hamilton, Ontario, Canada

Raman Mundi MD MSc
McMaster University
Hamilton, Ontario, Canada

S Rajasekaran MS DNB FRCS(Ed) MCh (Liverpool) FACS PhD
Chairman
Ganga Hospital
Coimbatore, Tamil Nadu
India

Sarah Resendes MPH
Grand River Hospital
Waterloo, Ontario, Canada

Shakir Ahamed BSc
University of Western Ontario
London, Ontario, Canada

Sohail Sheriff MD
McMaster University
Hamilton, Ontario, Canada

Steve Rocha MS (Ortho)
Hand Surgeon
Sancheti Institute for Orthopaedics and Rehabilitation
Pune, Maharashtra, India

Tahira Devji PhD (Cand)
McMaster University
Hamilton, Ontario, Canada

Thuva Vanniyasingam PhD (Cand)
McMaster University
Hamilton, Ontario, Canada

Vijay Shetty MS (Ortho)
Fellow, Cambridge Hip and Knee Unit, Cambridge (UK)
Hiranandani Othopaedic Medical Education (HOME)
Dr L H Hiranandani Hospital
Mumbai, Maharashtra, India

Yashama Anwar BSc
McMaster University
Hamilton, Ontario, Canada

Ydo V Kleinlugtenbelt MD
Deventer Hospital
Deventer, Overijssel
The Netherlands

Zenon Sirko BSc (Cand)
University of Western Ontario
London, Ontario, Canada

Zohaib Ansari MD
University of Perpetual Help System
Biñan, Laguna, Philippines

Preface to the Second Edition

Since its inception approximately 26 years ago, evidence-based medicine (EBM) has become a standard part of many educational curricula worldwide. The concepts of EBM empower us to formulate appropriate clinical questions, appraise the literature using the hierarchy of evidence, and apply the study results to their practice. The application of evidence-based medicine is not easy. It requires a fundamental understanding of research methodology and critical appraisal. Critical concepts for health care providers include the strengths and limitations of meta-analyses, randomized trials, cohort studies and case series.

Although we may perceive that evidence-based medicine mandates a strict adherence to randomized trials, it more accurately involves informed and effective use of all types of evidences (from meta-analysis of randomized trials to individual case series and case reports). With the ever-increasing amount of available information, we must consider a shift in paradigm from traditional practice to one that involves question formulation, validity assessment of available studies and appropriate application of research evidence to individual patients.

The highly successful *Clinical Research Made Easy* has now been updated and revised in its Second Edition to offer a one-stop resource developed for the busy health care provider in mind.

We have assembled a group of leading researchers, surgeons and physicians with the aim of providing high quality content to our readers. Whether a practising surgeon, physician, physiotherapist, student or allied health care provider, this book bridges your knowledge gaps and facilitates practical application of EBM and clinical research. Led by practising physicians and researchers, we understand the challenges in research and provide simple guidelines for success. We distil complexities of clinical research into simple facts. Our question and answer format uses commonly asked questions in each topic area and provides focused summaries. We have further added new content including a summary of reporting guidelines, a more advanced discussion of sample size calculations and subgroup analyzes, additional details on ethics approval and consent forms, a new chapter about who does what on a study (study roles), and additional information on what happens after a study is completed, e.g. how to submit papers for publication, knowledge translation, and summaries of recommendations (GRADE).

In an emerging era of innovation in medicine and health care we have a responsibility to engage in the process of research acquisition, conduct and dissemination. We should no longer consider clinical research as only occurring in high profile institutions around the world, but rather occurring in every health care setting in all environments. Clinical research must be made easy to become widely accessible and widely applied.

Our vision towards a complete embrace of EBM comes one step closer with this second edition. We feel proud to support the new generation of evidence users and evidence providers with Clinical Research Made Easy!

Mohit Bhandari
Parag Kantilal Sancheti

Preface to the First Edition

Since its inception approximately 20 years ago, evidence-based medicine (EBM) has become a standard part of many educational curricula worldwide. In his original document to trainees at McMaster University, Professor Gordon Guyatt described EBM as an attitude of 'enlightened scepticism' toward the application of diagnostic, therapeutic, and prognostic technologies in their day-to-day management of patients." The concepts of EBM empower us to formulate appropriate clinical questions, appraise the literature using the hierarchy of evidence, and apply the study results to their practice. The application of evidence-based medicine is not easy. It requires a fundamental understanding of research methodology and critical appraisal. Critical concepts for health care providers include the strengths and limitations of meta-analyses, randomized trials, cohort studies and case series.

Although we may perceive that evidence-based medicine mandates a strict adherence to randomized trials, it more accurately involves informed and effective use of all types of evidence (from meta-analysis of randomized trials to individual case series and case reports). With the ever-increasing amount of available information, we must consider a shift in paradigm from traditional practice to one that involves question formulation, validity assessment of available studies and appropriate application of research evidence to individual patients.

For those of us wishing to produce high quality evidence to guide patient care, the good research practice is paramount. From beginning to end, the development of a quality study protocol, an appropriate statistical evaluation of sample size, the use of a valid outcome measure and sound ethical practices are basic requirements.

With the ever-increasing demands to adopt evidence-based medicine in practice, health care providers require educational resources that present the concepts of the EBM, research methodology and guides to publishing medical research in a simple and easy-to-understand format.

Clinical Research Made Easy is one resource developed with the busy health care provider in mind. We have assembled a group of leading researchers, surgeons and physicians with the aim of providing high quality content to our readers. Whether a practising surgeon, physician, physiotherapist, student or allied health care provider, this book bridges your knowledge gaps and facilitates practical application of EBM and clinical research. Led by practising physicians and researchers, we understand the challenges in research and provide simple guidelines for success. We distil complexities of clinical research into simple facts. Our question and answer format uses commonly asked questions in each topic area and provides focused summaries.

In an emerging era of innovation in medicine and health care we have a responsibility to engage in the process of research acquisition, conduct and dissemination. We should no longer consider clinical research as only occurring in high profile institutions around the world, but rather occurring in every health care setting in all environments. Clinical research must be made easy to become widely accessible and widely applied.

We hope this book provides one step in the right direction—and stimulates a new generation of evidence users and evidence providers!

Mohit Bhandari
Parag Kantilal Sancheti

Contents

SECTION 1: THE BASICS

1. **The Origins of Evidence-based Medicine**   3
   Mohit Bhandari, Parag Kantilal Sancheti
   - What is Evidence-based Medicine (EBM)? *3*
   - Through the Ages of EBM *4*
   - EBM and Modern Era *7*

2. **Why do we Need Evidence-based Medicine?**   9
   Hamza Jalal
   - Case Example *9*
   - What is EBM? *10*
   - Why do we Need EBM? *10*

3. **Tips to becoming an Evidence-based Clinician**   14
   Ilyas Aleem
   - Evidence-based Medicine (EBM) *14*
   - The PICO Question *15*
   - Conducting a Literature Search *16*

4. **Quality of Evidence—Has it Improved?**   21
   Enal Hindi
   - What are the Various Forms of Medical Literature Available? *21*
   - What is Current Medical Literature Used for? *22*

SECTION 2: CHOOSING THE RIGHT STUDY DESIGN

5. **Levels of Evidence—A Quick Guide**   33
   Yashama Anwar
   - What is the Hierarchy of Evidence? *33*
   - Levels of Evidence *34*
   - Types of Study Designs *34*
   - Different Types of Evidence *35*

6. Level 1 Evidence—Randomized Controlled Trials — 40
Zohaib Ansari, Hiba Mannan
- Hierarchy of Evidence: Level 1 *40*
- Key Features *41*
- Blinding *42*

7. Level 2 Evidence—Prospective Cohort Studies — 53
Sohail Sheriff
- What is a Prospective Cohort Study? *53*
- Where do Cohort Studies Rank in the Hierarchy of Evidence? *55*
- What are the Limitations of Prospective Cohort Studies? *55*
- How do we Select an Appropriate Cohort? *56*
- What Types of Bias Should we be Aware of? *57*

8. Level 3 Evidence—Case-control Studies — 63
Raman Mundi
- What is a Case-control Study? *63*
- Important Learning Points *69*

9. Level 4 Evidence—Clinical Case Series — 72
Shakir Ahamed
- What is a Clinical Case Series? *72*
- What are the Strengths of a Clinical Case Series? *73*
- What are the Limitations of a Clinical Case Series? *74*
- What Makes a Good Case Series? *76*

10. Level 5 Evidence—Surveys — 79
Arnav Agarwal
- What is a 'Survey'? *79*
- How are Surveys Important in Clinical Research? *80*
- How are Surveys Developed? *80*
- How are Surveys Administered? *83*
- How are Survey Results Reported? *84*
- What are Limitations of Survey Research? *85*
- How can Researchers Ensure Optimal Response Rates? *86*
- How can I Assess the Quality of Survey Research? *87*

SECTION 3: SPECIAL DESIGNS AND TOPICS

11. The Basics of Systematic Reviews and Meta-analysis — 95
Alonso Carrasco-Labra, Lyubov Lytvyn
- What is a 'Systematic Review'? *95*
- What is a 'Meta-analysis' and How it is Conducted? *100*
- How to Identify Credible Systematic Reviews *103*

12. The Basics of Economic Evaluation — 110
Manraj Kaur, Feng Xie, Tahira Devji
- What is Health Economics and Health Economic Evaluation? *110*
- Why should one Conduct an Economic Evaluation of Healthcare Interventions? *111*
- What are the Different Types of Health Economic Evaluation? *111*
- What are the Key Things to Consider When Conducting an Economic Evaluation? *116*
- Critically Appraising a Published Economic Evaluation *124*

13. The Basics of a Diagnostic Test Study — 133
Kathleen G Dobson, Alonso Carrasco-Labra, Raman Mundi, Steve Rocha
- What is a Diagnostic Test Study? *133*
- Why do we Need to Conduct Studies of a Diagnostic Test? *134*
- What Should be Considered to Conduct an Ideal Study of a Diagnostic Test? *135*
- What Results of the Diagnostic Test Study Should be Reported? *136*
- How are LR of a Diagnostic Test Incorporated into Clinical Practice? *141*
- Receiver Operating Characteristic (ROC) Curves *143*
- How do you Appraise a Study of a Diagnostic Test? *144*

14. The Basics of Reliability — 149
Chloe Bedard, Anil jain
- What is 'Reliability'? *149*
- What are the Different Measures of Reliability? *153*

- What are the Characteristics of a Reliability Study? *155*
- How do I Critically Appraise a Reliability Study? *159*

15. Quick Guide to Assess Risk of Bias in Randomized Controlled Trials — 163
Alonso Carrasco-Labra, Kathleen G Dobson
- Bias in Randomized Controlled Trials *163*
- Assessing Risk of Bias in RCTs *170*

16. GRADE—Understanding Grades of Healthcare Recommendations — 176
Mark Phillips, S Rajasekaran
- Overview of the GRADE Approach *176*
- Research Questions and Determining Important Outcomes *177*
- Factors to Increase the Quality of Evidence Rating *182*
- Formulating Recommendations from the Evidence *184*

SECTION 4: THE RESEARCH PROTOCOL

17. First Things First—The Research Proposal — 191
Andrew Duong, Chuan Silvia Li
- What is a Clinical Research Proposal? *191*

18. Choosing the Outcome—A Primer — 200
Alisha Garibaldi, Gurava Reddy
- What is an Outcome in a Clinical Study? *200*
- Why is Choosing the Right Outcome Important in Clinical Research? *200*
- How Many Outcomes can I Choose? *201*
- How do I Choose an Outcome for my Study? *201*
- What are Patient-important Outcomes? *202*
- What is a Measuring Instrument? *202*

19. Common Quality of Life and Health Utility Outcome Tools — 205
Rajeev Jetly, Ydo V Kleinlugtenbelt
- What is a 'Life and Health Utility Outcome Tool'? *205*

20. An Introduction to Sample Size — 217
Christopher Scott Smith, Ashok Shyam, Thuva Vanniyasingam

- What is Sample Size and Why does It Matter? *217*
- What should be Considered before Calculating Sample Size? *218*
- What is Needed to Calculate Sample Size for a Clinical Trial? *218*
- What are Some Common Pitfalls When Calculating Sample Size? *221*
- How do I Report Sample Size Calculations? *223*

21. Estimating an Appropriate Sample Size—Advanced Concepts, Formulae and Examples — 227
Thuva Vanniyasingam, Lawrence Mbuagbaw, Christopher Scott Smith

- What Basic Components are Needed for Sample Size Estimations? *227*
- What are the Basic Steps for Sample Size Estimation? *228*
- What are the three Types of Comparisons Made in Randomized Controlled Trials? *228*
- Why is Hypothesis Testing Important in RCTs? *229*
- How do I Manually Estimate Sample Size? *230*
- What Programs are Available for Sample Size Estimation? *236*

22. Planning your Analysis—Keep it Simple — 241
Kerry Tai, Kim Madden, Ashok Rajgopalan

- Types of Data *241*
- Descriptive Statistics *243*
- Hypothesis Testing *246*
- How to Analyze your Data *246*
- Statistical Significance vs Clinical Significance *249*

23. What are Subgroup Analyses and How should You Interpret Them? — 252
Erika Arseneau, Jean-Eric Tarride

- What is a Subgroup Analyses? *252*
- What does a Well-designed Subgroup Analysis Consist of? *253*

- Why do Subgroup Analyses have Such a Bad Reputation? *254*
- A Classic Example of Subgroup Analysis Gone Wrong *257*
- How are Subgroup Analyses Performed? *257*
- How are Subgroup Analyses Reported? *258*
- Guidelines for Interpretation and Application of Subgroup Analysis *258*
- Can you Compare Results of Subgroup Analyses from Different Studies? *259*

SECTION 5: DOING RESEARCH

24. Study Roles—Who does What? 265
Mark Gichuru, Madhav Borate
- What are the Roles of a Principal Investigator? *265*
- What do I Need to Become a Principal Investigator? *267*
- What are the Roles of the Research Coordinator? *267*
- What do I Need to Become a Research Coordinator? *269*
- What are the Roles of the Clinical Trial Monitor? *269*
- What do I Need to Become a Clinical Research Associate/Assistant? *270*
- What are the Roles of the Clinical Research Nurse? *270*

25. Research Ethics Approval—A must Before any Clinical Trial 275
Zenon Sirko, S Rajasekaran
- What is 'Research Ethics' and Why is it Important? *275*

26. Why do we Need Patient Consent? Designing a Good Consent Form 283
Chuan Silvia Li, Madhav Borate
- What is Patient Informed Consent? *283*
- What are the Key Steps in the Informed Consent Process? *285*
- What are the General Guidelines on Designing Patient Informed Consent Forms (ICFs)? *286*

Contents

27. Collecting Data—It all Begins with a Good Data Form — 297
Nikhita Singhal, Steve Rocha
- What is a Data Form and Why is it Needed? *297*

SECTION 6: GETTING THE WORD OUT—PRESENTATION AND PUBLICATION

28. Creating an Impactful Slide Presentation — 309
Colm McCarthy, Mandeep Dhillon
- What is a Slide Presentation? *309*
- What is a Great Slide Presentation? *310*

29. Writing a Good Clinical Research Paper — 316
Sarah Resendes, Ashok Shyam
- Why is Scientific Writing Important? *316*

30. Making Sense of Reporting Guidelines — 324
Akhila Rachakonda, Kim Madden
- Why do we Need Reporting Guidelines and Checklists? *324*

31. Submitting a Paper for Publication—A Guide to Success — 331
Patrick Thornley
- How do I Select Which Journal to Submit my Research Paper to? *331*
- How do I Prepare my Manuscript for Submission? *333*
- How do I Navigate the Online Submission Process? *335*
- How do I Effectively Respond to Reviewers' Comments? *337*

32. Knowledge Translation 101—Maximizing Impact — 339
Austin MacDonald, Vijay Shetty
- What is Knowledge Translation? *339*

Glossary — 345

Index — 363

1

The Basics

Section Outline

1. The Origins of Evidence-based Medicine
2. Why do we Need Evidence-based Medicine?
3. Tips to becoming an Evidence-based Clinician
4. Quality of Evidence—Has it Improved?

1
The Origins of Evidence-based Medicine

Mohit Bhandari, Parag Sancheti

Key Objectives

- Become familiar with the concepts behind evidence-based medicine.
- Understand the history of evidence-based medicine with various examples.
- Learn how evidence-based medicine is used in the modern world.

What is Evidence-Based Medicine (EBM)?

Evidence-based medicine is a term that was coined by Professor Gordon Guyatt in 1990 at McMaster University in Hamilton, Ontario while he was preparing a document for applicants to the International Medicine Residency Program.[1] Even though the term EBM may seem to be fairly new, its overall teachings and fundamentals have been around for many centuries.

Evidence-based medicine is defined as the systematic approach for finding and analyzing the best available evidence and using it for the basis of clinical decision-making.[1,2] This concept is very important for physicians and other healthcare workers as they are required to use current research findings and data to diagnose and treat patients. Due to the rapid pace of modern day research, however, keeping up with current research findings may be a daunting task. This is where EBM comes in, as it effectively bridges the gap between the best available evidence and the physician.[1]

Essentially, EBM is about asking important questions based on the patients' needs, findings and appraising the relevant data, then using the data for best patient care.

Through the Ages of EBM

There are three main periods in the development of EBM, each of which made a unique contribution to the modern day approach of EBM. The periods are as follows:

Ancient Era

The ancient era involved the use of anecdotes, transmitted primarily through authoritative means and stories. The concept of EBM was loosely termed during this time period.[2] An example can be seen in biblical accounts of healing:

Then Daniel said to the guard, 'Eat only vegetables and drink only water for 10 days. Then compare your looks with that of young men and be guided in your treatment by what you see.' The guard listened to what Daniel said and tested it for 10 days. At the end of the 10 days he looked healthier and was better nourished than all the young men.[2]

In this example, one can loosely see the modern teachings of EBM through biblical accounts. Daniel is providing a treatment to the guard's disease based on the guard's symptoms.

Renaissance Era

The renaissance era began during the 17th century and coincided with challenges and objections to popular theories.[2] Also, during this time period, one could see the development of journals and textbooks which contained various conclusions of research findings. From this period of time, the two examples of EBM include ***bloodletting*** and ***scurvy***.

- ***Bloodletting:*** Bloodletting is the removal of high quantity of blood from an individual to help, prevent or cure disease. The concept dates back to the Egyptian era and it spread to the Greeks and Romans.[3] This concept started to be questioned near the 17th century. Despite the disputes, challenges, and conflicting data over bloodletting;

brochures and pamphlets were still being written regarding its use and advantages.[2,3] Near the end of the 19th century, the practice of bloodletting vanished as it was deemed an ineffective tool against disease.[3]

- It is very important to realize the connection between bloodletting and EBM. Through the 16th and 17th century, bloodletting was a common tool used to cure disease and illness, though once research refuted its claims, the practices diminished. Most importantly, due to conflicting evidence, physicians stopped the use of bloodletting.[2] This shows the importance of keeping current with new findings in research.
- Interestingly enough, even though evidence against bloodletting was found in the 17th century, it was still used until the late 19th century. This brings about another important characteristic of EBM, which deals with the fact that evidence is neither easily nor rapidly translated into practice. Once again, it is ultimately up to the physician to keep up with current research findings.

- ***Scurvy:*** Today, we know that scurvy is a disease caused by prolonged deficiency of vitamin C. It is a disease that can lead to anemia, ulceration of the gums, and hemorrhages into the skin.[4] The discovery, prevention and cure of the disease is an interesting example of EBM in the renaissance era.

  - Scurvy was interestingly discovered and cured at sea during the 1700s by a physician turned sailor known as Dr James Lind.[2,5] While at sea, there was lack of fruits and vegetables to eat and thus, the sailors did not get the proper nutrients that they needed.[2] Most often, the sailors had rotting gums, weak knees, and were often very sick. Lind then decided to experiment on his fellow crew members by giving each of them something different to eat. Some were given nutmeg, while others were given lemons and oranges.[2,5] After 6 days of duty, Lind saw sudden and visible positive effects on the patients who ate lemons and oranges.[5] From this simple experiment he concluded that lemons and oranges were the best treatment for distemper (scurvy) at sea.

- **How does this relate to EBM?** At first, due to a lack of data, the use of lemons and oranges as a cure for scurvy was limited and remained speculative. However, due to his discovery, clinical trials were conducted and evidences were gathered. Scurvy was better understood and treatments were incorporated in clinical practice.[2] This was one of the first moves away from clinical expertise and towards EBM.

Transitional Era

The transitional era began during the mid to late 19th century and lasted till the 1970s. A very important individual in this era was Ernest Amory Codman who has been called the pioneer of EBM.[5]

Codman was important in the development of a concept known as 'the end result'.[2] Essentially, the idea behind the end result was that hospitals should follow-up with patients who have been treated, for long enough, to determine if the treatment was successful.[2,6] If the treatment was unsuccessful then the physician should ask themselves why the treatment was unsuccessful. With the overall goal of preventing failures in the future, Codman's methodology worked by the development of 5–8 inch cards that surgeons would use to write characteristics of the patient before and after the treatment.[6] These cards were then brought back to the hospital 1 year later and the treatment was evaluated on the terms of overall success. This was extremely important as this provided hospitals a method to compare the various treatments given by surgeons and physicians to determine which treatments were the most effective and successful.[2,6]

Initially, Codman's ideas were very controversial due to the fact that a surgeon's success was measured by status and seniority rather than the outcomes of surgery and success rate. In modern medicine, however, Codman's concepts were nothing short of brilliant in the development of EBM. Due to Codman's work, registries were created to record outcomes of research and establish important standards. This was very important in the modern era of EBM.

EBM and Modern Era

The modern era of EBM began during the mid to late 20th century with the involvement of two important figures: Archie Cochrane and David Sackett. This era was very important for EBM as it lead to the biggest development of what we now know as ***randomized controlled trials (RCT)***.[2,7] Cochrane was effectively the first to show the importance, significance, and effectiveness of using RCTs for assessing treatments.[2] His work led to the formation of the Cochrane Center, which later was known as the ***Cochrane Collaboration***. The Cochrane Collaboration is very important in evaluating, monitoring, and producing RCTs in almost all areas of medicine.[2] Also, as you will learn later in this book, the Cochrane Collaboration is very important in the further evaluation and production of systematic reviews of healthcare interventions as well as the promotion for the use of clinical trials.

Another key figure in the modern era of EBM is David Sackett. He is effectively credited for defining the use and applicability of EBM in clinical practice.[2] As we will see in coming chapters, Sackett proposed that EBM is a clinical tool, to be used as a guide to supplement conventional methods of decision-making in healthcare. It cannot be used in isolation without consideration of the values and ideas of the individual patient, nor is it a substitute for clinical expertise.[2]

Important Learning Points

- The term 'EBM' was coined by Gordon Guyatt at McMaster University in Hamilton, Ontario.
- There are three main eras of EBM—the Ancient era, Transitional era and Renaissance era.
- The modern era of EBM involved two important figures, namely Archie Cochrane and David Sackett.

Definitions

Cochrane Collaboration: A non-profit organization that aims to provide current and readily available healthcare information worldwide.

Randomized controlled trials: A study designed to determine a cause-effect relationship between treatment groups and/or control group. RCTs involve a randomization process to assign patients to each group.

REFERENCES

1. Bhandari M, Joensson A. Historical perspectives of clinical research. Clinical Research for Surgeons. Thieme Publishing Group, New York. 2009.
2. Claridge JA, Fabian TC. History and development of evidence-based medicine. World J Surg. 2005;29(5):547-53.
3. Power D. The decay of bloodletting 1909. Practitioner. 2009; 253(1717):20.
4. Glouberman S. Knowledge transfer and the complex story of scurvy. J Eval Clin Pract. 2009;15(3):553-7.
5. Doherty S. History of evidence-based medicine. Oranges, chloride of lime and leeches: barriers to teaching old dogs new tricks. Emerg Med Australas. 2005;17(4):314-21.
6. Kaska SC, Weinstein JN. Historical perspective. Ernest Amory Codman 1869–1940. A pioneer in evidence-based medicine: the end result idea. Spine. 1998;23(5):629-33.
7. Worrall J. What is evidence in evidence-based medicine. Philosophy of Science. 2000;69:316-30.

2 Why do we Need Evidence-based Medicine?

Hamza Jalal

Key Objectives

- Demonstrate that evidence-based medicine is an important component of the clinical decision making process
- Understand the benefits of EBM including the tools to critically evaluate new clinical knowledge; providing a standardized approach; enabling information consolidation and facilitating ongoing medical education.

Case Example

Individuals with atherosclerotic disease of the heart vasculature are vulnerable to sudden occlusion syndromes such as myocardial ischemia. Those with severe disease can undergo bypass surgery, which circumvents the diseased vessel, in order to maintain viable heart function. Likewise for brain vasculature, it was hypothesized that individuals with symptomatic atherosclerotic disease of the internal carotid artery may benefit from bypass surgery of the extracranial and intracranial arteries, again circumventing the problematic portion of the vessel, in order to prevent future cerebral ischemic events. A randomized controlled trial (RCT) by Barnett et al. (1985) not only failed to demonstrate the benefit of surgery, it in fact, demonstrated substantially worse outcomes when compared to the non-surgical group.[1] This example neatly illustrates the virtues of evidence-based medicine (***EBM***).

What is EBM?

The term EBM was coined by Gordon Guyatt in 1990[2] but has its origins extending all the way to the ancient times (see previous chapter). A widely used definition is that EBM is the 'integration of clinical expertise, patient values, and the best research evidence into the decision of making process for patient care'.[2]

It is worth highlighting that EBM is a clinical tool, used as a guide to supplement conventional methods of decision-making. It is not used as a cookbook approach to medicine, and it certainly cannot be used in isolation without consideration of the values and ideas of the individual patient. Therefore, finding research studies and evaluating data with respect to specific clinical inquiries is simply one, though vital, aspect of EBM.

Why do we Need EBM?

EBM vs Conventional Medicine

Conventional medicine, especially prior to the advent of EBM, was often grounded on intuition, guesswork and personal experiences. With time, this knowledge was increasingly predicated on advances in the basic sciences such as anatomy, physiology, biochemistry and genetics, among others. Ultimately, significant medical breakthroughs and advances were made owing to this flourishing expertise. A good example would be the discovery of penicillin, discovered entirely by accident, but with wide clinical application that initially was borne of observations at the basic science level.[3] Later studies would extend its use to many conditions and spawn a myriad of newer antibiotic drugs.

Yet, expertise can be misleading too, as is illustrated poignantly in the case example discussed earlier. Grounded in physiology and anatomy, with an entirely rational analogy using the heart, the hypothesis that bypass surgery of the intracranial and extracranial vasculature would lead to decreased cerebral outcomes made sense. The surgery was performed in many hospitals throughout the world. Yet, through the application of the principles of EBM, it was clear that the hypothesis was incorrect, and unfortunately, even more harmful than conservative approaches.

Once again, it is worth highlighting that expertise and EBM are not mutually exclusive. In fact, as in the case of penicillin, although expertise initially introduced the drug, it was the principle of EBM that helped to refine its use to specific patient indications and pathogens.

Alternative to EBM

The amalgamation of clinical expertise and EBM provides a powerful and transparent method to observe, evaluate, and ultimately benefit patients and advance scientific knowledge. In spite of this, however, certain practitioners of alternative and complementary medicines such as homeopathic physicians, traditional Chinese medics and bonesetters may have a tendency to rely on personal experience, anecdotal evidence, authority figures and tradition.[4] It is not within the scope of this book to evaluate each of these professions, however, as a general statement, these approaches often lack transparency and do not allow for appropriate hypothesis testing. In this respect, it resembles the pre-EBM conventional medicine practice, which was illustrated earlier and can be easily misguided. The principles of EBM require the aggregation and collection of a wide body of evidence, from many different sources, for valid conclusions to be formed with a reasonable degree of confidence. In its absence, there is little objective evidence to provide confidence in the claims of a health practitioner, and thus the patient is vulnerable to harm.

EBM Guidelines to Evaluate the Quality of Evidence

As just mentioned, claims are useful to an extent that a reasonable degree of confidence can be ascertained. One of the functions of EBM is to provide the appropriate methodology to evaluate the quality of the evidence in a systematic manner. Literature can be evaluated based on a hierarchy of the strength of evidence. For example, case reports would rank lower in strength when compared to observational studies, which, in turn would rank lower than an RCT. This will be further explored in the following chapters.

Moreover, within each type of study, there are specific, standardized statistical measures that best approximate the size of an effect, the significance of the data, and the precision and accuracy associated with them. Thus, not only are the types of studies themselves important, but also the specific data gathering and analysis within each study, which together provide objective and measurable ways to assess quality of evidence.

EBM Provides a Common Language and Consolidates Information

Ours is an exciting time to be in medicine. With the tremendous and rapid advancement in technology and communication, every region of the world is actively contributing new medical observations and evidences, and with wide global access just a few clicks away. EBM not only provides the tools to critically evaluate these data, but also standardizes their presentation and reporting. This allows aggregation of data, and in turn, facilitates new discoveries while enabling cross-collaboration. The enabling of a standardized language is also useful in the creation of guidelines and standards against which performance of individual physician, therapies and interventions can be assessed. This has important implications for guideline development, quality improvement, medico-legal issues, education and research.

EBM Facilitates Continuing Medical Education

Medical knowledge is expanding at an exponential speed and it is impossible for an individual physician or healthcare worker to stay current with the daily stream of new studies and discoveries. Fortunately, EBM provides the tools and hierarchy of evidence that can facilitate learning and education to stay up-to-date, without individually investing the time and effort required. For example, systematic reviews provide the highest level of evidence, and summarize the accumulation of trials, case reports and observations pertaining to a specific clinical question. Thus, whether vitamin C supplements are helpful in treating common cold requires a simple literature search for systematic reviews, which within a few moments will provide a summary of the best available evidence and thus facilitates clinical decision-making, all without having to conduct your own trials or analyzing numerous individual studies.

Summary

EBM is a useful tool to help guide clinical decision-making, supplementing, and incorporating medical expertise with patient values and preferences. It is an objective and transparent methodology to critically assess the quality of evidence. Through standardized and systematic methodology, it facilitates advancement in medical knowledge by enabling collaboration, information consolidation and ongoing education.

Definition

Evidence-based medicine: The integration of clinical expertise, patient values and the best research evidence into the decision making process for patient care.

REFERENCES

1. Barnett. Failure of extracranial-intracranial arterial bypass to reduce the risk of ischemic stroke. Results of an international randomized trial. The EC/IC Bypass Study Group. N Engl J Med. 1985;313(19):1191-200.
2. Fleming A. On the antibacterial action of cultures of a penicillium, with special reference to their use in the isolation of B. influenzae. 1929. Bull World Health Organ. 2001;79(8):780-90.
3. Guyatt G., Rennie, D. Users' guides to the medical literature: a manual for evidence-based clinical practice. AMA press Chicago, IL. 2002.
4. Goldacre B. Bad Science: Quacks, Hacks, and Big Pharma Flacks. 2010.

3 Tips to becoming an Evidence-based Clinician

Ilyas Aleem

Key Objectives

- Understand the concepts behind practicing evidence-based medicine in the clinical setting.
- Learn the role of the physician in evidence-based medicine.
- Become familiar with the overall process of incorporating the principles of evidence-based medicine in daily practice.

Evidence-Based Medicine (EBM)

Evidence-based medicine aims to improve the quality of care through the integration of best research evidence with clinical expertise and patient preferences.[1] The next section discusses the application of EBM into daily practice, with an example from orthopedic surgery. In 2005, Akobeng introduces the five-step EBM model.[2]

1. Identify the problem and convert the information required into an answerable question.
2. Search the literature for relevant clinical articles to answer the question.
3. Evaluate (critically appraise) the evidence with regards to its validity and applicability to the current clinical question.
4. Apply the appraised evidence to the clinical and patient context.
5. Evaluate/audit performance and improve the above mentioned steps.

Consider the case of a middle-aged patient presenting to an orthopedic spine surgeon after an isolated burst fracture of the thoracolumbar spine. The patient has no neurological deficits. His computed tomography (CT) scan shows 20 degrees of kyphotic deformity and 30% retropulsion of bone into the canal. The patient has considerable back pain and the orthopedic spine the orthopedic spine surgeon will decide whether to proceed with conservative or surgical treatment.[3] Surgical stabilization and possible decompression may result in earlier mobilization, reduced time to hospital discharge, and faster return to work[4], but it may also involve higher early complication rates, increased risk for subsequent revision surgery and greater overall healthcare costs.[4] Non-operative management that involves symptomatic pain control, mobilization as tolerated, and possibly a brace may be an acceptable alternative in properly selected patients.[5, 6] The orthopedic spine surgeon is deciding what would be the best treatment option for this patient.

The PICO Question

Given that this patient is presenting with a thoracolumbar burst fracture and is neurologically intact, it is important to ask a relevant ***research question*** to initiate the EBM approach. The question, arguably the most important step of the EBM process, can relate to diagnosis, prognosis, treatment, harm, quality of care or health economics.[7] When deciding on a question, it is important to ask questions that pertain to the specific needs of the patient.[2] Five components have been suggested for an appropriate clinical question:[8, 9]

1. ***Patient population:*** Specify the patient population, considering gender, age or disease factors that may be relevant.
2. ***Intervention:*** Specify the treatment, exposure or maneuver that is being evaluated.
3. ***Comparison:*** Specify the comparison group, which may be another intervention, sham/placebo, the previous gold standard, or no treatment.
4. ***Outcome:*** This should ideally be an endpoint important to patients, consisting of a primary outcome, secondary outcome or composite outcome.
5. ***Time:*** Specify the time at which the outcome of interest will be assessed.

Furthermore, it is important to first analyze the important characteristics that the patient possesses and try to formulate a question that is appropriately specific. The key features of this patient is that she is presenting with an acute thoracolumbar burst fracture of the spine, is neurologically intact, and has a CT scan showing a kyphotic deformity of the spine with some retropulsion of bone into the canal. An appropriate question which gives this clinical scenario would be, 'In a neurologically intact patient presenting with a thoracolumbar burst fracture, does surgical versus non-surgical treatment result in superior clinical outcomes?'

Conducting a Literature Search

After formulating a clear and concise question, the next step is to conduct a comprehensive literature search and find the best evidence in order to properly treat the patient. After converting the clinical problem into an answerable question, Akobeng suggests several strategies to appropriately conduct a literature search. These are as follows:

- ***Generate appropriate keywords:*** Based on the clinical question, an appropriate word list can be generated. For example, from the clinical question presented here, the following keywords could be used for the search: thoracolumbar burst fracture (patient or problem); neurologically intact (patient or problem); surgical treatment (intervention).
- ***Choose a bibliographic database:*** Numerous online databases are available, including MEDLINE, EMBASE, and the Cochrane Library databases. A combination of databases may also be used.
- ***Conduct the search:*** The search can be run using the keywords in the various databases, usually combined with Boolean operators such as 'AND' and 'OR'.[11]

Now back to the example: a recent ***Cochrane Review*** is found in the literature evaluating outcomes of surgical versus non-surgical treatment after thoracolumbar burst fractures without neurologic deficit.[12] Authors performed a systematic review and meta-analysis of two randomized or quasi-randomized controlled trials (total, n = 87) for comparing surgical treatment with non-surgical treatment. Quasi-randomized trials use non-random methods of allocation such as alternation to assign participants to the comparison group. They raise the possibility of selection bias because the treatment allocation can be predicted before potential patients are enrolled.[13] Functional outcomes were reported according to the Roland-Morris Disability Questionnaire (RMDQ), a well-validated, patient-reported outcome measure for back pain.[14] However, the RMDQ does not address psychological or social dysfunction and is most useful when the disability level is only low to moderate.[15, 16]

Critically Appraising Literature

The next step is to ***critically appraise*** the studies which were found in order to determine their clinical relevance and accuracy. The physician has to be able to discern whether an article can be relied on to give clinical guidance. Unfortunately, a large portion of published medical literature is not relevant or does not have adequate methodology, so is unreliable.[17] ***Critically appraising literature*** involves the use of asking key questions about the validity of the evidence and its relevance to a specific patient population. Several easy-to-use guides and checklists have been developed to aid the physician in critically appraising studies and determining quality such as the JAMA User's Guide. Tools used in orthopedic surgery include the Oxman and Guyatt Index which is used to evaluate the scientific quality of a systematic review.

Upon further appraisal of the Cochrane review, it is found that substantial clinical heterogeneity and a general lack of randomized trials limited the ability of the authors to provide definitive treatment recommendations. One of the included studies by Siebenga et. al.[18] compared surgical treatment with short-segment posterior only stabilization followed by a Jewett hyperextension orthosis, whereas the other randomized controlled trial by Wood et al. used posterior or anterior fusion and instrumentation.[19] This meta-analysis was not able to address other controversial management issues such as the level and classification of thoracolumbar fractures, the optimal timing of surgery in spinal trauma, surgical approach, or the role of bone graft in addition to fusion. Based on the limited evidence, however, it was concluded that operative treatment of thoracolumbar burst fractures without neurologic deficit did not appear to cause any significant advantage over non-operative treatment. A more recent review done by Gnanenthiran et al. included two additional trials and had the same conclusions; although operative management of thoracolumbar burst fractures without neurologic deficit may improve residual kyphotic deformity of the spine, no improvement in pain, function or return to work was noted at an average of 4 years after injury.[20] Furthermore, surgery was associated with higher complications and costs.

In the context of limited healthcare resources and to minimize patient risk, clinicians must carefully allocate healthcare resources to patients who would likely benefit from a given intervention. Given the results of these two reviews suggesting equivocal outcomes after surgical and non-surgical treatment of this fracture, a discussion ensued with the patient regarding the results and limitations of the best available evidence taking into account clinician experience and patient preferences. The patient proceeded with non-operative treatment with symptomatic pain control and mobilization as tolerated and close follow-up. Appropriate follow-up in subsequent appointments showed that the patient responded well to non-operative treatment with near complete resolution of pain and return to full activity.

Important Learning Points

- Formulating a research question is a key step in the EBM process. The question can relate to diagnosis, prognosis, treatment, iatrogenic harm, quality of care or health economics.
- Search the literature using a comprehensive and thorough search strategy.
- Critically appraise the studies found in order to determine the clinical relevance and accuracy of the literature.
- When applying the evidence to patient care, take into consideration clinician expertise and patient preferences.

Definitions

Critical appraisal: Systematically judging the validity, applicability and methodological quality of research.

Research question: The question that the investigator(s) intend to answer using research methodology. Developing a clear research question is the first step in conducting a research project.

REFERENCES

1. Sackett DL, Rosenberg WM, Gray JA, et al. Evidence-based medicine: what it is and what it isn't. BMJ. 1996;312(7023):71-2.
2. Akobeng AK. Principles of evidence-based medicine. Arch Dis Child. 2005;90(8):837-40.
3. Aleem IS, Nassr A. Cochrane in CORR: Surgical versus non-surgical treatment for thoracolumbar burst fractures without neurological deficit. Clin Orthop Relat Res. 2016;474(3):619-24.
4. Thomas KC, Bailey CS, Dvorak MF, et al. Comparison of operative and nonoperative treatment for thoracolumbar burst fractures in patients without neurological deficit: A systematic review. J Neurosurg Spine. 2006;4(5):351-8.
5. Bailey CS, Urquhart JC, Dvorak MF, et al. Orthosis versus non-orthosis for the treatment of thoracolumbar burst fractures without neurologic injury: A multicenter prospective randomized equivalence trial. Spine J. 2014;14(11):2557-64.
6. Cantor JB, Lebwohl NH, Garvey T, et al. Nonoperative management of stable thoracolumbar burst fractures with early ambulation and bracing. Spine. 1993;18(8):971-6.
7. Richardson WS, Wilson MC, Nishikawa J, et al. The well-built clinical question: A key to evidence-based decisions. ACP J Club. 1995;123(3):12-3.
8. Wyatt J, Guly H. Identifying the research question and planning the project. Emerg Med J. 2002;19(4):318-21.
9. Stone PW. Popping the (PICO) question in research and evidence-based practice. Appl Nurs Res. 2002;15(3):197-8.
10. Haynes RB, Sackett DL, Guyatt GH, Tugwell P. Clinical epidemiology: how to do clinical practice research, 3rd edition. Philadelphia: Lippincott Williams & Wilkins; 2006.
11. Craig JV, Smyth RL. The evidence-based manual for nurses, 3rd edition. London: Churchill Livingstone Elsevier; 2012.
12. Abudou M, Chen X, Kong X, et al. Surgical versus non-surgical treatment for thoracolumbar burst fractures without neurological deficit. Cochrane database syst rev. 2013;6:CD005079.

13. Kunz R, Vist G, Oxman AD. Randomization to protect against selection bias in healthcare trials. Cochrane Database Syst Rev. 2007;18(2):MR000012.
14. Roland M, Morris R. A study of the natural history of back pain. Part I: development of a reliable and sensitive measure of disability in low-back pain. Spine. 1983;8(2):141-4.
15. Deyo RA, Battie M, Beurskens AJ, et al. Outcome measures for low-back pain research. A proposal for standardized use. Spine. 1998;23(18):2003-13.
16. Roland M, Fairbank J. The Roland-Morris disability questionnaire (RMDQ) and the Oswestry Disability Questionnaire. Spine. 2000;25(24):3115-24.
17. Rosenberg W, Donald A. Evidence-based medicine: An approach to clinical problem-solving. BMJ. 1995;310(6987):1122-6.
18. Siebenga J, Leferink VJ, Segers MJ, et al. Treatment of traumatic thoracolumbar spine fractures: A multicenter prospective randomized study of operative versus nonsurgical treatment. Spine. 2006;31(25):2881-90.
19. Wood K, Buttermann G, Mehbod A, et al. Operative compared with nonoperative treatment of a thoracolumbar burst fracture without neurological deficit. A prospective, randomized study. J Bone Joint Surg Am. 2003;85(5):773-81.
20. Gnanenthiran SR, Adie S, Harris IA. Nonoperative versus operative treatment for thoracolumbar burst fractures without neurologic deficit: A meta-analysis. Clin Orthop Relat Res. 2012;470(2):567-77.

4

Quality of Evidence—Has it Improved?

Enal Hindi

Key Objectives
- Learn about the various forms of medical literature.
- Learn about the uses of medical literature.
- Understand the issues with regards to assessing the quality of the medical literature.
- Understand the ongoing challenges and solutions of incorporating evidence based medicine into clinical practice.
- Understand the unique challenges in surgical research.
- Learn about different ways to assess and evaluate the quality of evidence in surgical research.

What are the Various Forms of Medical Literature Available?

There are many different forms of literature used by the medical community for the transfer of information. These include scientific journal articles, medical textbooks and meeting abstracts. Journals are frequently released publications of a collection of related research articles in a particular area. Medical practitioners in all specialties are now faced with the concept of integrating personal clinical expertise with the best external clinical evidence from very up-to-date and validated medical research.[1] Journals that are of utmost importance to the medical community are peer-reviewed journals. This means that each article has been reviewed by experts in the field to ensure that the research findings that are being published are relevant, appropriate and they meet the standard criteria for publication.

Journal articles give medical professionals easy access to current available evidence from research studies that may be used in clinical practice. This evidence comes from research studies that are being conducted to test various hypotheses about new drugs, treatment procedures, or general concepts about medical conditions. Current research can come in the form of summaries of individual studies, systematic reviews, and evidence-based clinical guidelines. Systematic reviews are useful as a comprehensive review of evidence from several different studies conducted on a particular topic.

Books and meeting abstracts are other examples of medical literature. Textbooks published on various medical topics can be used as reference material to gain in-depth knowledge on various topics. One disadvantage of referring to the textbooks for information on medical topics is that the time it takes to get published, the material may become dated. While textbooks, guidebooks, and instructional manuals are valuable for gaining a basic understanding of a topic, consider using other forms of literature for current medical research (e.g. scientific journals) where information is both accessible and up-to-date. Meeting abstracts are documents that summarize the discussions from a meeting or conference about a specific topic, and may also provide up-to-date summary of discussions that took place at medical meetings and conferences.

What is Current Medical Literature Used for?

In medical practice today, the vast amount of information available in the medical literature has led to a growing need for understanding and using the principle of evidence-based medicine (EBM). As a result, medical practitioners must consider a paradigm shift from traditional practice to a new approach that involves formulation of questions, validity assessment of study findings, and suitable application of current evidence to clinical practice.[1] Though plenty of medical literature may be available, it is important to be able to draw upon high quality, helpful evidence to use in clinical practice. All published research is not of the same quality, and even more importantly, not all findings are directly applicable to patient treatment. In the hierarchy of evidence, findings reported from randomized controlled trials are considered to be the most helpful and of the highest quality (i.e. least biased).[2] An example of a resource for EBM is the Cochrane Database, which is an online database containing a wide-ranging collection of systematic reviews on various topics.[1]

Another use of medical literature is to serve as an up-to-date educational resource for the medical community, students, public health organizations, as well as the general public. Apart from application in patient treatment, medical professionals can also use medical literature to keep themselves updated with the latest research surrounding their own field of work, or other fields of personal interest. Similarly, public health organizations may rely on medical literature to be the supportive evidence which is used for improving old policies or developing new policies regarding current health concerns. Members of the general public who have an interest in medical topics for educational purposes may also access the medical literature either by free public access to some databases, or via registration within an institution that subscribes to various sources of medical literature.

How can we Assess the Quality of the Medical Literature?

One matter of concern with regards to medical literature is the quality of the study from which evidence is being extracted for use in clinical practice. Some factors to look out for include study design, sample size of a study, and agreement of evidence with other similar studies wherever available.[2] Randomized controlled trials are considered to be the highest level of evidence but are fairly complex in nature. These large scale studies are much more common today, but are complex because they are generally involve in the participation of several medical institutions, organizing committees and ethics management and strict adherence to the protocol to limit bias in the assessment of outcomes.[3] With such complexity, it is a natural concern that there is more room for error.

Another important issue is conflicts of interest surrounding research findings that are presented in the medical literature.

Financial conflicts of interest are fairly common in medical research due to the fact that the funding source can have a significant influence on a clinical trial. For example, investigators of clinical research who have a conflict of interest may be more likely to arrive at positive conclusions from a biased study design, suppress negative outcomes, there may be preferential funding for projects likely to succeed, or analyze findings in a biased manner. Academic institutions, such as universities, have policies regarding conflicts of interest but the influence of industry on medical research is difficult to monitor. Although, it would be ideal if research was conducted without profit-minded motivations, healthcare systems often depend heavily on industry to drive the development of new drugs and devices for public access.[4] Industry is able to provide substantial amounts of funding for clinical research but does require the input of physicians to guide their work. The collaboration is inevitable and necessary but there should be a set of guidelines for how to limit and supervise the research when conflicts of interest are present.

Evidence-based Medicine and Clinical Practice

The important principle of *evidence-based medicine* (EBM) has changed the assessment of evidence in clinical research. EBM introduces new standards of quality in the field of science and medicine, as well as more objective way to measure the effects of a particular treatment. Furthermore, EBM offers a unifying platform for physicians and investigators to collaborate, share knowledge, improve their findings, and ultimately offers the best possible treatment for their patients.[5,6] Although very promising in the research field, EBM confronts the inevitable challenge of being easily integrated into clinical practice.

What are the Challenges of Incorporating the Evidence into Clinical Practice?

This section will discuss some of the challenges of incorporating the best available evidence into clinical practice, with a focus on the orthopedic surgery literature. The incorporation of evidence-based clinical guidelines into practice, bridges the gap of physicians acting both as clinicians and scientists in the treatment of their patients. The essential question is: 'Although Randomized Controlled Trials (RCTs) are being performed, are the results being applied to clinical practice?[5,6]

Consolidated Standards of Reporting Trials (CONSORT) published a checklist for reporting on RCTs in 1996, which was revised in 2001 and in 2010.[7] The checklist includes clear guidelines for reporting on the design of the trial, conduct, analysis, and interpretation, and assessment of the cogency of the results. CONSORT has standardized RCT reporting and now 600 journals and editorial groups endorse it.[6,7] This checklist was further developed into the Checklist to Evaluate a Report of Non-Pharmacological Trial (CLEAR NPT) to acknowledge the distinctions between surgical and medical trials. Although, this checklist was designed to unify the guidelines for RCTs, Bhandari et. al. found that on average published orthopedic trials followed only 32% of the CONSORT standards.[7,8]

Regardless of advances in RCTs, many investigators recognize challenges that are unique to surgical research. Some of these challenges include blinding, patient preferences, differences in individual surgical techniques from surgeon to surgeon, and the overall heterogeneity in surgical practice. This often differs from RCTs with medications, which can be more easily standardized across practitioners.[8,9]

Although the number of RCTs in the orthopedic literature is growing, before 2000, only 3% of studies were of RCTs.[5-7] In fact, much of orthopedic research is derived from uncontrolled studies, including case-control studies, case series, and expert opinion. Furthermore, Wright et al. suggested that there is a culture in orthopedic practice that may potentially hinder further RCTs in orthopedics. This includes the current model of training, in which younger surgeons learn the celebrated techniques of their attendings, often without support from EBM or controlled studies. Therefore, Wright et al. suggested that there is a strong hesitancy to accept any uncertainty in knowledge, and thus surgeons would practice the successful and well-established techniques acclaimed by their institution instead of newer ones emerging from

EBM.[8-10] RCTs have many benefits including providing statistical data and unbiased results. Uncontrolled case studies have played an important role in medicine, but with mere comparisons of techniques, do not offer the same benefits of unbiased statistical data.

One major challenge that was recognized in surgical trials is the difficulty associated with blinding participants to surgical treatments.[11] Medical treatments are often appropriate for blinding patients. In surgical trials, however, either the patient will know which arm they were randomized to (e.g. surgical vs nonsurgical), or the surgeon will know which arm the patient is randomized to (e.g. surgery vs sham procedure). This poses an inherent threat to the validity of the study, because patient or surgeon preference may result in differential treatment or assessment of outcomes. Poor reporting also contributes to the low quality evidence in orthopedic RCTs. The imbalance in surgeons' expertise and reporting on their respective techniques can directly influence the outcome of the treatment.

Moreover, of the 72 (from 1988 to 2000) RCTs that Bhandari et al. examined, 60% of them were considered to be low quality, with a quality score of less than 75%.[11] By examining these studies, three statistics about the lack of structure and organization in RCTs in orthopedic surgery were noted: ***first***, 61.2% of the studies did not identify the study as an RCT in the title. ***Second***, less than 8% of the studies incorporated a structured abstract. And ***last***, about 90% of the studies did not state the planned subgroup or covariate analysis a priori.[11]

One consistent issue in surgical trials is with regards to patient preferences. Many patients are hesitant to decide their treatment randomly, and may end up either enrolling in observational arms of a study or crossover to the alternative treatment. A prime example of this is the Spine Patient Outcomes Research Trial (SPORT). The SPORT study examined surgical versus nonsurgical treatment for intervertebral disc herniation, spinal stenosis, and degenerative spondylolisthesis. Patients in SPORT were given a choice of whether they wanted to enroll in a randomized arm or an observational arm. If the patient chose not to be randomized, they were able to decide between surgical and nonsurgical treatment in the observational arm. This study provided ample observational information, by not having a completely randomized design. Patients had the option to choose which treatment they would prefer, and thus treatment arms (including the randomized arm) began to cross over due to patient preferences. Crossover defeats the primary purpose of randomization as it allows patients to flow from one treatment type to another, instead of being allocated randomly to one treatment type. In effect, 50% of patients who were randomized to nonsurgical treatments ultimately received surgery.[11,12] This of course, introduces bias into the analysis. This high crossover rate exemplifies the intrinsic complexity of randomization in surgical trials. Strong patient preference poses a drastic limitation, especially, as evidenced in SPORT, when other treatment options are available outside the randomization arm.[11,12]

One way to overcome strong patient preference and patients' hesitancy to join a randomized trial for their treatment is educating patients about their options in healthcare. Investigators and physicians can offer options and educate their patients about the various ways to receive treatments. They can also encourage patients to be proactive about their health and make informed decisions about the benefits and also about the risks of randomized trials, and the possible outcomes of EBM. Physicians can draw on evidence when speaking to their patients and emphasize the role of evidence in medicine and future medical treatments. The decision ultimately belongs to the patient, yet knowledge, education and recommendations based on evidence are key to not only ease patient preference, but to also improve loss to follow-up in trials.

The rise in RCTs and focus on higher quality evidence in the past few decades shows a promising trend. Recognition of the unique challenges that differentiate surgical trials from medical trials is an important step in improving the overall quality of the evidence presented. The use of standardized guidelines would also improve the overall quality of RCTs.[13,14] Measures that can improve the quality of RCTs include blinding, allocation concealment, a priori subgroup analyses and sample size calculations and abiding by the intention to treat principle. Furthermore, greater transparency in reporting may increase efficiency and ensure rapid access to clinicians and evidence users.[13]

Important Learning Points

- Currently available medical literature includes scientific journals, textbooks and meeting abstracts.
- Peer-reviewed journals are a valuable source of expert-reviewed information on current medical topics.
- Textbooks are a good source of information for basic and well-understood topics but use with caution when dealing with very current medical information.
- Medical literature may be used for many purposes including EBM practice, clinical guidelines, policy and education.
- When incorporating EBM into clinical practice, it is essential that physicians incorporate their patients' values, clinical expertise and the best available evidence to treat their patients.
- As the number of RCTs is on the rise, there is also a need for a more standardized set of guidelines to regulate and assess the quality of RCTs.

Definition

Evidence-based medicine (EBM): The integration of clinical expertise, patient values and the best research evidence into the decision making process for patient care.

REFERENCES

1. Bhandari M, Giannoudis PV. Evidence-based medicine: What it is and what it is not. Injury. 2006;37(4):302-6.
2. Zlowodzki M, Jönsson A, Bhandari M. Common pitfalls in the conduct of clinical research. Med Princ Pract. 2006;15(1):1-8.
3. Bhandari M, Pape HC, Giannoudis PV. Issues in the planning and conduct of randomized trials. Injury. 2006;37(4):349-54.
4. Okike K, Kocher MS, Mehlman CT, et al. Industry-sponsored research. Injury. 2008;39(6):666-80.
5. Sackett DI, Rosenberg WM, Gray JA, et al. Evidence-based Medicine: What it is and what it isn't. BMJ. 1996;312:71-2.
6. Guyatt G, Cook D, Haynes B. Evidence-based medicine has come a long way. BMJ. 2004;329(7473):990-1.

7. Begg C, Cho M, Eastwood S, et al. Improving the quality of reporting of randomized controlled trials. The CONSORT statement. JAMA. 1996;276(8):637-9.
8. Bederman SS, Wright JG. Randomized Trials in Surgery: How far have we come? J Bone Joint Surg Am. 2012;94:2-6.
9. Chaudry H, Mundi R, Singh I, et al. How good is the orthopaedic literature? Indian J Orthop. 2008;42(2):144-9.
10. Oxman A, Guyatt GH, Cook D, et al. Users' guides to the medical literature: A manual for evidence based clinical practice. Chicago: AMA Press; 2002. p.155–73.
11. Bhandari M, Richards RR, Sprague S, et al. The quality of reporting of randomized trials in the Journal of Bone and Joint Surgery from 1988 through 2000. J Bone Joint Surg Am. 2002;84(3):388-96.
12. Hanzlik S. Mahabir RC, Baynosa RC, et al. Levels of evidence in research published in the journal of bone and joint surgery (American Volume) over the last thirty years. J Bone Joint Surg Am. 2009;91(2):425-8.
13. Wright JG, Katz JN, Losina E. Clinical trials in orthopaedics research. Part I. Cultural and practical barriers to randomized trials in orthopaedics. J Bone Joint Surg Am. 2011;93(5):15.
14. Bhandari M, Guyatt GH, Lochner H, et al. Application of the Consolidated Standards of Reporting Trials (CONSORT) in the Fracture Care Literature. J Bone Joint Surg Am. 2002;84:A(3)485-9.

2 Choosing the Right Study Design

Section Outline

5. Levels of Evidence—A Quick Guide
6. Level 1 Evidence—Randomized Controlled Trials
7. Level 2 Evidence—Prospective Cohort Studies
8. Level 3 Evidence—Case-control Studies
9. Level 4 Evidence—Clinical Case Series
10. Level 5 Evidence—Surveys

5

Levels of Evidence— A Quick Guide

Yashama Anwar

Key Objectives
- Learn about the different types of study designs
- Understand the levels of evidence and their respective ranks in the hierarchy of evidence.

What is the Hierarchy of Evidence?

Evidence-based medicine (EBM) is defined as the conscientious, explicit and judicious use of current evidence in making decisions about the care of individual patient, incorporating the best available evidence with patient's values.[1] Among other tools, physicians use the hierarchy of evidence to help guide clinical-decision making.

The *hierarchy of evidence* helps to display the various strengths of the types of research. In the ranking process a variety of factors are considered, including study design and methodology, validity and quality of research. The ranking system consists of 5 levels, 1st being the highest quality of evidence and 4th or 5th being lowest quality evidence. There are three types of studies that can be ranked using the hierarchy of evidence. Randomized controlled trials (RCTs) rank at the top of the hierarchy, observational studies are found in the middle and case series/expert opinion is ranked the lowest.[2] In order to ensure the validity of the research being completed, controls are often used. These controls include concurrent controls, sequential controls, and historical controls. This ensures that factors such as bias and other confounding variables do not play any role in the conclusion obtained.[1] Throughout this chapter, we will be discussing about the overall design of studies, the different types of evidence as well as their ranking. Different types of studies will be compared to one another. The advantages and disadvantages of each study will also be analyzed.

Levels of Evidence

The levels of evidence describe various studies in terms of their quality and validity. Generally speaking, the higher the study is on the hierarchy of evidence, the more confidence we can place in the study results. Level 1 evidence is at the top of the hierarchy and is considered to be the highest quality of evidence and is the most reliable. Level 5 is the lowest on the hierarchy of evidence and is of low quality thus the least reliable.

High-quality Evidence

High-quality evidences are both internally and externally valid and can be confidently applied to clinical practice. High-quality evidence is based upon the design of the study completed with an emphasis on RCTs and meta-analysis of RCTs.[1,2,3,4,5] Overall, high quality evidence provide confidence, a high degree of validity and sound methodology.

Low-quality Evidence

Low-quality evidence is categorized as not being very reliable and thus should be applied with caution to clinical practice. Observational studies, animal research, narrative reviews and *in vitro* research are all ranked under low quality evidence.[1,2]

Types of Study Designs

There are two broad types of study designs—descriptive and analytical studies.[5] Descriptive studies focuses on the distribution of a disease in relation to factors such as age, location and sex. Cross-sectional studies and case reports are examples of descriptive studies.[5] Analytical studies test a specific hypothesis about the relationship of a disease to a putative cause, by relating a particular exposure of interest to the disease of interest. Analytical studies are further divided into two types: observational and experimental studies. The difference between the subtypes of studies is the role the investigator plays in each type of study. In observational studies, the investigator does not play an active role with regards to manipulating the intervention; in experimental studies, the investigator actively manipulates the intervention.

A passive role would require that the investigator observes all the actions in a study without intervening while an active role would require the investigator to intervene in the actions of the study. Case-control studies and cohort studies fall under observational studies, while RCTs fall under experimental studies.

It is also important to differentiate between retrospective and prospective studies. Retrospective studies allow for the investigator to follow-up with patients even after the desired outcome. Prospective studies however, ensures that the investigator examines the patients before the desired outcome.[6] This will be important when classifying a particular study design under the types of evidence, which will be further discussed later in this chapter.

Different Types of Evidence

Level 1 Evidence—RCTs and Meta-analysis

Randomized Controlled Trials (RCTs)

RCTs are considered the gold standard of medical evidence and if well conducted are considered to be extremely reliable and valid. They have strong methodology, randomization and blinding.[2,4,5,7] In an RCT, patients are randomly assigned to either an experimental group or a control group. Patients in the control group may or may not receive a known and accepted treatment, while in the experimental group patients receive the specific intervention of interest.[7]

Researchers that conduct RCTs tend to evaluate the events or outcomes that arise, or are absent, after the patient receives the specific intervention. Like many other study designs, it is important to look at the methodology of an RCT before applying it to clinical practice—in a poorly conducted RCT, validity may be compromised.[2]

Meta-analysis

Like RCTs, meta-analysis of randomized trials are considered the highest form of evidence. Meta-analysis of RCTs takes data from numerous individual studies and statistically pools the results, allowing for increased generalizability.[2] It is important to note that the quality of the meta-analysis depends on the RCTs that are being included. High-quality trials lead to high-quality meta-analysis and low-quality trials lead to low-quality meta-analysis.[8]

Level 2 Evidence—Cohort Studies

Cohort studies involve following groups of patients with and without an exposure of interest, forward to determine if a specific outcome of interest develops.[9] These patients may be compared with other individuals who are healthy, do not have the disease or have not been exposed to the treatment. Both groups are then followed over the time to determine the rate of development of a specific disease or condition.[2] In cohort studies the follow-ups with patients are thoroughly examined in order to make sure the results and reports are as accurate as possible.

Cohort studies can be retrospective or prospective.[9] If the study is prospective in nature then the groups of individuals are followed up with in the future to determine if the desired outcome presented itself.[9] A prospective cohort study allows the investigator to accurately track progress of patients over time to determine which factors are related to the development of the outcome.

Cohort studies can also be retrospective in nature. In retrospective cohort studies, patients are treated by examining past medical records and the investigator works backwards in time, in order to determine the factors that could have caused the outcome. A retrospective design may be far more time efficient than a prospective design however, they may be limited by missing or incomplete data.[9]

Data collection in rigorously conducted. Cohort study is usually very accurate and reliable and thus ranks closer to the top of the hierarchy of evidence.[9] However, there are limitations to cohort studies specifically, the long time span to conduct prospective cohort studies as well as high expenses associated with these studies.[9]

Level 3 Evidence—Case-control Studies

Case-control studies are studies where a patient that already presents with a specific condition is compared with other people who do not have that condition.[10] These studies rely on medical records, databases, and patient recall for data collection. They compare factors that are similar between the patients with and patients without the disease and then infer what factors are associated with the presentation of the disease.[2,5,10] For example, if an investigator wants to determine factors causing heart disease, he would conduct a test in which one group would consist of patients with heart disease and one control group with healthy patients without the disease. The investigator would then compare patient histories and determine possible factors that may be related to disease occurrence. These types of studies are often less reliable because a correlation between two factors does not necessarily mean causation.

Case-control studies are retrospective studies because they look back in time to determine all the possible factors that may have caused the specific outcome.[10] There are limitations associated with case control studies due to the possibility of missed information or confounding variables that may skew the results and misleading conclusions. Although testing is done for each possible factor there is always a chance for error.

Level 4 Evidence—Case Reports and Case Series

Case reports and case series are collection of reports of the treatment of an individual patient. These studies have limited statistical inference and do not use a control group to compare their collected data to. Case reports and case series examinations are descriptive study designs and are retrospective in nature.[2] These types of studies may be subject to be biased and generalized[2,5] due to incomplete follow-up, loss to follow-up or missing data. Even though these studies are not considered as reliable evidence they are still valuable in hypothesis generation. [2, 5]

Level 5 Evidence—Expert Opinion

Expert opinion is at the bottom of the hierarchy of evidence. Expert opinions are generally uncontrolled and have limited reliability. They may be useful in situations of very rare conditions or outcomes, or in the description of specific surgical techniques. Examples of expert opinion studies include surveys, which may been used to determine how appropriate a therapy can be.[2,5]

Important Learning Points

- There are two types of studies—analytical studies and descriptive studies.
- Analytical studies are further divided into observational and experimental studies.
- The hierarchy of evidence ranks the levels of evidence into five categories with level 1 being the highest and level 5, the lowest. An understanding of these levels will help guide clinicians to the applicability of study results to their specific patient population.

Definitions

Analytical studies: Studies that test a specific hypothesis about the relationship of a disease to a putative cause, by relating a particular exposure of interest to the disease or outcome of interest.

Descriptive studies: Studies that focus on describing the distribution of a disease in relation to factors such as age, location and sex.

Hierarchy of evidence: A ranking system for health case research where a variety of factors are considered, including study design, methodology, validity and quality of research. The ranking system consists of 5 levels, 1st being the highest quality of evidence and 4th or 5th being low quality evidence.

REFERENCES

1. Kocher MS, Zurakowski D. Clinical epidemiology and biostatistics: a primer for orthopaedic surgeons. J Bone & Joint Surgery. 2004;86-A(3):607-20.
2. Petrisor B, Bhandari M. The hierarchy of evidence: levels and grades of recommendation. Indian J Orthop. 2007;41(1):11-5.
3. Bhandari M, Joensson A. Hierarchy of research studies: from case series to meta-analyses. In: Bhandari M and Joensson A (Eds). Clinical Research for Surgeons. Germany: Thieme Publishing Group; 2009.
4. Bhandari M, Giannoudis PV. Evidence-based medicine: what it is and what it is not. Injury. 2006;37(4):302-6.
5. Brighton B, Bhandari M, Tornetta P 3rd, et al. Hierarchy of evidence: from case reports to randomized controlled trials. Clin Orthop Relat Res. 2003;(413):19-24.
6. Bhandari M, Joensson. Various research designs and classficiations. In: Bhandari M and Joensson A (Eds). *Clinical Research for Surgeons*. Germany: Thieme Publishing Group; 2009.
7. Bhandari M, Joensson A. The randomized trial. In: Bhandari M and Joensson A (Eds). *Clinical Research for Surgeons*. Germany: Thieme Publishing Group; 2009.
8. Bhandari M, Joensson A. The prospective cohort study. In: Bhandari M and Joensson A (Eds). *Clinical Research for Surgeons*. Germany: Thieme Publishing Group; 2009.
9. Bhandari M, Joensson A. The case-control study. In: Bhandari M and Joensson A (Eds). *Clinical Research for Surgeons*. Germany: Thieme Publishing Group; 2009.
10. Bhandari M, Joensson A. The clinical case series. In: Bhandari M and Joensson A (Eds). *Clinical Research for Surgeons*. Germany: Thieme Publishing Group; 2009.

Level 1 Evidence—Randomized Controlled Trials

Zohaib Ansari, Hiba Mannan

Key Objectives

- Learn the key characteristics of Level I evidence, such as randomization, blinding of subjects and investigators, sample size and analysis
- Understand the advantages and limitations associated with randomized controlled trials (RCTs).

Hierarchy of Evidence: Level 1

Analytical research designs are used to evaluate the safety and effectiveness of new medical approaches to prevent, screen for, diagnose or treat a disease.[1] There are two basic kinds of analytical studies: observational and interventional. An observational study (such as a case-control or cohort study) is done to observe natural associations and make statistical inferences between risk factors and certain health outcomes.[2] Observational studies will be discussed further in the following chapter.

RCT is considered to be the most rigorous research design[3] and the most powerful tool in modern clinical research.[4] An RCT is an epidemiologic experiment in which subjects in a population are randomly allocated into groups to receive (experimental group) or not receive (control group) an intervention. The term 'intervention' usually refers to ***treatment*** however, it can be used in a much wider sense to include any clinical intervention offered to study participants that may have an effect on their health status. Clinical interventions may include prevention strategies, screening programs, diagnostic tests, interventional procedures, healthcare settings and educational concepts. Furthermore, the 'control group' may receive a placebo/sham intervention, alternate intervention or no intervention at all. Interventions are also controlled to ensure consistent participant treatment across all study groups (except for the factor that is unique to their group, i.e. the type of intervention they receive). ***Outcomes*** are then compared between experimental and control groups using various statistical measures.[5,6]

Key Features

Sample Selection

The sample is defined as a group of participants selected for the study. The sample should be a close representation of the population of interest. A broadly representative sample would enable the findings to be generalized to a diverse population. It may also allow the investigators to explore whether the treatment appears more or less effective with some population subgroups. ***External validity,*** i.e. the real-world relevance and applicability of a study can also be enhanced by having the study sample include representation of a range of important demographic characteristics such as gender, ethnicity and socioeconomic status.[7]

Things to Consider are

Balance of prognostic factors: Maintaining a balance of prognostic factors between the treatment and control group minimizes bias and tests with better estimation, the hypothesis of a potential association between the intervention and treatment effect as opposed to some extraneous confounding factor.[8]

Size matters: The size of the expected effect of the intervention is the main determinant of the sample size necessary to conduct a successful trial.[9] The smaller the expected effect of the intervention, the larger the sample size needed to be able to conclude, with enough power, that the differences are unlikely to be due to chance.[10]

In keeping with this there has been an appropriate shift away from undertaking small inconclusive RCTs assessing surrogate outcomes, towards conducting appropriately designed, larger (and sometimes simple) RCTs that evaluate the effects of treatments on major clinical outcomes.[11]

Random Assignment

Randomization is a key characteristic of high quality RCTs. This process involves assigning eligible patients to a treatment group and/or a control group through a random process. The goal of randomization is to reduce the risk of serious imbalance in an important known and unknown variable that may influence the clinical course of the participants and affect the study outcomes. These variables are also known as ***confounding factors***. Randomization achieves this goal by giving all participants an equal chance of being in the treatment or control arm.[12]

The preferred method of randomization involves a 'blinded' third-party member (i.e. someone not involved in any other way with the study) who generates numbers from a table or computer program. Such a process eliminates even unconscious ***bias*** from the assignment process. Many times the participants would leave the study before the intervention has even begun. To avoid this situation the randomization process should take place as close as possible to the initiation of the intervention. This is important because every participant who is randomized, whether those who drop out or continue till the end, will ideally be included in the study's outcome analyses. This practice is called an ***intention to treat analysis***.[7]

Control Group

The choice of a control group usually depends on the specific question being asked and the state of existing knowledge about the intervention under study.[7] Different scenarios are depicted in Table 6.1.

Blinding

Blinding is the purposeful concealment of the patients' intervention group allocations. Blinding patients eliminates any psychological expectation, also known as the placebo

Table 6.1: Various control group options

- ***No-treatment comparison condition:*** Patients randomly assigned to receive the new treatment are compared to those patients assigned to receive no treatment at all.
- ***Wait list comparison:*** Patients randomized to receive a new treatment are compared to those randomized to be on a wait list to receive the new treatment.
- ***Treatment as usual comparison (TAU):*** Patients randomized to receive a new treatment are compared to those randomized to receive treatment as usual (i.e. whatever intervention is prevalent and standard practice).
- ***Relative efficacy/comparative effectiveness:*** A direct comparison between two or more treatments to assess the best practice or standard of care.
- ***Parametric/dose finding:*** Usually done early in the development of a new treatment in order to determine the optimal 'dose' or format of treatment. Different forms of the intervention varying on factors such as the number, length, or duration of treatment comprise the conditions to which patients are randomly assigned.
- ***Treatment dismantling:*** Also called 'component analysis', in this approach, patients randomized to receive the full efficacious intervention are compared to those randomized to receive a variant of that intervention minus one or more parts of it.

effect, which has a significant impact on the measured outcome.[8] The best way of avoiding this is to keep patients unaware of whether they are assigned to the intervention or control group. Being ***single-blinded*** means that only the patient is unaware of the group he/she is part of. In a ***double-blind study***, neither the participants nor the investigator know the participants' treatment assignment.[13] This level of blinding also reduces ***ascertainment bias,*** i.e. the influence of expectations held by participants or by research staff about which treatment will have a better effect on the outcome.[6]

The effect of not blinding the groups can systematically bias endpoint evaluations. In some clinical trials, such as surgical trials, it is impossible to 'blind' the physician from the treatment group. However, one way to overcome the biases associated with this is to blind the research staff that will be doing the follow-up and analysis of the data.[13]

Adequacy and Concealment of Allocation

The adequacy of the patient allocation process is dependent on how well extraneous variables are controlled. A study has an adequate allocation sequence when researchers are unable to influence or predict their patients' group assignments.[8] Concealment means that the individuals enrolling patients into the RCT are unaware of the upcoming treatment assignments. The allocation sequence must be 'concealed' from the researchers as well to avoid bias in the selection process. Otherwise, researchers may selectively place patients with more severe symptoms in the treatment group, downsizing the treatment effect or vice versa.[14]

Note: Concealment of randomization may be compromised when non-random methods of treatment allocation (e.g., admission date, hospital number and alternate assignments) are utilized.[11]

Patient Follow-up

During a clinical trial, investigators are interested in patients' outcome measures regardless of the group they were assigned to. Patients with unknown data are classified as 'lost to follow-up'. High losses to follow-up decrease the ***internal validity*** of a study. If the study has fewer subjects with complete data than originally planned, the study may be under-powered. This means the study does not have enough subjects in order to show that the difference between the groups is statistically significant, even though it may be clinically important. Care must always be taken to minimize missing responses and to follow-up those who withdraw from treatment.[15]

Intention-to-treat Analysis

In the clinical researcher's perfect world, every patient entered into RCT would satisfy all eligibility criteria, complete their allocated treatment as described in the protocol and contribute data records which were complete in all respects. In practice, it is doubtful if this ideal is ever achieved; hence, strategies have been developed for analysis that seek to protect the inferential basis of a study from consequent biases. Such a strategy is called 'intention to treat' analysis (ITT).[16] Analysis is done on all randomized patients in the groups to which they were randomly assigned, regardless of their compliance with the entry criteria, the treatment they actually received, and whether they withdrew from treatment midway or deviated from the study guidelines.[17] ITT analysis preserves the prognostic balance of groups that was achieved through randomization and also minimizes *type I error*.[18,31] However, a full application of the intention to treat approach is possible only when complete outcome data are available for all randomized subjects. In case of patient losses to follow-up, various imputation methods may be used to estimate the missing responses such as using the patient's last observed response (carry forward) or assuming that all missing responses were constant.[19]

Study Designs

The usefulness of a trial depends on the extent to which a causal relationship can be inferred (i.e. the experimental treatment caused an outcome). The ability to make valid inferences depends on how well the investigator designed, conducted and reported various procedures to minimize bias in the study. Table 6.2 highlights some of the common RCT study designs.

Analysis

There are two important aspects of analyzing an RCT. First, a list of outcomes that will be analyzed should be outlined prior to the beginning the clinical trial. This is known as *a priori* analysis.[13] A priori analysis will reduce potential bias as the collected data would not influence the aspects of the outcome that one chooses to analyze. Another important part of a good analysis is the intention-to-treat design as discussed earlier. One of the important ways to ensure patient safety is by:

Interim Analysis

It is a planned analysis at certain points in the clinical trial, which examines certain factors of the treatment groups. As per the ethics of conducting RCTs, if there are indications that one of the treatment groups is receiving an inferior intervention the clinical trial must be terminated. This is known as a *stopping rule* and is a part of this interim analysis. An interim

Table 6.2: Common RCT study designs

Classified according to the different aspects of interventions evaluated

Efficacy Vs effectiveness: Efficacy refers to interventions carried out under ideal circumstances, whereas effectiveness evaluates the effects under circumstances similar to those found in daily practice. Efficacy trials are sometimes called explanatory trials, whereas effectiveness trials are also known as pragmatic trials.[20]

Phase 1, 2, 3 and 4 trials: These terms describe the different types of trials used for the introduction of a new intervention, traditionally a new drug.

    Phase 1: To document the safety of the intervention in humans.
    Phase 2: Evaluating efficacy in a small group of real patients.
    Phase 3: RCTs conducted to evaluate effectiveness.
    Phase 4: Post-marketing studies of the intervention.[9]

Classified according to participants' exposure and response to the intervention.

Parallel design: Most common design where each group of participants is exposed to only one of the study interventions. Results are analyzed by comparing groups.[21]

Factorial design: Two or more experimental interventions are not only evaluated separately but also in combination and against a control. Design generates four sets of data to analyze—data on patients who received none of the interventions, patients who received treatment A, patients who received treatment B, and patients who received both A and B.[21]

Crossover design: Each of the participants is given all of the study interventions in successive periods. The order in which the participants receive each of the study interventions is determined at random.[21]

Cluster design: Whole groups of participants (e.g., schools, clinics, worksites) are randomized to intervention or control. The unit of randomization is a group rather than an individual.[22]

Classified according to the number of participants.

N-of-one trials: RCT with only one participant. Trials that involve thousands of patients and limited data collection are called 'megatrials'.[21]

Sequential design: The number of participants is not specified beforehand; the investigators continue recruiting participants until a clear benefit of one of the interventions is observed or until they become convinced that there are no important differences between the interventions.[21]

Fixed trials: The investigators establish deductively the number of participants (sample size) that will be studied. This number is decided arbitrarily or can be calculated using statistical methods.[9]

analysis should be planned before the initiation of the clinical trial. It should include[23]:
- Standard operating procedure that outlines possibility of an early termination.
- Define who will have the authority to stop the trial early.
- Outline the actions that would be taken to protect the subjects and their information.

Note: That many studies do not require an interim analysis and repeated monitoring of a study may compromise study results in many cases.

Data and safety monitoring board (DSMB): It is appointed to examine the data at various points of the trial and to determine if it is safe to continue the study. The following factors are usually considered by the DSMB[24]:
- Any safety issues identified in the collected data
- If the assumptions made initially in the trial remain appropriate for the clinical trial
- If it is likely to detect a treatment difference with this study design
- If there is a strong statistical power to favour continuation of the study
- If there are any observations that should be presented to the sponsors and/or patients.

Reporting

Awareness concerning the quality of reporting RCTs and the limitations of the research methods of RCTs is growing. A major barrier hindering the assessment of trial quality is that, in most cases, we must rely on the information contained in the written report. A trial with a biased design, if well reported, could be judged to be of high quality, whereas a well-designed but poorly reported trial could be judged to be of low quality. Spurred on by the recognized importance of RCTs in the world of evidence-based medicine, the 'Consolidated Standards of Reporting Trials' (CONSORT) working group published their checklist on the recommendations for reporting RCTs in 1996. The checklist was subsequently revised in 2001 and most recently in 2010. This checklist attempts to ensure a clear reporting of trial design, conduct, analysis, and interpretation as well as the assessment of the validity of the results of

Table 6.3. The CLEAR NPT purports that the ten quality items should be assessed in the design and reporting of non-pharmacological trials:

- Adequate allocation sequence
- Concealed allocation
- Details of intervention for each group
- Appropriate skill/experience of providers in each group
- Participant adherence (not applicable for one-time surgical treatments)
- Blinded participants
- Blinded providers
- Blinded assessors
- Same follow-up for each group
- Intention-to-treat analysis

checklist.[25] Recognizing the differences between surgical and medical trials, this group additionally developed the 'Checklist to evaluate a report of a nonpharmacological trial (CLEAR NPT)', outlined in Table 6.3.[26]

Merits and Concerns

Ethical Concerns

It is not ethical to design a trial in which, before enrollment, evidence suggests that patients in one arm of the study are more likely to benefit from enrollment than patients in the other arm.[27] When conducting a clinical trial with a placebo group, it is unethical to deprive patients of necessary treatment by giving them placebo medicines. RCTs are not a panacea to answer all clinical questions; for example, the effect of a risk factor such as smoking cannot ethically be addressed with RCTs.[2,8]

Limitations

RCT may not be appropriate for the assessment of interventions that have rare outcomes or have effects that take a long time to develop.[27] Furthermore, in many situations RCTs are not feasible, necessary, appropriate, or ethical to help solve important problems. In other cases, RCTs may not be feasible because of financial constraints or because of the

Table 6.4: Advantages and disadvantages related to RCT

Advantages	Disadvantages

• Allows rigorous evaluation of a single variable
• Prospective design (data is collected on events that happen after you decide to do the study)
• Uses hypothetic-deductive reasoning (seeks to falsify, rather than confirm, its own hypothesis)
• Potentially eradicates bias by comparing two otherwise identical groups
• Allows for **meta-analysis** (combining the numerical results of several similar trials at a later date)
	• Expensive and time consuming; hence:
	  ▫ Many RCT are never done
	  ▫ Are performed on too few patients or
	  ▫ Are undertaken for too short of a time period
	• Most are funded by large research bodies (university or government sponsored) or drug companies, who ultimately dictate the research agenda
	• Surrogate endpoints are often used in preference to clinical outcome measures and may introduce 'hidden bias' especially through:
	  ▫ Imperfect randomization
	  ▫ Failure to blind assessors to randomization status of patients

expectation of low compliance or high dropout rates.[29] Table 6.4 highlights the advantages and disadvantages of RCTs.

Definitions

A priori: A method of defining the aspects of the treatment and outcomes that will be analyzed, prior to beginning a clinical trial.[13]

Ascertainment bias: Occurs when the results or conclusions of a trial are systematically distorted by knowledge of which intervention each participant is receiving.[6]

Bias: Systematic deviation from the underlying truth because of a feature of the design or conduct of a research study.[8]

Confounding variable: A variable or factor that is correlated with both the outcome and exposure. It therefore may appear to be directly causing the outcome because its value fluctuates in synchrony with the causative exposure.[12]

Data and safety monitoring board: An independent group of experts that monitors and assess collected data for patient safety and determine if it is safe for the clinical trial to continue.[24]

Double-blinded study: A clinical trial in which both the patient and physician/investigators are masked from knowing which treatment group the patient is receiving.[13]

External validity: The extent to which a study can be generalized to other populations or situations.

Intention-to-treat analysis: Includes all randomized patients in the groups to which they were randomly assigned, regardless of their adherence with the entry criteria, regardless of the treatment they actually received and regardless of subsequent withdrawal from treatment or deviation from the protocol.[16]

Internal validity: Internal validity is the ability of the study results to support a cause-effect relationship between the treatment and the observed outcome. In other words, the observed difference in outcome between groups is attributable only to the effect of the intervention under investigation.[30]

Meta-analysis: Statistically combining quantitative data from several studies to yield a single pooled summary estimate.[32,33]

Outcome: An indicator of health status that will be used to assess the difference between the treatment and/or control groups.[6]

Single-blinded study: A clinical trial in which only the patient is unaware of the treatment group he/she is part of.[13]

Stopping rule: Is a part of the interim analysis and is used as a guide to terminate the clinical trial as soon as there is an indication for one of the treatment groups being inferior to the other.[23]

Type I error: Incorrect rejection of the null hypothesis and concluding a relationship exists between two variables when in fact it does not. Also known as a spurious result.

Type II error: Incorrect acceptance of the null hypothesis and concluding no relationship exists between two variables when in fact it does.

REFERENCES

1. Clinical Trials: Key to medical progress. NIH Medline Plus. Summer 2008 Issue: Volume 3 Number 3 Pages 4 – 5. http://www.nlm.nih.gov/medlineplus/magazine/issues/pdf/summer2008.pdf. Accessed: March 26, 2015
2. Grimes DA, Schulz KF. An overview of clinical research: the lay of the land. Lancet. 2002;359(9300):57-61.

3. Norman GR, Striener DL. Biostatistics: the bare essentials. St. Louis: CV Mosby, 1993.
4. Silverman WA. Gnosis and random allotment. Control Clin Trials 1981;2(2):161-4
5. Last JM. A Dictionary of Epidemiology, 4th edition. Oxford University Press; 2001.
6. Jadad AR. Randomised controlled trials: a user's guide. London, England: BMJ Books; 1998.
7. West A, Spring B. (2007). Randomized controlled Trials. [online] EBBP website. Available from www.ebbp.org/course_outlines/randomized_controlled_trials/. [Accessed March 2015].
8. Brian Chan, Bernd Robioneck, Anders Joensson. User's guide to the orthopaedic literature: How to use an article about a randomized trial? Indian J Orthop. 2008;42(2):118-25.
9. Stolberg H, Norman G, Trop I. Fundamentals of Clinical Research for Radiologists. American Journal of Radiology. 2004;183(6):1539-44.
10. KB Freedman, S Back, J Bernstein. Sample size and statistical power of randomized, controlled trials in orthopaedics. J Bone Joint Surg Br. 2001;83(3):397-402.
11. Devereaux PJ, Yusuf S. The evolution of the randomized controlled trial and its role in evidence-based decision making. J Internal Med. 2003;254(2):105-13.
12. McDonald, J.H. Handbook of Biological Statistics, 3rd edition. Baltimore, Maryland: Sparky House Publishing; 2014.
13. Chung KC, Burns PB. A guide to planning and executing a surgical randomized controlled trial. J Hand Surgery Am. 2008;33(3):407-12.
14. Schultz KF, Grimes DA. Allocation concealment in randomized trials: defending against deciphering. Lancet 2002;359(9306):614-8.
15. Streiner DL. Sample size and power in psychiatric research. Can J Psychiatry. 1990;35(7):616-20.
16. Lewis JA, Machin D. Intention to treat-who should use ITT? Br J Cancer. 1993;68(4):647-50.
17. Fisher LD, Dixon DO, Herson J, et al. Intention to treat in clinical trials. In: Pearce KE, ed. Statistical issues in drug research and development. New York: Marcel Dekker. 1990; pp. 331–350
18. Fergusson D, Aaron SD, Guyatt G, et al. Post-randomisation exclusions: the intention to treat principle and excluding patients from analysis. BMJ. 2002;325:652-4. Available from www.ncbi.nlm.nih.gov/pmc/articles/PMC1124168/ [Accessed March 2015].
19. DL Sackett, WS Richardson, WM Rosenberg, et al. Evidence-based medicine: what it is and what it isn't. 1996;312(7023):71-2.
20. Schwartz D, Lellouch J. Explanatory and pragmatic attitudes in therapeutical trials. J Clin Epidemiol. 2009;62(5):499-505.

21. Greenhalgh T. How to read a paper. Getting your bearings (deciding what the paper is about). BMJ. 1997;315(7102):243-6.
22. Puffer S, Torgerson D, Watson J. Evidence for risk of bias in cluster randomised trials: review of recent trials published in three general medical journals. BMJ. 2003;327(7418):785-9.
23. Emerson SS, Kittelson JM, Gillen DL. Bayseian evaluation of group sequential clinical trial design. Stat in Med.26. 2007;26(7):1431-49.
24. Delgado-Herrera L, Anbar D. A model for interim analysis process: a case study. Control Clin Trials. 2003;24(1):51-65.
25. Begg C, Cho M, Eastwood S, et al. Improving the quality of reporting of randomized controlled trials. The CONSORT statement. JAMA. 1996;276(8):637-9.
26. Boutron I, Moher D, Tugwell P, et al. A checklist to evaluate a report of a nonpharmacological trial (CLEAR NPT) was developed using consensus. J Clin Epidemiol. 2005;58(12):1233-40.
27. Duffy SW. Interpretation of the breast screening trials: a commentary on the recent paper by Gotzsche and Olsen. Breast. 2001;10(3): 209–212.
28. Alejandro RJ, Murray WE. Randomized Controlled Trials: Questions, Answers and Musings, 2nd edition. BMJ Books/Blackwell Publishing; 2007.
29. Achilleas Thoma, Sheila Sprague, Claire Temple, et al. The Role of the Randomized Controlled Trial in Plastic Surgery. Clin Plastic Surg. 2008;35(2):275-84.
30. Bhandari M, Guyatt GH, Swiontkowski MF. User's guide to the orthopaedic literature: how to use an article about a surgical therapy. J Bone Joint Surg Am. 2001;83-A(6):916–26.
31. Banerjee A, Chitnis UB, Jadhav SL, et al. Hypothesis testing, type I and type II errors. Ind Psychiatry J. 2009;18(2):127-31.
32. Mulrow CD. Rationale for systematic reviews, Chapter 1. In: Chalmers I, Altman DG, eds Systematic Reviews. London: BMJ Publishing Group, 1995; 1–8
33. Montori V, Guyatt G. Summarizing the evidence: publication bias, Chapter 2E. In: Guyatt G, Rennie DR, eds Users' Guides to the Medical Literature. United States of America: AMA Press, 2002; 529–38

Level 2 Evidence— Prospective Cohort Studies

Sohail Sheriff

Key Objectives

- Understand the definition of a cohort study and the contexts for its use
- Understand the place of cohort studies in the hierarchy of medical evidence
- Be able to compare and contrast a cohort study with a randomized controlled trial (RCT)
- Understand the limitations associated with a cohort study
- Understand how to select an appropriate cohort
- Understand sources of bias that can arise in cohort studies such as: confounding bias, observer expectancy, sampling bias, the Hawthorne effect and loss to follow-up.

What is a Prospective Cohort Study?

"All we know is, that his legions were organized in cohorts, that as in the days of Marius the cohort was the tactical unit.[1]" Julius Caesar, general of the Roman army and a pivotal figure during the rise of the Roman Empire, strategically used cohorts to create an imposing military presence. Although, Caesar is not credited for inventing cohorts himself, the idea of a cohort have ancient Roman military roots.[2] Similar to the Roman military, but more applicable to today's use in clinical research, a cohort can be thought of as a group of subjects with similar characteristics. These subjects possess some sort of variable, and are monitored for the *incidence* of outcomes of interest. Cohorts are grouped based on the presence of a risk factor or variable that is being investigated, known as an

exposure. As such, cohort studies provide a framework and a means for researchers to assess particular exposures and their association to the onset of various diseases, known as ***outcomes***. It is important to note that cohort studies can be conducted either prospectively or retrospectively.

In a ***prospective cohort study***, the researcher is interested in a particular exposure but unaware of the outcome at the time when the study is conducted. To understand how a prospective cohort study works, let us consider a researcher interested in studying diseases associated with infants born to mothers who are addicted to smoking. In this simple example, the exposure would be secondhand smoke during pregnancy and the condition of the infants at birth would be the outcome. The researcher could construct a cohort, consisting of pregnant mothers who identify themselves as smokers and then monitor them throughout their pregnancy to see if they give birth to infants presenting with the disease or not. Similarly, the researcher could also construct an alternative cohort consisting of pregnant mothers who are non-smokers, for comparison as a control group. If the incidence of the outcome is higher in the exposure group than in the control, this would indicate a positive association between the exposure and outcome.[3] In this manner, cohort studies can help to uncover the etiology and risk factors of diseases. Once we know that a factor/exposure is associated with an outcome, we can study it more rigorously to establish the presence or lack of causality. It is very important to note that an association between an exposure and outcome itself is not necessarily evidence of causation.

Furthermore, in a ***retrospective cohort study***, the researcher is already aware of a specific outcome and is interested in studying a particular exposure associated with that outcome. To understand how a retrospective cohort study works, let us consider an example where a researcher is interested in studying risk factors of developing lung cancer during childhood. The researcher could construct a cohort consisting of children recently diagnosed with lung cancer in 2015 and collect all their medical history since 2010. Beginning with health records from 2010, researchers could move chronologically in time and look for exposures up until their actual diagnosis of cancer (the outcome) in 2015.[4]

Where do Cohort Studies Rank in the Hierarchy of Evidence

Cohort studies are classified as Level 2 evidence within the hierarchy of medical evidence. On examining why they are classified as Level 2, it is helpful to compare cohort studies to RCTs. RCTs are considered to be the gold standard in terms of clinical research and are thus classified as Level 1. However, there are instances where an RCT is not possible to implement. There are often cases where the exposure of interest is putatively harmful and thus it would be unethical to knowingly put a subject in harm way.[5] For example, it would not be ethical to randomize non-smokers to a smoking group if we wanted to study the association between smoking and lung cancer. In such cases, we may employ a cohort design which is very similar to an RCT design but lacks randomization. In both types of studies, there is a control group and an exposure group and the incidence of the outcome of interest in each group is recorded. RCTs should never be confused with cohort studies. The key to understanding the difference between them lies in distinguishing experimental studies from observational ones. An experimental study is one in which investigators intervene and introduce a variable to the subjects, such as in RCTs. Conversely, in observational studies investigators follow exposed and unexposed groups over a specified period of time.

What are the Limitations of Prospective Cohort Studies?

Without randomization, we significantly weaken the internal validity of the study. Randomization is the best way to balance both known and unknown *prognostic factors* between the groups in a study. Prognostic factors are characteristics that may have an influence on the outcome. How can we be sure that if there is in fact a difference in outcomes between the exposed and non-exposed groups, it is not due to some other factor? We can measure characteristics that we think may have an effect on the outcome and check that they are balanced between the groups. But even then, we are not accounting for all unknown prognostic factors. Randomization, in principle, takes care of all of these and is thus more rigorous than the cohort study.[6] Since cohort studies do not employ randomization, they are susceptible to **prognostic imbalance**. This may result in what is known as **confounding bias**, which will be elaborated later in this chapter. For now, understand that bias occurs when there is a systematic deviation in the results from the truth due to the unintentional introduction of external factors into the study.[5]

Another significant disadvantage of cohort studies is long follow-up times associated with rare outcomes of interest.[7] Such outcomes could potentially take decades to present, for example a rare form of cancer. These types of studies could become very expensive to sustain for such an extended period of time, as resources are required longterm.[7] Furthermore, many participants may not even go on to develop the rare outcome at all, making the study highly inefficient in the end.[7]

Furthermore, there are also several different types of bias that limit the effectiveness of cohort studies and these will be discussed later in this chapter.

How do we Select an Appropriate Cohort?

The proper selection of cohorts prior to embarking on a study is essential to the quality of results. All patients in both cohorts (exposure and non-exposure groups) should be free from the outcome or disease of interest at the beginning of the study. We want to see how many people in each group develop the disease (incidence) and if some subjects already have the disease the results will be skewed.[6]

Additionally, subjects in each group should have an equal chance of developing the outcome of interest in all regards, besides one group having the exposure of interest. This reduces the possibility that any association between outcome group that we see in the results is not due to the some factor other than the exposure of interest.[5]

In other words, we must ensure that all potential prognostic factors/characteristics (besides the exposure of interest) are reasonably balanced between the groups at the start of the study. If this is not the case, statistical adjustment

Table 7.1: A fictional table showing baseline characteristics of an exposed (exercise regimen) and non-exposed group of patients with chronic myofascial pain syndrome (musculoskeletal disorder).

	Exercise regimen group	No exercise group
Mean Age	45	47
Male/Female ratio	57:43	55:45
Baseline pain score (Visual analogue scale)	7.2	7.4
Average number of years with diagnosed disorder	4	15

must be used to compensate for these baseline imbalances.[5] This adjustment would be necessary as ***sampling bias***, discussed in further detail later in this chapter, could occur and potentially affect the outcomes observed. In most of the studies, the first table presented will give an overview of the baseline characteristics of the study groups (e.g. mean age, gender, baseline pain scores, etc.) (Table 7.1). We must scrutinize such tables to ensure proper attention was given to this matter—without proper baseline balance, the basis of the study results may be weak.

Even so, as mentioned earlier, there will always be prognostic factors and characteristics that may have a bearing on the outcome but are unknown to the investigator. This is known as ***residual confounding***, a problem that cannot be remedied without randomization.[5]

We see the baseline characteristics are similar between the groups, except for average number of years with disorder. If the investigators find a greater improvement in pain scores in the exercise group, we may worry that the imbalance in duration of the disease between groups may be influencing the results.

What Types of Bias Should we be Aware of?

Confounding Bias

A confounder is an independent variable associated with both the exposure and outcome and may not be identified

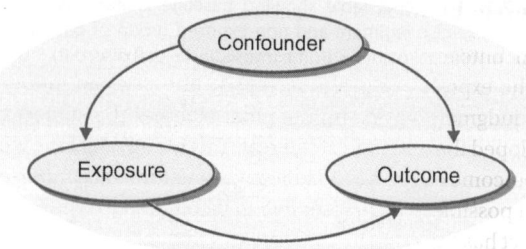

Fig. 7.1: Relationship between confounder, exposure and outcome

by investigators initially (Figure 7.1). Failing to identify a confounder can falsely lead an investigator to believe there is evidence of causation between an exposure and an outcome.[4] The concept of a confounder can be difficult to understand at first but can be quite easily illustrated if we consider a very simplified example. Let us consider a scenario, where an investigator was studying a population of elderly retired shipyard workers and discovered a high incidence of lung cancer. Initially, solely based on the findings of the study, the investigator would be inclined to conclude that working in a shipyard causes lung cancer. However, a closer look would reveal that it was not simply working in a shipyard that caused lung cancer, it was the high level of asbestos present in old shipyards that caused the development of cancer. Thus in this example, asbestos would be considered a confounder.

Furthermore, ***confounding bias*** arises from imbalances in known and unknown baseline characteristics and prognostic factors between groups. In randomized trials, the process of random allocation takes care of balancing characteristics between groups.[3] We will never be able to totally safeguard against confounding bias in cohort studies. This is due to the inescapable residual confounding from unknown prognostic factors that we cannot foresee.[5] Thus, confounding bias limits our ability to make causal inferences from cohort studies.[8]

A confounder is an independent variable associated with both the outcome and exposure. Inability to identify confounders can result in falsely concluding that there is an evidence of causation between exposure and outcome.[4]

Observer Expectancy

When outcome assessors are aware of whether a subject has the exposure (e.g. risk factor) or not, this can influence their judgment in determining that whether the subject has developed the outcome of interest. This is a special case when the outcome of interest is subjective in nature. It is important, when possible, for the assessors to be blinded to whether the subject has the exposure in order to avoid this bias.[3]

Additionally, if the assessor is aware of which group is exposed to the factor of interest first, they may follow and examine that cohort more diligently since, they expect the outcome of interest to develop. This is known as ***surveillance bias*** and can lead to spurious associations and over-estimates of risk.[5] For example, a non-blinded assessor may look more carefully for development of cancer in a smoking group than in the control non-smoking group. They may detect cases in the smoking group that might otherwise have gone unnoticed if equal attention was given to each group. Blinding can be implemented to ameliorate this problem.

Sampling Bias

It is a common occurrence in cohort studies and realistically, in many cases, unavoidable. A sampling bias occurs when both groups in a cohort study differ in something other than just the exposure.[2] To explain this further, let us consider an example where a researcher is investigating the effects of a low-sugar diet on the incidence of type 2 diabetes. One cohort would consist of subjects who adhere to a strict diet with low-sugar, while the other cohort would continue on with no dietary restriction (control group). Ideally, the only difference between both the groups should be the amount of sugar in their diet. Realistically, however, the low-sugar group would probably also differ in other lifestyle choices such as exercise and overall fitness, which would likely affect the outcomes observed.[2] Being able to eliminate all potential differences between groups in cohort studies is nearly impossible; therefore, selection bias should always be kept in mind.[2]

Hawthorne Effect

The ***Hawthorne effect***, also known as the 'observer effect,' is a common phenomenon that occurs in clinical trials.[9] It can be described as the alteration of one's behavior when aware of being monitored.[5] The investigators unintentionally influence participants to modify their behavior and as a result, this weakens the validity of conclusions drawn from variables being studied.[9] One way to reduce this unwanted effect is to blind the subjects to the purpose/hypothesis of the study, however, it is important to remember that this does not eliminate the effect altogether.[9]

Loss to Follow-up

Loss to follow-up occurs when a participant drops out of a study and fails to complete it. This is a common occurrence in large studies or studies that span over longer period of time, as consistent participation over an extended period is difficult to sustain. Loss to follow-up can potentially have a significant effect on the outcome as it occurs while the study is well underway.[10] It is important for investigators to be able to recognize the bias caused by loss to follow-up. A difference in the proportion of participants lost in each of the groups being studied is also indicative of bias which is caused by loss to follow-up.[10]

Important Learning Points

- In a cohort study, ***exposed and non-exposed group*** are followed and the incidence of the outcome of interest in each group is determined.
- ***Prospective and retrospective cohort studies*** are both observational study designs. Whereas, retrospective studies start at the outcome and work backward towards the exposure, cohort studies follow exposed and unexposed patients forward in time.
- Cohort studies are less rigorous than randomized trials due to the possibility of prognostic imbalance between the groups. Thus, they may be plagued by ***confounding bias***, hampering our ability to make causal inferences from them.

- There are several types of bias to watch out in cohort studies, including confounding bias, observer expectancy, sampling bias, the Hawthorne effect and bias due to loss to follow-up.

Definitions

Confounding bias: This type of bias is due to spurious associations resulting from imbalance in prognostic factors between groups.

Exposure: Something which patients are exposed that may affect their health. This could either be a putatively harmful intervention, or a beneficial one.

Hawthorne effect: Refers to the phenomenon where subjects tend to improve specific behaviors when they know they are being studied.

Incidence: The number of new cases of disease or outcome as a percentage of the total number of subjects in the group.

Outcome: An indicator of health status that will be used to assess the difference between the treatment and/or control groups.

Prognostic factors: Baseline factors or characteristics of a subject which may influence their risk of developing the outcome of interest. These can unfortunately act as confounders when they are not balanced between the groups in the study.

Prognostic imbalance: A lack of similarity of prognostic characteristics between the groups being studied. For example, if age is a prognostic factor then great differences in the age distribution of participants between the two groups would be considered prognostic imbalance.

Residual confounding: Refers to the fact that some unaccounted for prognostic characteristics remain unbalanced even after statistical adjustment and attempts to balance between groups. It is due to the presence of prognostic factors unknown to the investigator; this is inevitable in cohort studies.

Surveillance bias: Occurs when the assessors follow and examine one cohort more closely than the other. This can be avoided by blinding assessors to which group is receiving the exposure.

REFERENCES

1. Fuller, J. (1965). Julius Caesar: man, soldier, and tyrant (pp. 81-82). New Brunswick, N.J.: Rutgers University Press.
2. Grimes DA, Schulz KF. Cohort studies: marching towards outcomes. Lancet. 2002;359(9303):341-5.
3. Gordis L. Epidemiology, 3rd edition. Philadelphia: Elsevier and Saunders. pp. 149-158.
4. Kestenbaum B, Adeney K, Weiss N, Shoben A. (2009). Epidemiology and biostatistics (pp. 33-100). Dordrecht: Springer.
5. Guyatt G, Rennie D, Meade M, et al. Users' guides to the medical literature, 2nd edition. USA: McGraw-Hill companies; 2008.
6. Haynes RB, Guyatt G, Tugwell P, et al. Clinical epidemiology, 3rd edition. Philadelphia: Lippincott Williams & Wilkins; 2006.
7. Fletcher RH, Fletcher SW, Fletcher GS. Clinical epidemiology: The Essentials, 5th edition. Baltimore: Lippincott Williams & Wilkins; 2012. pp. 65-7.
8. Hulley S, Cummings S, Browner W, et al. Designing clinical research- an epidemiologic approach, 3rd edition. Philadelphia: Lippincott Williams & Wilkins; 2007.
9. Salkind NJ. Encyclopedia of research design. Los Angeles: SAGE publication Inc; 2010. pp. 561-3.
10. Bryant DM, Willits K, Hanson BP. Principles of designing a cohort study in orthopaedics. J Bone Joint Surg Am. 2009;91(Suppl 3):10-4.

8

Level 3 Evidence—Case-control Studies

Raman Mundi

Key Objectives

- Be able to define what a case-control study is
- Understand when it is reasonable to use case-control studies
- Understand some of the key components in the design of case-control studies
- Determine how to distinguish high quality from low quality case-control studies
- Understand some of the limitations of the case-control design.

What is a Case-control Study

It is a study design in which a group of people with a certain disease state or condition (i.e. 'cases') are identified first and then compared to a group without the disease state or condition (i.e. 'control').[1] The study compares these two groups to look for whether the cases have an exposure that controls do not, which could possibly represent a cause or risk factor. Case-control studies are considered *retrospective* studies because the cases already have the disease or condition of interest and the investigators are looking retrospectively for the factors that are associated with this outcome. This is completely opposite to the prospective study design [i.e. observational cohort studies and randomized controlled trials (RCTs)] in which exposure or risk factors are identified first and then patients are followed *prospectively* in time to track that who develops the disease and who does not.

An example of a case-control study would be a study looking to determine whether hip fractures in elderly people were associated with benzodiazepine use.[2] All patients presenting to the emergency department with a hip fracture were considered *cases*, whereas patients presenting with other acute illnesses were considered *controls*. Both groups were evaluated using retrospective indicators of benzodiazepine use (e.g. questionnaires, previous medical records). The study determined that only lorazepam, but no other benzodiazepines were associated with increased risk of hip fractures in elderly people.

How Can I Use This Type of Study Design?

The Oxford Center for Evidence-based medicine (EBM) classifies case-control studies as Level 3 evidence, which is one level above the patient case-series and one level below observational cohort studies.[3] RCTs are considered the best primary study design and should be used whenever feasible. However, in spite of being so low on the hierarchy of evidence, there is remain instances where case-control studies are either the most feasible study design to use, or where it is impractical to use higher levels of evidence.

The case-control design is often the only reasonable option when studying in a very rare conditions, as it allows for an appropriate ratio of cases to controls.[4] For instance, if a condition has only a few hundred new cases per year, one would have to recruit hundreds to thousands of patients to generate enough statistical *power* in a prospective cohort study. A similar argument can be made for diseases that have a very long *latency period* between exposure and onset of symptoms.[4] It is often impractical to prospectively follow a group of patients with a certain risk factor or exposure for 10, 20 or 30 years. In this scenario, selecting known cases upfront and employing a case-control design is more cost-efficient and practical. Because conducting case-control studies is relatively cost-efficient and time-efficient, the other instance where case-control studies are appropriate is in generating preliminary hypothesis or preliminary data with the intent of following-up these studies with higher level studies in the future.[4] Generating hypothesis or data may be useful to researchers when trying to narrow down that what exposures or risk factors to study in a prospective trial. This information is also useful in providing preliminary data when writing grant proposals. Finally, case-control studies are useful when an RCTs is unethical. For example, one cannot randomly assign patients to inhale cigarette smoke or asbestos as it is clearly unethical. Because the case-control design is retrospective in nature, one is able to follow the patients who have already undergone exposure to see if it is a causative factor.

How do I Design a Case-control Study?

As with any study, a case-control study begins with a hypothesis. Typically, this involves asking whether a certain outcome is associated with a particular exposure or risk factor. The next step involves determining on how both the outcome of interest and the exposure will be defined. Will the definitions be based on objectively documented data sources or self-reported measures? Something as simple as a patient's cholesterol levels may be defined objectively, such as LDL-c (low-density lipoprotein) levels over the past year as documented in a patient's medical chart, or more subjectively, such as by asking the patient whether he/she has suffered from cholesterol issues in the past. How the outcome and exposure are defined will have implications for the quality of the results by either introducing or minimizing potential for bias.

The next step involves selecting cases for one's study. Once the definition of the outcome of interest has been established, as just discussed, screening for cases should be relatively straightforward. However, determining where to draw the cases from, it requires some consideration. Will the cases be drawn from the general population—a somewhat ideal approach but one that presents significant logistical challenges or will the cases be drawn from a university hospital? In the latter case, the patients may actually have more comorbidities than cases in the general population or at a community hospital and thus not very representative of the community. Ultimately, a decision that takes into account logistical, financial and practical considerations needs to be made. The limitations of approach that is adopted, is taken should be acknowledged by the investigators. As a general rule of thumb, ***incident cases*** are also better to use than ***prevalent cases***.[5] This increases the likelihood that the exposure(s) being studied is actually associated with the development of the outcome.

Following this, an appropriate control group needs to be selected. The control group, by definition, is simply a group of individuals who do not suffer from any disease. This appears to be a relatively easy task, as there are millions of people who do not suffer from the disease being studied. However, two criteria should be considered when selecting the control group.[5] Firstly, the control group should part of a population that is reasonably 'at risk' of acquiring the outcome being studied. It does not make much sense to use healthy young athletes as a control group if the outcome of interest is an osteoporotic hip fracture. Secondly, the exposure status or risk factors of the controls should be measurable as accurately as they are measurable in cases. It would not be appropriate, for instance, to use controls from a population that does not frequently a primary care practitioner if the exposure is being measured using a family physician's charts. Generally, to fulfil both these criteria as well as to ensure rigorous results, four techniques are commonly used[4]:

1. The control group is selected from the same setting as the cases are, such as from in-patients at a community hospital.
2. Both the control group and cases are selected from the general population within a particular geographical or alternately defined boundary.
3. The control group is selected randomly from the general population, even though the cases have not been. However, the control group has been 'matched', meaning that it has similar characteristics in terms of age, gender, height, and other ***confounding variables***.
4. Two control groups are selected from different populations. For example, in a large case-control study of the risk of myocardial infarction in obese individuals, one control group was selected from amongst relatives of cardiac patients and the other came from hospital in-patients with non-cardiac conditions.[6]

In selecting cases and controls, ideally a 1:1 ratio is used. However, this approach is often not adequate in generating appropriate statistical power when the disease being studied is very rare. In such instances, investigators may choose to use four or five controls in one case. Any ratio beyond this is often not worthwhile in terms of increasing statistical confidence in the results.[5]

How do I Collect and Analyze the Data?

As mentioned earlier, data collected can be subjective or objective. **Subjective data** includes patient self-reported exposures or risk factors and it is often not reliable. Relying on patient recall often introduces bias in the results because patients with a disease are more likely to remember an exposure than the control subjects (so-called recall bias). If feasible, partial blinding may be used, whereby both case and control are not aware of the study hypothesis.[4] However, this is not always possible, especially considering most of the cases know that they have a disease and most controls know that they do not. Ideally, objective data—includes data derived from previous medical charts, previous radiographs/imaging, government records, etc. is better. Nevertheless, the use of objective data often also proves problematic because the data was never originally intended for research use. Investigators may find that records are incomplete, reporting is variable or simply illegible and/or access to the data is limited.

The ultimate goal of any study that looks into exposures and resultant outcomes is to numerically define the risk of developing the outcome in someone who is subjected to a specific exposure. For binary data (i.e. exposed versus not exposed) in case-control studies only a measure known as an **odds ratio**, can be calculated.[7] Fortunately, the odds ratio tends to closely approximate **relative risk**, especially for diseases with low incidence/prevalence. Statistical methods can also be used to control for known confounding variables. A detailed discussion of statistical analysis is beyond the scope of this chapter.

How Can I Critically Appraise Case-control Studies?

Distinguishing high from low quality studies has been discussed throughout this chapter. Some further points for consideration are made in this section.

Right from the beginning, there should be an evident hypothesis that is made *a priori*. There should also be an evidence of a sample size calculation to ensure adequate statistical power. Cases and controls should be reasonably similar as well. 'Table 1' of a study should typically compare the characteristics of the cases group and control group. Factors such as age, gender, and other confounding factors should be reported and reasonably similar between the groups. The reader should also make a judgment as to whether there was a reasonable attempt made to account for all major confounding variables or not. The reader should also be aware of 'overmatching'—are the groups so similar that the control group may actually have experienced the exposure being investigated to some degree. This may actually lead to the study which underestimating the magnitude of the effect.

High quality case-control studies also generally make a concerted effort to minimize biases. One of these biases, ***recall bias***, was discussed above. Another frequent bias results when equal rigour is not applied to the exposure measurement between cases and controls. For instance, consider a theoretical case-control study of lung cancer (outcome) and its association with smoking (exposure). Patients in the 'cases' group may be considered chronic smokers at lower thresholds, whereas controls may be interrogated more rigorously before being considered positive for chronic smoking. This is called ***surveillance bias***. Readers must be aware of other sources of unequal treatment between cases and controls.

What are Some of the Limitations of Case-control Design?

There are some inherent limitations to the case-control design that cannot be avoided even with the most rigorously conducted studies. Most importantly, causal relationships cannot be definitively proven using the case-control design. Cause-and-effect relationships can only be proven in well-designed prospective trials that have limited all biases. With case-control studies, it is often impossible to prove a temporal relationship between exposure and outcome—a key requirement in proving causality. Even when the temporal relationship is clear—for example, the exposure occurred years, earlier at a single and identifiable point in time such as might occur in a nuclear accident—it is still impossible to control for all the other intermittent exposures and all possible confounding variables. Controlling for these variables also relies to some degree on human judgment and therefore is prone to the introduction of bias. Thus, one should be sceptical of any authors purporting a causal relationship in a case-control study. For this same reason (i.e. all biases can never be controlled) and because retrospective data is being relied on, even the most well-conducted case-control studies will never hold more weight than the most well-conducted prospective studies. Therefore, higher levels of evidence should always be sought out if feasible.

Important Learning Points

- The case-control study is a retrospective study design in which individuals with a condition (cases) are compared to individuals without the condition (controls) to determine associated exposures or risk factors.
- Case-control studies are appropriate for rare conditions, conditions with long latency periods and for generating hypothesis or preliminary data.
- Designing a case-control study involves the generation of a hypothesis, adequately defining both outcome and exposure/risk factors, appropriate selection of both cases and controls, collecting the data, analyzing the data and reporting the results.
- The appropriate selection of cases and controls is one of the most difficult, yet most important, aspects of a case-control study.
- Investigators and readers should be aware of the many biases and confounding variables that may impact accuracy of the results of a case-control study.
- Case-control studies cannot prove cause-and-effect relationships.

More to Read

Bhandari M & Joensson A. Historical perspectives of clinical research (Eds). Clinical Research for Surgeons. Thieme Publishing Group, New York; 2009.

Definitions

Case-control study: A study design in which a group of people with a certain disease state or condition are identified first and then compared to a group without the disease state or condition.

Confounding variables: A variable or factor that is correlated with both the outcome and exposure. It therefore, may appear to be directly causing the outcome because its values fluctuates in synchrony with the causative exposure.

Incidence: The number of new cases of disease or outcome as a percentage of the total number of subjects in the group.

Latency period: The period of time between a specific exposure and the development of symptoms of a disease.

Odds ratio: A ratio of the odds of an outcome in an exposed group to the odds of the same outcome in a non-exposed group.

Power: The probability of rejecting a false null hypothesis. It is inversely proportional to Type II error (β).

Prevalence: The total number of cases of a disease that exist at a given point in time.

Relative risk: The ratio of the risk of disease in exposed individuals to the risk of disease in non-exposed individuals.

REFERENCES

1. Mihailovic A, Bell CM, Urbach DR. Users' guide to the surgical literature. Case-control studies in surgical journals. Can J Surgery. 2005;48(2):148-51.
2. Pierfitte C, Macouillard G, Chaslerie A, et al. Benzodiazepines and hip fractures in elderly people: case-control study. BMJ. 2001;322(7288):704-8.
3. Phillips B, Ball C, Sackett D, et al. (2009). Oxford Centre for Evidence-Based Medicine. Levels of Evidence. [online] CEBM website. Available from www.cebm.net/oxford-centre-evidence-based-medicine-levels-evidence-march-2009/ [Accessed March 2009].
4. Mann CJ. Observational research methods. Research designs II: cohort, cross sectional, and case-control studies. Emerg Med J. 2003;20(1):54-60.
5. Coggon D, Rose G, Barker DJP. Case-control and cross sectional studies. Epidemiology for the uninitiated. BMJ. 1997.

6. Yusuf S, Hawken S, Ounpuu S, et al. Obesity and the risk of myocardial infarction in 27,000 participants from 52 countries: a case-control study. Lancet. 2005;366(9497):1640-9.
7. Jaeschke R, Guyatt G, Barratt A, et al. Measures of association. In: Guyatt G, Rennie D (eds). The users' guides to the medical literature: a manual of evidence-based clinical practice. AMA. 2002;351-68.

9
Level 4 Evidence— Clinical Case Series

Shakir Ahamed

> **Key Objectives**
> - Understand how to identify a clinical case series study
> - Learn about the strengths and weaknesses of a clinical case series study design
> - Learn how to critically appraise evidence from a clinical case series.

What is a Clinical Case Series?

Clinical case series are under the category of descriptive studies, which are examples of an observational study design and are used to collect the general disease characteristics of a person, place and time.[1] A ***case series*** is comprised of a collection of related case reports. A ***case report*** is a detailed description of the clinical experience of an individual patient, intervention or outcome, as opposed to using statistical measures. A case series may describe the experience of a group of people with a similar disease or treatment.[2] Case series are unique compared to other studies. As opposed to testing a hypothesis, they are generally hypothesisgenerating.[1,3] Although case series are Level IV evidence, above only expert opinion, they may still be a very valuable resource. Randomized controlled trials (RCTs) are not suitable for all cases because of technical or ethical reasons. For example, in the treatment of open fractures, it would be unethical to randomly assign patients' early or delayed treatment. In this case, an observational study may be more appropriate.

What are the Strengths of a Clinical Case Series?

Novel Procedure or Treatment

The first obvious strength of a case series is that they are often the first data available on a novel disease or treatment. For the same reasons they can also be used for assessing rare conditions.[1] Consider a researcher who wishes to conduct a case series on patients undergoing a new minimally-invasive treatment for spinal deformity surgery. The researcher can obtain valuable information by recording medical or surgical outcomes by enrolling these patients in a case series and collecting detailed descriptions of postoperative follow-up details and adverse effects. New techniques, such as minimally-invasive spine surgery, require highly specialized surgeons and initially it may not be practical to conduct a large scale RCT to investigate surgery outcomes. Therefore, case series provide an easy alternative to investigate outcomes of new techniques and procedures.

Hypothesis Generation

The primary purpose of a case series should be the generation of a hypothesis, which can then be further tested in a more complex study design.[1] Using the same example of minimally-invasive spinal deformity surgery, if the researcher finds that out of 100 patients in the case series, 5 developed wound complications, then data collected in the case series will likely not be able to provide a clear answer to whether these patients developed wound complications as a result of the surgery or whether there is in fact some other factor in these individual patients that caused them to develop a wound complication. As a result, the findings of the case series can lead to further investigation to test the hypothesis that wound complications are a side effect of minimally-invasive deformity surgery.

Pragmatic Reflection of Clinical Practice

In case series as well as all observational studies the investigator does not control which intervention(s) the patient receives. Because of this, the results of a case series study more accurately represents clinical practice and could therefore be considered more relevant. A secondary benefit of not controlling the treatment decision is that the surgeons are not forced to perform an operation in which they are less experienced.[1]

Efficient Study Design

The simple design of a case series makes it an efficient and cost-saving design due to the lack of a ***comparison group*** and the lack of randomization.[1] A major benefit of this design is that you can easily obtain a detailed account of clinical experience of the particular topic.[2] Not only is the data easily obtained, but also it is easy to understand.[4]

Ethically Sound

Another big advantage of a case series is that they generally lack any major ethical dilemma, which may involve issues of patient identification, or confidentiality. Since it is an observational study, there is no randomly assigned treatment group, thus the ethics of ***placebo*** or sham treatment is avoided.[1] For example, consider a researcher who wants to look at the effects of a new blood pressure medication by comparing three groups: treatment, standard of care and placebo. It would not be ethically sound to have someone on a placebo because if a patient really requires medication to reduce their blood pressure, it would be dangerous to their health to be receiving no medication at all via the placebo. In such cases, it is more ethically acceptable to conduct a clinical case series on patients who have elected to try the new medication in place of their old one, and then record any adverse events for future research.

If done correctly, the data of multiple case series can be combined, allowing for more accurate and reliable hypothesis to be formulated.[4] Important points to keep in mind in order to write a good case series will be discussed later in this chapter.

What are the Limitations of a Clinical Case Series?

Lack of a Comparison Group

The biggest limitation of a case series is the lack of a comparison (control) group. Without a control group, it is impossible to determine whether outcomes are due to the treatment or to other patient characteristics. Therefore casual relations should not be made between the treatment and the outcomes.[1] As stated before, only hypothesis can be made which should be tested by a more complex study design. For example, you are conducting a case series on 10 basketball players by recording, how well each player performs after having an energy drink before playing. If your results show that 8 of the players play extremely well in the game, there is no way of knowing whether this high performance was due to the fact that they had the energy drink, or whether it was because of some other reason, unique to each player. Therefore, case series are not well suited for research questions that involve evaluating a treatment effect.

Retrospective Design

Another limitation is that most case series are retrospective studies (i.e. data is collected after the event that is being studied has already taken place).[1] The problem with retrospective design is that there is no control over each case and therefore variables are not kept constant between each case. Well-developed protocols and a single dedicated investigator are absent in retrospective design. This results in incomplete and non-standard data collection leading to an increase in biased measurement.[1] Also, biased measurement may arise when different measurement methods are used.

Selection Bias

Many types of observational studies are also subject to selection bias. Selection bias is when patients who experience better or worse outcomes are less likely to be included in the follow-up data. For example, in many cases, only patients available for a follow-up of a certain time length are included in the study. If a patient dies, or changes hospital before the follow-up time is complete they will not be included. As a result there will be bias as some patients that experienced a worse outcome have been exempted.[1] Consider a case series that is done on several hundred people enrolled in a smoking cessation program. If the follow-up point for the study is at 6 months into the program, then all the people who did not make it to the 6-month mark are excluded. Therefore, even if the study shows positive outcomes for the smoking cessation program, the selection of research participants is biased because those who had a worse outcome (i.e. left the program) are not considered. Selection bias in case series may also lead to inaccurate assumptions about a treatment, as well as findings that are not generic to the general population.

What Makes a Good Case Series?

Clearly Defined Question

The first characteristic of a good case series is a clearly defined question. Due to the nature of case series, they should avoid comparison questions, such as 'is one treatment better than another', or 'whether a certain treatment is effective in treating a disease'. The question of a case series should be very focused, for example, how a particular treatment is utilized in healthcare, or the functional status of patients after receiving a particular treatment?[3] In short, the question of the study should list the population, the intervention, and the primary outcomes.[1]

Well-described Study Population and Intervention

The next characteristic is a well-described study population & intervention. The reader of a case series should be able to compare their patients with the patients described in the case series; this is done by using standardized (or explicit) definitions. They should also use standard descriptive information (i.e. age, gender and socioeconomic status) when describing patients. This allows the reader to easily compare their case.[3] It is also important to outline detailed procedure or treatment so that another center(s) can replicate the study.[3]

Well-described Results and Follow-up

It is also important to have well described results. During follow-up, not all patients will be able to be studied. For example, a number of patients may decide to switch to other treatments, or a few of the patients may die, as a result, the total number of patients lost follow-up should be reported.[3] It is also important to take care that the results from the follow-up are not misleading. For example, let's consider a case that has variable follow-up time. In this hypothetical case, the majority of the patients had a short follow-up time (around 9 months) and most of them had no side effects, while a smaller proportion of the population was followed for a longer time, and almost all of the developed a side effect. From this data it may suggest that the occurrence of side effects is low; to describe the situation more accurately, a *rate* should be used.[4]

Following these guidelines mentioned in the above paragraphs will make a case series more accurate and useful.

Conclusions

Despite its simple nature, a case series is a very important type of study. Case studies can be used when other studies are unfeasible (either due to funding, sample size, or other variables). It is important to remember that the main function of a case series it to formulate a hypothesis and not to prove a causal relationship. This formulated hypothesis can then be a foundation for more advanced and complex studies. Although case series will not provide all the information needed, it is often a very good first step.

Important Learning Points

- Clinical case series are descriptive studies that consist of a collection of multiple related patient case reports containing observations made by a physician regarding a particular clinical scenario.
- The main purpose of a case series is hypothesis generation.
- Case series are advantageous because they are often the first study on a novel procedure or treatment, they are useful in hypothesis generation, they are a pragmatic reflection of clinical practice, they are an efficient study design, and they are ethically sound.
- Limitations include lack of a comparison group, the retrospective nature of the design and selection bias.
- A good case series includes a clearly defined question, well-described population, intervention and results.

Definitions

Case report: A detailed description of the clinical experience of individual study subjects.[2]

Case series: A collection of related case reports, consisting of patients with similar diagnosis undergoing the same treatment.[2]

Comparison group: A group in RCT that receives no treatment.

Placebo: Biologically inert substance that is as similar as possible to the active intervention. Placebo allows implementing blinding.

Rate: The number of events in those at risk for the event divided by the total follow-up person time.[3]

REFERENCES

1. Kooistra B, Dijkman B, Einhorn TA, et al. How to design a good case series. J Bone Joint Surg Am. 2009;91(Suppl 3):21-6.
2. Kestenbaum, Bryan. Epidemiology and biostatistics, 1st edition. New York: Springer-Verlag; 2009.
3. Carey TS, Boden SD. A critical guide to case series reports. Spine. 2003;28(15):1631-4.
4. Jabs DA. Improving the reporting of clinical case series. Am J Opthamol. 2005;139(5):900-5.

10

Level 5 Evidence— Surveys

Arnav Agarwal

Key Objectives

- Understand the purpose and importance of surveys in clinical research
- Learn about the development, administration and reporting of surveys
- Learn tips on acquiring optimal response rates
- Learn how to assess the quality of survey research.

What is a 'Survey'?

The term 'survey' refers to the standardized collection of information from a group of people belonging to a ***population of interest*** in order to make inferences about that population at a specific time.[1,2] Surveys aim to gather reliable and unbiased data from a representative sample of respondents.[3] Types of information that can be collected includes demographics, socioeconomic and health characteristics, attitudes, opinions, past or present personal circumstances, knowledge and behaviours.[2,4] The population of interest can be patients, learners, researchers, colleagues etc. Common modes of survey administration used in clinical research include ***self-administered*** postal, fax and web surveys, as well as face-to-face or telephone interviews. Survey objectives, methodology, data analysis and results are typically reported in a scholarly article or report.

Surveys can be characterized as descriptive, explanatory or evaluation based. Descriptive surveys provide information about characteristics, behaviours and attitudes of a particular group and may estimate specific parameters in a population or describe cross-sectional associations between population characteristics and behaviours. Explanatory surveys move beyond simple description, typically involving a longitudinal design to identify the direction of associations and draw inferences between sets of variables or constructs.[5] This survey strategy is often used in cohort, panel and trend study designs.[2,4] Evaluation surveys assess effects of a planned change on a group of people.[6]

How are Surveys Important in Clinical Research?

Surveys have an advantage over other research strategies in their utilization of empirical data, greater generalizability than some other approaches based on data collection from a representative sample and their low-cost, short-duration and large-scale data collection nature. This research strategy can use clinical practice data to stimulate new research questions and impact clinical practice through its findings. In the political spectrum, it may serve as a source of reference for policy development, evaluation of recent developments and strategic planning.[2]

How are Surveys Developed?

There are four general steps involved in the development of surveys (Fig. 10.1). The first step is figuring out its purpose or in other words, framing the ***research question***. This can be rooted in questions posed by others in the literature or in an issue that the researcher is simply interested in.[7] Researchers use existing literature, personal experience and the advice of other researchers and healthcare practitioners to develop and refine their research question.[1,2] Framing the research question involves determining a clear objective with a specific topic, respondents and primary and secondary research focuses to be addressed. Identifying a representative and appropriately generalizable sampling frame with due consideration to response rates, survey objectives and available resources is also important in framing the question.[5] Good research questions are specific, clear, simple and answerable.[1,4] This step shapes the design, content and evaluation of the survey instruments.[2]

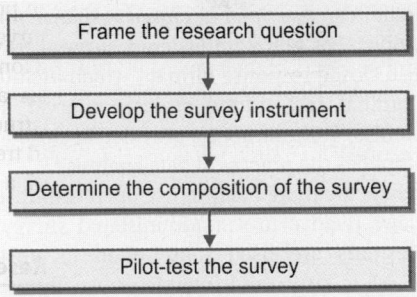

Fig. 10.1: Four general steps in survey development

The next step is survey ***instrument development.*** Researchers may choose to create their survey independently, modify a survey developed by another author or use a combination of both methods.[4] Survey development typically involves item generation, considering all potential ideas and concepts related to themes or categories addressing the research question for inclusion. Literature reviews, interviews, focus groups, respondent or expert input and the Delphi process represent mediums for idea generation.[4,5,8] Item generation is followed by defining constructs, classifying items into domains, formulating questions within each domain and subsequent item reduction to minimize respondent burden without eliminating entire domains or constructs.[4,5,8,9,10] When constructing or modifying survey ***items***, the researcher needs to consider two components: the ***stem*** and ***response format***. Good stems are shorter than 20 words, relevant, easily interpretable, unbiased and clear.[4,5,7] Questions that are vague, double-barrelled, condescending, judgemental, socially or culturally insensitive, contain more than one variable and double negatives are usually avoided as they may confuse or discourage respondents.[4,5,7,10] The perspective from which questions are addressed, language used, response format and ordering and question-stem synthesis and presentation, have been reported to influence survey completion and types of responses received as well.[3,4,5,11,12,13] Response formats provide a framework for answers to posed survey questions.[4,5]

The researcher can use ***open*** or ***closed response formats*** for the questions.[4] For self-administered surveys, researchers typically use closed response formats, which include binary, nominal ordinal (e.g. rating scales), interval and ratio measurements.[5,7,14] The structure provided in closed response formats simplifies the process of data analysis.[4,15]

Researchers are more likely to use open response formats for interviews relative to self-administered surveys. Open-ended questions are used more often in unstructured interviews, while structured interviews usually use closed-ended questions with closed response formats (e.g. list of questions asked in specified order, with list of pre-coded answers for closed-ended questions). Semi-structured interviews have less rigid planning and ordering of questions.[1] Investigators determining response options should also consider whether or not to include indeterminate response options to acknowledge uncertainty, avoiding ***floor and ceiling effects*** by providing more response options to increase discrimination among responses and including "other" response options for elaborations or unique response entries. [3,4,5,7,11,16,17] ***Determining survey composition*** is the third step in survey development. A personalized cover letter containing the survey's objective, why potential respondents were selected, academic institutional affiliations, a time estimate for survey completion and affirmation of the respondent's participation, should be included.[5,18,19] The instrument with the survey's rationale highlighted should be placed inside a selected envelope with the cover letter, return envelope and incentive, if provided. Investigators may consider a booklet format for long questionnaires, coding of surveys before administration if multiple stages are involved and "opt-out" responses to identify respondents who were incorrectly identified or do not have an interest in participating.[5,11,16] Question numbering and organizing, question ordering on the basis of content, clear requests for either single or multiple responses in the question stem—clear instructions, operational definitions and attention to spatial arrangement, color, brightness and visual presentation consistency, are also recommended.

Following a pretesting stage to revise questions based on appropriateness and whether they are interpreted as intended, the last step in survey development is ***pilot-testing***. Pilot-testing the survey with a group of individuals from the target population assesses the instrument in a semi-structured interaction, assessing flow, salience, acceptability, relevance, language, redundancy and time to and ease of completion. Pretesting and pilot-testing minimize question misinterpretation, misrepresentation of participant responses and facilitate further item reduction. Assessments may be conducted to determine whether response formats are easily understandable, how much appropriate and comprehensive items are, whether the instrument addresses the study objective and topic of interest and how effectively questions are able to differentiate between respondents such that similar participants respond consistently and vice versa.[4,5]

How are Surveys Administered?

The optimal mode of administration for a particular survey depends on its subject matter, time and resources available to the investigator, the amount and type of data to be gathered and whether test properties are established.[5,16] Surveys can be self-administered, such as postal, fax and web surveys.

Postal surveys are sent by mail and incur costs of postage and stationery. Fax surveys require both parties to have access to fax machines. Web surveys are sent via Email either in the body of the message, attached to the message or in an online survey software for which a hyperlink is provided in the Email message. Web surveys have the lowest cost, fastest response process and do not require manual recording of data.[20] However, several studies have reported lower response rates with web surveys relative to postal administration.[5,21,22,23] This mode of survey administration requires that both parties have computers with internet access and may require skilled information technologists, server space and electronic software for survey development and analysis. Advance noticed preceding administration of the survey instrument, an electronic cover letter and electronic incentives provided as necessary, are other strategies investigators should consider with web survey administration.[5] Other modes of survey administration include face-to-face and telephone interviewing. These modes are advantageous in that they provide an opportunity for the researcher to clarify and probe deeper with questioning.[24] The face-to-face interview involves the interviewer personally approaching respondents to ask for their participation in the survey. The interviewer asks questions and notes responses. Telephone interviews involve the researcher approaching and surveying respondents over the phone. Telephone interviewing is cheaper and more time-efficient than face-to-face interviewing.[1]

The different dynamics of researcher respondent interaction in each mode of administration can affect the responses of participants.[25,26] For example, respondents answering health self-assessment questions over the telephone have been found to use more positive and extreme answers compared to those asked via mailed questionnaire.[26] Different modes of survey administration present varying levels of pressure to give socially desirable answers and differ in the wording of questions and response formats.[25,27] These factors, among others, lead to mode-dependent influences on participant responses.

Investigators should choose a mode of administration based on both convenience grounds and on scientific and ethical grounds. Due consideration to respondent needs and preferences, retention, accuracy of questions and response options, research team skills and resources and the nature of the study (short-term versus long-term, pilot versus large-scale) should supplement an assessment of ease of delivery and related expenses.[28]

How are Survey Results Reported?

Survey results are usually reported in a scholarly article or report and this is done in different ways according to the type of publication and intended audience.[2] Some key elements of a survey report are as follows[1]:
- The research questions
- Background information from existing literature
- Details about the research method

- Who the respondents are and how they were selected?
- Description of the survey and its development process
- The response rate
* Details about the data collection and analysis procedures
* Results
* Discussion of the findings
* Limitations of the study
* Conclusion and recommendations.

What are Limitations of Survey Research?

Surveys as research instruments, have several limitations (Table 10.1). Many of these limitations can bias survey results and efforts should be made to minimize this bias whenever possible. For example, a respondent's inclination to give culturally appropriate responses to sensitive topics may bias results.[4] Researchers asking about sensitive topics may choose to use self-administered surveys instead of the more personal modes to reduce this bias. Also, responses may be biased if the wording order or format of the questions causes respondents to misunderstand or misinterpret what is really being asked.[4,15] This can be avoided by ensuring that questions are written at an appropriate reading level and by accommodating the language preferences of the respondents.[4] *Sampling error* can also bias the result.[1,15] Sampling error can never be eliminated in full, but its magnitude can increased or decreased depending on the *sampling technique* that is used. For survey research, *random sampling* would be optimal to reduce sampling error.[1] The most important type of bias that concerns survey researchers is *non-responder bias*. Non-responder bias occurs when the response rate is too low, casting doubt on the generalizability of the results.[4] The researcher can compare the demographic data of responders and non-responders in an effort to prove that the two groups do not differ, but this is challenging and the information is usually difficult to obtain.[15] A minimum 70% response rate is generally considered sufficient, although no specific response rate guarantees an unbiased representation of the population.[4,15] Other types of bias pertaining to survey development include[29]:

- ***Question design:***
  - Problems with wording (described earlier)
  - ***Missing or inadequate data:*** Failure to identify a common starting time for exposure or illness, collection of degraded data and use of an insensitive measure
  - ***Inappropriate scale:*** Limited response categories, missing or overlapping response choice intervals
  - ***Leading questions:*** Negative or guiding phrases leading to specific selections
  - ***Intrusiveness:*** Selective suppression of information with self-reporting, refusal to respond, inaccuracy of responses to sensitive questions
  - ***Inconsistency:*** Differences in case definitions, change of measurement scale, changes in wording and diagnostic terminology.
- ***Survey design:***
  - ***Formatting:*** Horizontal versus vertical formats, juxtaposed versus independent scales, left versus right alignment
  - ***Length:*** Selection of *yes* or *no* for all questions, quality of responses with open questions, respondent fatigue
  - ***Structure:*** Logical errors in question flow, errors in skipping sequence of questions.
- ***Survey administration:***
  - ***Interviewer bias:*** Subconscious or conscious gathering of selective data, non-blinding
  - ***Respondent bias:*** Avoiding end-of-scale responses, providing skewed positive responses to questions addressing satisfaction, falsely appearing sick to qualify for support, over reporting of socially desirable responses and under reporting of socially undesirable exposures or conditions, biased responses to subsequent questions based on initial responses, responding based on perceived knowledge of the study hypothesis, soliciting information from proxies, inaccuracies or incompleteness in recalling information.

How can Researchers Ensure Optimal Response Rates?

High response rates increase the precision of estimates, reduce selection bias risk and enhance the validity of study findings.[3,5,21] A major factor affecting response rates is the choice of administration mode used for the survey. Face-to-face interviews have the highest reported response rates, followed by telephone, postal, Email and web surveys.[1,30,31] For physicians, however, it has been reported that postal surveys yield higher response rates than do telephone interviews.[32] A 'mixed mode' method of survey administration has also been shown to increase response rates, although there are concerns over the effect of administration mode on responses.[33]

Other factors that affect response rates involve survey lay-out and format. These factors are specific to self-administered surveys. Lengthy surveys can reduce response rates, so it is recommended that 25 or fewer items are used.[4,14] Also, surveys that appear to be lengthy due to formatting (e.g. booklet) have lower response rates than more compact formats.[34] Surveys that are concise, easy to understand and have the most relevant questions placed at the beginning have the highest response rates.[1,34] The cover letter can also be used to encourage respondents to take part in the study.[14] Cover letters should include the purpose of the survey, details of how and why the respondent was chosen to complete it, the importance of their participation, the name and contact information of the researcher, any potential benefits or harm inherent in participation and assurance of confidentiality.[1,4] Ensuring confidentiality, including a self-addressed, stamped envelope and personalizing the cover letter with a signature are other techniques to increase response rates.[14,35] Also, the researcher can provide monetary or non-monetary incentives with the survey and follow-up with phone calls, repeat mailings and reminders.[1,2,5,7,36,37,38,39,40,41,42]

How can I Assess the Quality of Survey Research?

When assessing the quality of survey research, it is important to consider potential biases and the researcher's effort to minimize those biases. This usually involves examining the methodology of survey development, administration and sample selection, as described above earlier. Another important consideration is the *sample size*. Generally, larger sample sizes reduce the likelihood of any of the inferences drawn being a product of chance and have better statistical quality and precision as a result.[1] Sample sizes tend to be limited, however, by the resources and time the researcher has available data for collection and analysis.[1] **Validity** and **reliability** are other important considerations in assessing survey research quality.[2]

Important Learning Points

- Survey research provides us with important information about patients, researchers, healthcare practitioners and learners.
- The key to developing a good survey is crafting a clear and refined research question.
- The best choice for administration mode is unique to the type of survey and the resources available to the researcher.
- Surveys have a number of limitations, but steps can be taken to reduce the bias they introduce to the results.
- Quality surveys are valid, reliable and have minimum bias.

More to Read

- Calder J. (1998) Survey research methods. **Medical Education** 32, 638-652.
- Passmore C, Dobbie AE, Parchman M *et al.* (2002) Guidelines for constructing a survey. **Family Medicine** 34, 281-286.
- Burns KEA, Duffett M, Kho ME *et al.* (2008) A guide for the design and conduct of self-administered surveys of clinicians. **Canadian Medical Association Journal** 179, 245-252.
- Boynton PM, Greenhalgh T. (2004) Selecting, designing and developing your questionnaire. **British Medical Journal** 328, 1312-1315.
- Boynton PM. (2004) Administering, analysing and reporting your questionnaire. **British Medical Journal** 328, 1372-1375.
- Choi BCK, Pak AWP. (2005) A catalog of bias in questionnaires. **Preventing Chronic Disease** 2, 1-13.

Definitions

Closed response format: A survey response format that provides pre-coded responses for the respondent to choose from.[1,4]

Item: A question in a survey. It is comprised of two components: stem and response format.[4]

Non-responder bias: When difference in the characteristics of responders and non-responders [4] leads to inaccurate results and inferences. This is usually a concern when response rate is too low.

Open response format: A survey response format that allows the respondent to respond in their own words.[1,4]

Pilot-testing: Administering the survey to a sample of the target population to identify any changes that need to be made. This is done before the main administration takes place.

Population of interest: The specific group of people that the researcher is interested in making inferences about from the study.[1]

Random sampling: A sampling technique in which individuals for a study sample are selected by chance.[1]

Reliability: The consistency of the data and its interpretation.[2]

Research question: The question that the investigator(s) intend to answer using research methodology. Developing a clear research question is the first step in conducting a research project.

Response format: The component of a survey item that provides the framework for the answer.[4]

Sample size: The number of participants or experimental units included in a clinical research study.

Sampling error: The probability that the sample is not representative of the population from which it is drawn.[1]

Sampling technique: The method employed by the researcher for selecting individuals for the study sample.

Self-administered survey: Surveys that are administered with no personal interaction between the surveyor and respondent while being conducted.

Stem: The question or statement component of an item in a survey.[4]

Validity: How well the data collected by the survey instrument reflects what the researcher set out to measure.[2]

REFERENCES

1. Kelley K, Clark B, Brown V, et al. Good practice in the conduct and reporting of survey research. Int J Qual Health Care. 2003;15(3):261-6.

2. Calder J. Survey research methods. Medical Education. 1998;32:638-52.
3. McColl E, Jacoby A, Thomas L, et al. Design and use of questionnaires: a review of best practice applicable to surveys of health service staff and patients. Health Technol Assess. 2001;5(31):1-256.
4. Passmore C, Dobbie AE, Parchman M, et al. Guidelines for constructing a survey. Fam Med. 2002;34(4):281-6.
5. Burns KE, Duffett M, Kho ME, et al. A guide for the design and conduct of self-administered surveys of clinicians. CMAJ. 2008;179(3):245-52.
6. Kelley K, Clark B, Brown V, et al. Good practice in the conduct and reporting of survey research. Int J Qual in Health Care. 2003;15(3):261-6.
7. Sierles FS. How to do research with self-administered surveys. Acad Psychiatry. 2003;27(2):104-13.
8. Ehrlich A, Koch T, Amin B, et al. Development and reliability testing of a standardized questionnaire to assess psoriasis phenotype. J Am Acad of Dermatol. 2006;54(6):987.
9. Fox J. Designing research: basics of survey construction. Minim Invasive Surg Nurs. 1998;8(2):77-9.
10. Dillman DA. Mail and other self-administered questionnaires. In: Rossi PH, Wright JD anderson AB (Eds). Handbook of Survey Research. 1983;359-76.
11. Stone DH. Design a questionnaire. BMJ. 1993;307(6914):1264-6.
12. Woodward CA. Questionnaire construction and question writing for research in medical education. Med Educ. 1988;22(4):345-63.
13. Guyatt GH, Cook DJ, King D, et al. Effect of the framing of questionnaire items regarding satisfaction with training and its effects on residents responses. Acad Med. 1999;74(2):192-4.
14. Wall CR, DeHaven MJ, Oeffinger KC. Survey methodology for the uninitiated. J Fam Pract. 2002;51(6):573.
15. Rubenfeld GD. (2004) Surveys: An introduction. Respiratory Care. 49, 1181-1185.
16. Henry RC, Zivick JD. Principles of survey research. Fam Pract Res J. 1986;5(3):145-57.
17. O'Cathain A, Thomas KJ. "Any other comments?" Open questions on questionnaires- a bane or a bonus to research? BMC Med Res Methodol. 2004;4:25.
18. Dillman DA. Mail and Internet surveys: the tailored design method. 2nd edition. Hoboken (NJ): John Wiley & Sons. 2000.
19. Turocy PS. Survey research in athletic training: the scientific method of development and implementation. J Athl Train. 2002;37(4 suppl):S174-S179.

20. McMahon SR, Iwamoto M, Massoudi MS et al. (2003) Comparison of e-mail, fax, and postal surveys of pediatricians. Pediatrics 111, 299-303.
21. Leece P, Bhandari M, Sprague S, et al. (2004). Internet versus mailed questionnaires: a randomized comparison (2) [published erratum appears in J Med Internet Res 2004;6:e38; corrected and republished in. J Med Internet Res2004;6:e39]. Journal of Medical Internet Research 6, e30.
22. Kim HL, Hollowell CM, Patel RV, et al. (2000) Use of new technology in endourology and laparoscopy by American urologists: Internet and postal survey. Urology 56,760-5.
23. Raziano DB, Jayadevappa R, Valenzuela D, et al. (2001) E-mail versus conventional postal mail survey of geriatric chiefs. Gerontologist 41,799-804.
24. Giuffre M. (1997) Designing research survey design--Part Two. Journal of PeriAnesthesia Nursing 12, 358-362.
25. Dillman DA. (2006) Why choice of survey mode makes a difference. Public Health Reports 121, 11-13.
26. Feveile H, Olsen O, Hogh A. (2007) A randomized trial of mailed questionnaires versus telephone interviews: Response patterns in a survey. BMC Medical Research Methodology 7, 27.
27. Dillman DA, Sangster RL, Tarnai J et al. (1996) Understanding differences in people's answers to telephone and mail surveys. In: Braverman MT & Slater JK (eds.) Advances in Survey Research, New Directions for Program Evaluation Series. Jossey-Bass Publishers, San Francisco, 45-62.
28. Boynton PM. (2004) Administering, analysing, and reporting your questionnaire. British Medical Journal 328, 1372-1375.
29. Choi BCK, Pak AWP. (2005) A catalog of bias in questionnaires. Preventing Chronic Disease 2, 1-13.
30. Jones R, Pitt N. (1999) Health surveys in the workplace: Comparison of postal, email and World Wide Web methods. Occupational Medicine 49, 556-558.
31. Mavis BE, Brocato JJ. (1998) Postal surveys versus electronic mail surveys: The tortoise and the hare revisited. Evaluation and the Health Professions 21, 395-408.
32. Hocking JS, Lim MSC, Read T et al. (2006) Postal surveys of physicians gave superior response rates over telephone interviews in a randomized trial. Journal of Clinical Epidemiology 5, 521-524.
33. Burroughs TE, Waterman BM, Cira JC et al. (2001) Patient Satisfaction measurement strategies: a comparison of phone and mail methods. Joint Commission Journal on Quality Improvement 27, 349-361.
34. Mullner RM, Levy PS, Byre CS et al. (1974-1982) Effects of characteristics of the survey instrument on response rates to a

mail survey of community hospitals. Public Health Reports 97, 465-469.

35. Leece P, Bhandari M, Sprague S et al. (2006) Does flattery work? A comparison of 2 different cover letters for an international survey of orthopedic surgeons. Canadian Journal of Surgery 49, 90-95.
36. Church AH. (1993) Estimating the effect of incentives on mail survey response rates: A meta-analysis. Public Opinion Quarterly 57, 62-79.
37. Dillman DA. Mail and telephone surveys. The total design method. Hoboken (NJ): John Wiley & Sons; 1978.
38. Fischbacher C, Chappel D, Edwards R, et al. (2000) Health surveys via the Internet: Quick and dirty or rapid and robust? Journal of the Royal Society of Medicine 93, 356-9.
39. McLean SA, Feldman JA. (2001) The impact of changes in HCFA documentation requirements on academic emergency medicine: results of a physician survey. Academic Emergency Medicine 8, 880-5.
40. Schleyer TKL, Forrest JL. (2000) Methods for the design and administration of Web-based surveys. Journal of the American Medical Informatics Association 7, 416-25.
41. Nakash RA, Hutton JL, Jørstad-Stein EC, et al. (2006) Maximising response to postal questionnaires: a systematic review of randomised trials in health research. BMC Medical Research Methodology 6, 5.
42. Edwards P, Roberts I, Clarke M, et al. (2002) Increasing response rates to postal questionnaires: systematic review. British Medical Journal 324, 1183-91.

3

Special Designs and Topics

Section Outline

11. The Basics of Systematic Reviews and Meta-analysis
12. The Basics of Economic Evaluation
13. The Basics of a Diagnostic Test Study
14. The Basics of Reliability
15. Quick Guide to Assess Risk of Bias in Randomized Controlled Trials
16. GRADE—Understanding Grades of Healthcare Recommendations

The Basics of Systematic Reviews and Meta-analysis

Alonso Carrasco-Labra, Lyubov Lytvyn

Key Objectives

- Gain a better understanding of systematic reviews and meta-analyses
- Learn what is involved in conducting systematic reviews and meta-analyses
- Be able to identify the advantages and limitations of systematic reviews and meta-analyses
- Be able to distinguish high-quality systematic reviews from low-quality ones.

What is a 'Systematic Review'?

A *systematic review* is a research design that aims to collect, summarize and assess all available evidence that fits into specific eligibility criteria, with the purpose of objectively answering a well-defined clinical question related to the effect of an intervention (e.g. statins on risk of stroke), the accuracy estimates of a diagnostic test (e.g. sensitivity and specificity of a new diagnostic test strategy) or an estimation of association between an exposure and an outcome (e.g. smoking on risk of lung cancer). The main goal of a systematic review is to make this information more accessible to healthcare professionals and decision makers.[1]

Are all Reviews in the Literature Conducted Systematically?

The term *review* is widely used and their scope and method of development varies greatly. Generally, they can be classified as **narrative** and **systematic reviews**.

A **narrative review** is a summary that addresses a certain topic. Usually, this type of review is written with the purpose of presenting the point of view of the reviewers, with selective references to support their arguments. These reviews are prone to systematic error, known as **bias**,[2] as narrative reviews may or may not include all relevant studies in the particular clinical area. Instead, the reviewer selects articles based on their own interest and knowledge, which is likely to result in **selective citation bias** and may include specific case-based experiences dealing with a small number of patients, defined as **anecdotal clinical evidence**. The key limitations of these reviews are that methods to identify and select evidence are not transparent, and there is rarely an assessment of the quality of included studies. Without this quality assessment, readers cannot judge the level of trustworthiness of the reported evidence, which is a key element for decision-making.

A **systematic review** is a thorough and comprehensive process, and is considered one of the most relevant tools for informing clinical decision making.[2] When appropriately conducted, the reviewers follow rigorous, transparent and reproducible methods that aim to minimize the effect of bias. Table 11.1, comparison between narrative and systematic reviews.

Process of Conducting a Systematic Review

There are 8 key steps to take while conducting a systematic review.[3]

1. **Formulate the question:** Develop a focused and explicit clinical research question.
2. **Outline the eligibility criteria:** Define which studies are to be included based on the Patient, Intervention, Comparison, and Outcome (PICO) and the type of study design.
3. **Establish how to address heterogeneity:** Develop criteria to identify heterogeneity and a priori hypotheses to explain heterogeneity, if present.
4. **Design and conduct a search strategy:** Choose search terms with appropriate sensitivity and specificity to yield the information regarding the research question. It is expected that reviewers use multiple databases. Examples

Table 11.1: Comparison between narrative and systematic reviews

Narrative reviews	Systematic reviews
It is not a study design, it is a scholarly opinion about a topic. Partially summarizes the available evidence	Study design that aims to summarize all available evidence
Unclear and broad questions. May answer many questions, providing the reader with an overview rather than focused answer	Specific and focus research question(s)
The process for identifying included studies is unclear and not explicit	Clear, comprehensive and reproducible searching process
No explicit description of selection criteria for included studies. Usually, the authors cite studies familiar to them or look for studies supporting their argument/opinion on the topic	Explicit and detailed inclusion and exclusion criteria for primary studies. Eligibility usually conducted independently by two or more reviewers
Lack of assessment of the risk of bias of included studies	Reporting on the assessment of risk of bias of included studies using validated instruments
Qualitative and unsystematic methods to summarize the evidence.	Systematic qualitative and/or quantitative methods to synthesize all of the available evidence.

of relevant health science databases are EMBASE, MEDLINE and Cochrane Central. It is necessary also to search through *grey literature* to ensure that you are accessing all available relevant information.[4] Examples include contacting experts in the field, manually searching through key journals and searching conference/meeting abstracts. It is also recommended to check reference lists of included studies, in case any relevant studies were missed. This process is called as ***recursive search***.

5. ***Screen studies:*** First, titles and abstracts are reviewed for potentially eligible studies, then full text studies. These steps must be conducted independently and in duplicate by two or more reviewers.
6. ***Abstract data and assess the risk of bias:*** To guarantee that data is collected systematically, the use of standardized data-retrieval forms is desirable. The risk of bias of the included studies should be assessed using validated instruments for the specific study design. One example is the Cochrane Risk of Bias tool for randomized controlled trials (RCT's).[5]
7. ***Synthesize results:*** Both qualitative and quantitative methods can be used to summarize the available evidence. When appropriate, reviewers should conduct a ***meta-analysis*** to present a pooled estimate of all included studies. Other evidence summary tables can be included such as the summary-of-findings tables proposed by the grading of recommendations, assessment, development and evaluations (GRADE) working group.[6]
8. ***Assess the certainty in the evidence:*** The confidence in the estimates of effect should be assessed and reported in the manuscript. Aspects such as risk of bias, imprecision, indirectness, inconsistency and publication bias are proposed by the GRADE working group as the main domains to consider.[7]

What are the Advantages of Systematic Reviews?

The breadth of literature available on any health topic is often unmanageable for busy clinicians and health science researchers. This is when high-quality systematic reviews become particularly relevant.[8] The strongest advantage that systematic reviews offer to clinicians and researchers is that they summarize all available information in a single, comprehensive article. Secondly, if meta-analyses were conducted, these types of analyses also provide a single pooled estimate of the effect of an intervention, accuracy estimates of a diagnostic test or an estimation of association between an exposure and an outcome. Lastly, scientific evidence is cumulative and systematic reviews are a great foundation for other researchers to build upon or reorganize the research agenda.[8]

What are the Limitations of Systematic Reviews?

The main disadvantage of systematic reviews is that, similar to narrative reviews, they are susceptible to bias with the potential to distort the final result or conclusion of the review.[8] There are two potential sources of bias that can be described:
1. Inherent to the review process, including methods to identify, select, appraise and summarize the available evidence, and
2. Inherent to the body of evidence or group of included studies.

In the former category, we can find ***selective citation bias***, ***time lag bias*** and ***language/country bias***, among others.[9] Selective citation bias is much more common in narrative reviews, however, it may still occur in systematic reviews if the reviewer does not conduct an appropriate systematic search and study selection. Time lag bias may occur as a result of including articles from an extensive time period, or when the review is not published for a considerable time after its completion. This bias would only affect results that are time-sensitive, where they could differ depending on when they were collected. Finally, language/country bias occurs when only certain articles are included in the review, based on the reviewer's access to international research and appropriate translators. This would cause the review to not be fully representative of all the literature in the field and therefore potentially inaccurate. Another type of bias, this time affecting the body of evidence, is ***publication bias***. This occurs when the publication of research findings depends on the nature or direction of the results.[4] Although, reviewers can apply the most rigorous methods when searching for studies, we can suspect publication bias (e.g. small trials showing impressive results, all industry funded), but it cannot be eliminated.

What is a 'Meta-analysis' and How it is Conducted?

It is a common mistake that 'meta-analysis' is used as a synonym for 'systematic review'. A meta-analysis is a statistical technique that allows the reviewers to pool together the results from different primary studies with the aim of obtaining a single summary estimate. When conducting a meta-analysis, researchers can use aggregated or individual-patient data from the included studies. Importantly, a meta-analysis is only appropriate if studies are similar enough. Reviewers can meta-analyze dichotomous outcomes (e.g. event/non-event) or continuous outcomes (e.g. blood pressure, quality of life and other patient-reported outcomes). For dichotomous outcomes, both the relative and the absolute measures of effect should be provided. Two of the most common relative effect estimates reported are *relative risks (RR)* and *odd ratios (OR)*. The RR is defined as 'the ratio of the risk of disease in exposed individuals to the risk of disease in non-exposed individuals'.[10] The OR is defined as 'the ratio of the odds of development of disease in exposed individuals to the odds of development of disease in non-exposed individuals'.[10] RR is easier and more intuitive to interpret, however, there are situations preferring OR, especially in meta-analysis of observational data. For continuous outcomes, the *mean difference (MD)* is used when the outcome is measured with the same instrument and *standardized mean difference (SMD)* when the instruments differ. Since SMD is expressed in units without a clinical meaning (standard deviation units), translating back to a common and well-known instrument is highly desirable to facilitate interpretation of results.[11]

The most common way to present a meta-analysis is by a *forest plot*,[8] which is a graphic representation comparing the results from different studies and display an overall, statistical aggregate result. As an example, we created a hypothetical collection of data, presented in Table 11.2 and generated a forest plot in Figure 11.1. The left column lists the studies according to the first author's last name and the year of publication. The right column lists the three reported studies' results, which are represented graphically as a square and horizontal line, corresponding to the point estimate and 95%

Table 11.2: Hypothetical data for a meta-analysis

Study	Number of adverse outcomes in drug group	Number of patients in drug group	Number of adverse outcomes in placebo group	Number of patients in placebo group
Sprague 2008	35	80	15	80
Dattani 2009	65	180	30	178
Bhandari 2005	10	50	13	49

confidence interval (CI) respectively. The 95% CI is the range of values within which we are 95% sure that the true value lies and is a reflection of the sample size and the number of events, as well as the variance (i.e. individual patients' differences in responses) in the outcome measurement of the study. The size of the black squares shows how each study is ***weighted*** in the statistical analysis compared to other studies. The Dattani 2008 study contains a larger number of patients and events than the other two studies (Table 11.2) and thus has a bigger impact on the results. The vertical line in the middle, above the number one, is the line of no difference between the groups. Note that the first two studies indicate that the probability of experiencing the outcome is higher in the exposed or experimental group than in the non-exposed or control group. The Bhandari 2005 study point estimate suggests the opposite and thus is on the other side of the line of no difference in the forest plot. The diamond in a forest plot displays the pooled estimate and 95% CI after combining all primary studies' results. Figure 11.1 shows that according to our included studies, the RR of experiencing the outcome in the experimental group compared with the control group is 1.88. In other words, the risk of experiencing the outcome is 1.88 times greater in the experimental group than in the control group. Another way to interpret a RR that is more intuitive for clinicians is using the RR reduction. To calculate, subtract 1 from the RR and express as in a percentage. For

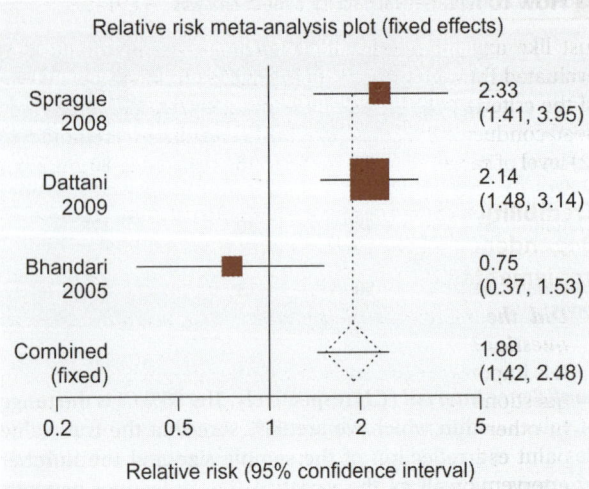

Fig. 11.1: Results from the hypothetical meta-analysis, graphed as relative risk data

example, Bhandari 2005 reports a RR of 0.75, which can be expressed as a RR reduction as follows: (1 − 0.75) × 100 = 25%. This means that there is a 25% RR reduction on the occurrence of the outcome in the experimental group compared to the control group. For the pooled estimate of the meta-analysis, the calculation is (1 − 1.88) ×100 = 88%. Since, now the RR is above one, it is interpreted as a RR increase in the outcome. This means that participants assigned to the experimental group have an 88% increase in the probability of experiencing the outcome.

The two most recognizable advantages of meta-analyses are their ability to increase precision and the benefit of providing a pooled estimate of all available evidence.[12] The precision with which a treatment effect can be estimated is highly dependent on the number of participants and events in a particular study. Conducting a meta-analysis allows reviewers to use data from all participants and all events reported, to obtain a single summary estimate, reducing ***random error*** and maximizing precision.[2]

How to Identify Credible Systematic Reviews

Just like any other scientific study, systematic reviews are evaluated through critical appraisal. The following are some of the criteria to determine whether a systematic review has been conducted in such a way that (1) results are credible and (2) level of certainty in the evidence has been determined.[3]

Credibility of Systematic Review Results in Dependency on the Rigor of the Methodology Implemented

- *Did the review explicitly address a sensible clinical question?*
  It is important to determine whether the review's research questions would effectively inform clinical practice. In other words, to what extent can we assume that the point estimates are similar across the range of patients, interventions, comparisons, and outcomes
- *Was the search for relevant studies exhaustive?*
  Systematic reviewers should incorporate all available evidence, published and unpublished, to make sure they provide the most accurate and unbiased summary estimate of effect. Furthermore, the search strategy should be reported in such a way that it can be easily reproduced.
- *Were selection and assessments of studies reproducible?*
  It is important that judgments regarding study eligibility should be conducted independently by at least two researchers. The same standard is expected for the assessment of the risk of bias among included studies.
- *Did the review present results that can be translated for clinical application?*
  Systematic reviewers should report all expressions of risk estimates to guarantee that the review will effectively inform clinical practice. When authors report only relative but not absolute estimates, clinicians and policy makers struggle to draw definitive conclusions and inform decision-making.
- *Did the review address confidence in estimates of effect (i.e. certainty in the body of evidence)?[13]*
  It is important that reviewers provide an assessment of how certain they are that the available evidence provides estimates that are close to the truth.

Certainty one can have on the Body of Evidence Depends on

- **How serious is the risk of bias in the body of evidence?**[14]
  Systematic reviewers should assess the limitations of the included study designs. When serious or very serious issues are identified, the risk of bias increases and consequently, the certainty in the evidence decreases.[1]

- **Are the results consistent across studies?**[15]
  It is important to determine to what extent the results included in the review are all describing similar situations. When authors determine that most or all studies' results are similar, they may feel more confident pooling them. On the other hand, when the studies show either clinical or statistical heterogeneity that cannot be explained, the certainty in the evidence diminishes.

- **How precise are the results?**[16]
  After pooling the results of all studies, it is still possible that the summary estimate of the meta-analysis is imprecise. This depends on the number of participants and events, and to what extent the extremes of the CI are informative to conclude about the potential effectiveness of an intervention or association with a risk factor. For example, picture an intervention that reduces the risk of postoperative infection by 30% [RR 0.70 (95% CI 0.30–1.10)]. The lower boundary of the 95% suggests a large benefit of 70% reduction, while the upper boundary suggests a 10% increase in the occurrence of postoperative infection, which can be considered large harm. Since both extremes of the 95% CI suggest clinicians to follow completely different courses of action, this interval is too wide for decision-making. Let's say that, with time, there were additional studies conducted on this intervention and outcome. Picture now a point estimate suggesting a 20% reduction in postoperative infections and narrower intervals [RR 0.80 (95% CI 0.70–0.90)]. The lower and upper boundaries of the 95% CI suggest a 30% reduction and a 10% reduction in the outcome, respectively. Although it's a smaller magnitude of effect, since the intervals both provide an important benefit, this CI is precise.

- **Do the results directly apply to my patients?**[17]

    It is important that review authors describe to what extent the identified studies match the research question that initiated the review process. In other words, can the retrieved studies directly answer the research question (PICO) of the review? When there are clinically relevant discrepancies between the components of the research question of the review and the identified studies, the certainty in the evidence is downgraded due to issues of indirectness. For example, a systematic review is interested in including studies conducted in pediatric population. However, only adult population studies are available to answer that question. Another example is related to the intervention under study, where the reviewers defined a specific dose or regimen for a drug. However, the available evidence reports the effect of the intervention at a much lower/higher dose or a different regimen. Finally, indirectness can also affect the certainty in the evidence when surrogate instead of patient-important outcomes are reported from the primary studies (e.g. blood pressure vs cardiovascular-related mortality).

- **Is there any concern about publication bias?**[18]

    Researchers conducting a systematic review should attempt to identify and include all available evidence. However, even if reviewers take all measures to find evidence (comprehensive search, thorough review of grey literature in all languages), some conducted studies are simply not published in the first place. This is often due to unimpressive results or in rare cases, potentially harmful results (e.g. side effects that are reported during long-term follow-up). When there is suspicion of publication bias, the certainty in the evidence diminishes.

- **Are there reasons to increase the confidence rating?**[19]

    If there are no issues in the risk of bias of included studies, the certainty in the evidence can increase for three reasons:
    (1) A large treatment effect or association is identified,
    (2) A dose response gradient has been established and
    (3) Even though there are antagonistic biases, a treatment effect or association is still detected.

We have presented different criteria to assess both the methodology of the review and the confidence in the evidence reported in it. It is important to note that rigorous systematic reviews can still provide low confidence in the evidence identified, while, on the other hand, poorly conducted systematic reviews can provide results that, although likely to be misleading, may still warrant high confidence in the estimates of effect.

Important Learning Points

- Reviews are a broad collection of articles, which includes narrative and systematic reviews.
- Systematic reviews may or may not include a meta-analysis and provides several advantages compared to narrative reviews for informing decision-making.
- Not all systematic reviews and meta-analysis are equal—some are better than others. Use critical appraisal methods to help identify the most credible ones. It is important to be critical about two aspects: (1) the rigor of systematic review methodology and (2) the level of certainty in the evidence.

More to Read

- Murad MH, Jaeschke R, Devereaux PJ, et al. The process of a systematic review and meta-analysis. In: Guyatt G, Rennie D (eds). Users' guide to the medical literature: A manual for evidence-based clinical practice, 3rd edn. United States:McGraw Hill;2015:459-69.
- Mollon B, da Silva V, Busse JW, et al. Electrical stimulation for long-bone fracture-healing: A meta-analysis of randomized controlled trials. J Bone Joint Surg Am. 2008;90(11):2322-30.

Definitions

Anecdotal clinical evidence: Case-based information on a small number of patients.

Bias: Systematic deviation from the underlying truth because of a feature of the design or conduct of a research study.

Certainty in the evidence: To what extent the estimates of effect or association for a particular outcome are close to the truth.

Confidence interval: The range of values within which there is a given probability that the true value lies. Usually a 95% confidence interval is provided.

Forest plot: Graphical presentation that illustrates the magnitude of treatment effect or association between an experimental and control group. It is the most common graphic representation of meta-analysis.

Grey literature: Reports that are produced by all levels of government, academics, business and industry in print and electronic formats but that are not controlled by commercial publishers.

Language/country bias: Bias due to only including in a systematic review studies published in certain languages or countries.

Mean difference (MD): Statistic that measures the absolute difference between the mean in two groups that are compared. This difference in means can be used as summary statistic in meta-analysis for continuous outcomes that were measured using the same scale among included studies.

Meta-analysis: Statistically combining quantitative data from several studies to yield a single pooled summary estimate.

Narrative review: An article that reviews literature (such as a book chapter) that is not conducted using methods to minimize bias and is not reproducible.

Odd ratios (ORs): The ratio of the odds of development of disease in exposed individuals to the odds of development of disease in non-exposed individuals.

Publication bias: Bias due to the selective publication of research depending on the direction of the study results and whether they are statistically significant.

Random error: Unavoidable influence of chance in any measure conducted. The larger the sample size, the smaller the random error and the more precise the results.

Recursive search: The process of reading the reference lists of studies included in a review to determine whether or not they should also be included in the review.

Relative risk (RR): The ratio of the risk of disease in exposed individuals to the risk of disease in non-exposed individuals.

Selective citation bias: Bias due to only including articles that contain certain results in a systematic review.

Standardized mean difference (SMD): A meta-analysis summary statistic used when the included studies assess the same outcome but measure them in a variety of ways. To solve this, it is necessary to standardize the results of the studies to a uniform scale to be combined. This statistic represents the effect size of the intervention expressed in standard deviation units.

Systematic review: The identification, selection, appraisal and summary of primary studies that address a focused clinical question using methods to reduce the likelihood of bias.

Time lag bias: The rapid or delayed publication of research findings, depending on the nature and direction of the results.

Weighted analysis: Taking into account the sample size and number of events of the studies included in a meta-analysis; bigger studies (or more events) have a greater effect on the overall result than smaller studies (or fewer events).

REFERENCES

1. Green S, Higgins JPT, Alderson P, et al. Chapter 1: Introduction. In: Higgins JPT, Green S (eds). Cochrane Handbook for Systematic Reviews of Interventions Version 5.1.0 (updated March 2011): The Cochrane Collaboration, 2011. Available from www.cochrane-handbook.org.
2. Guyatt G, Meade MO, Rennie D, et al. Users' guide to the medical literature: A manual for evidence-based clinical practice. 3rd edn. United States: McGraw Hill; 2015.
3. Murad MH, Jaeschke R, Devereaux PJ, et al. The process of a systematic review and meta-analysis. In: Guyatt G, Rennie D (eds). Users' guide to the medical literature: A manual for evidence-based clinical practice, 3rd edn. United States:McGraw Hill;2015:459-69.
4. Murad MH, Montori VM, Ioannidis JP, et al. How to read a systematic review and meta-analysis and apply the results to patient care: users' guides to the medical literature. JAMA. 2014;312(2):171-9.
5. Sterne JAC, Egger M, Moher D. Chapter 10: Addressing reporting biases. In: Higgins JPT, Green S (eds). Cochrane Handbook for Systematic Reviews of Intervention Version 5.1.0 (updated March 2011): The Cochrane Collaboration, 2011. Available from www.cochrane-handbook.org.
6. Higgins JPT, Altman DG, Sterne JAC. Chapter 8: Assessing risk of bias in included studies. In: Higgins JPT, Green S (eds) Cochrane Handbook for Systematic Reviews of Interventions Version 5.1.0 (updated March 2011): The Cochrane Collaboration, 2011. Available from www.cochrane-handbook.org.
7. Guyatt G, Oxman AD, Akl EA, et al. GRADE guidelines: 1. Introduction-GRADE evidence profiles and summary of findings tables. J Clin Epidemiol. 2011;64(4):383-94.

8. Guyatt GH, Oxman AD, Vist GE, et al. GRADE: An emerging consensus on rating quality of evidence and strength of recommendations. BMJ. 2008;336(7650):924-6.
9. Egger M, Smith GD, Altman DG. Systematic Reviews in Healthcare. 2nd edn. London: BMJ Publishing Group; 2001.
10. Song F, Eastwood AJ, Gilbody S, et al. Publication and related biases. Health Technol Assess. 2000;4(10):1-115.
11. Gordis L. Epidemiology. 4th edn. Philadelphia,PA: Saunders Elsevier; 2009.
12. Johnston BC, Thorlund K, Schünemann HJ, et al. Improving the interpretation of quality of life evidence in meta-analyses: The application of minimal important difference units. Health Qual Life Outcomes. 2010;8:116.
13. Balshem H, Helfand M, Schünemann HJ, et al. GRADE guidelines: 3. Rating the quality of evidence. J Clin Epidemiol. 2011;64(4):401-6.
14. Guyatt GH, Oxman AD, Vist G, et al. GRADE guidelines: 4. Rating the quality of evidence—study limitations (risk of bias). J Clin Epidemiol. 2011;64(4):407-15.
15. Guyatt GH, Oxman AD, Kunz R, et al. GRADE guidelines: 7. Rating the quality of evidence—inconsistency. J Clin Epidemiol. 2011;64(12):1294-302.
16. Guyatt GH, Oxman AD, Kunz R, et al. GRADE guidelines 6. Rating the quality of evidence—imprecision. J Clin Epidemiol. 2011;64(12):1283-93.
17. Guyatt GH, Oxman AD, Kunz R, et al. GRADE guidelines: 8. Rating the quality of evidence—indirectness. J Clin Epidemiol. 2011;64(12):1303-10.
18. Guyatt GH, Oxman AD, Montori V, et al. GRADE guidelines: 5. Rating the quality of evidence—publication bias. J Clin Epidemiol. 2011;64(12):1277-82.
19. Guyatt GH, Oxman AD, Sultan S, et al. GRADE guidelines: 9. Rating up the quality of evidence. J Clin Epidemiol. 2011;64(12):1311-6.

12
The Basics of Economic Evaluation

Manraj Kaur, Feng Xie, Tahira Devji

> **Key Objectives**
> - Understand the concept of health economics and its importance in healthcare
> - Compare and contrast four major types of health economic evaluation
> - Identify and summarize key factors that underline the design and analysis of health economic evaluation
> - Develop an insight on how health economic evaluation impacts policy decision-making

What is Health Economics and Health Economic Evaluation?

Economics concerns on how society allocates and uses resources.[1] The *scarcity* of the available resources underpins economic theory, from which three important questions arise:
1. What goods and services should be produced?
2. How should these goods and services be produced?
3. Who consumes these goods and services?

Health economics is a 'field of inquiry whose subject matter is the optimum use of *resources* for the care of the sick and the promotion of *health*. Its task is to appraise the *efficiency* of the organization of health services and to suggest ways of improving the organization.'[2] It is considered an applied field of economics in healthcare with its theoretical foundations in finance and insurance, industrial organization, labor and public finance.[3] Health economics strives to answer these questions mainly from the viewpoint of efficiency, that is, maximizing health ***benefits*** from available resources or in other terms, ensuring benefits gained exceed benefits forgone in healthcare.[4] Hence, in the face of limited healthcare resources and rapidly evolving intervention options, health economic evaluation uses economic methods to quantify costs and benefits of alternative ways of delivering healthcare. It produces evidence, specifically useful for healthcare resource allocation decision-making.

Why should one Conduct an Economic Evaluation of Healthcare Interventions?

When confronted with two competing interventions that vary in their ***health outcomes***, the choice is unambiguous—choose the one with better health outcomes. However, our healthcare system has been struggling to meet ever increasing needs with limited healthcare resources. Under such circumstances, both costs and health outcomes need to be considered when making a choice (Fig. 12.1). Health economic evaluations inform resource (budget) allocation decisions after considering the relative value of competing interventions[5] and in doing so it assists in maximizing benefits from healthcare expenditure. It provides information on the relative cost and health outcomes of different interventions or technologies allowing an empirically-driven, informed choice on funding decisions especially in the face of limited resources (e.g. physical infrastructure and human resources) to enhance population health.[5,6] A basic understanding of how to critically appraise and conduct health economic evaluation of surgical interventions, empowers surgeons to participate in funding and policy-making decisions in addition to choosing clinically and cost-effective interventions.

What are the Different Types of Health Economic Evaluation?

There are four main types of economic evaluation, depending on ***if*** and ***how*** the health outcomes (health benefits)[3] are considered:
1. Cost-minimization analysis
2. Cost-benefit analysis

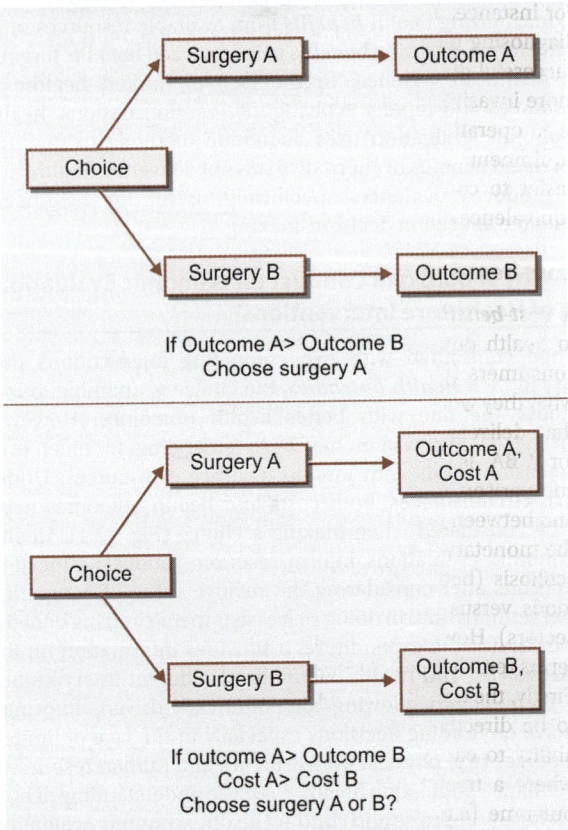

Fig. 12.1: Choosing between the two surgical interventions with different outcomes and costs

3. Cost-effectiveness analysis
4. Cost-utility analysis.

Cost-minimization Analysis

A *cost-minimization analysis (CMA)* is used when two comparative procedures are considered to have equivalent health outcomes but different costs.[7] Inevitably, when a CMA is conducted, the intervention with the lower cost is chosen.

For instance, a CMA may compare two different methods of diagnosing pancreatic cancer, where the health outcome of successful diagnosis is the same, but one procedure may be more invasive, resulting in higher consumption of resources (e.g. operating room, nurse, anesthetist, operating room equipment and supplies) and higher cost. It is relatively easier to conduct a CMA. However, the demonstration of equivalence of health outcomes is sometimes challenging.

Cost-benefit Analysis

A ***cost-benefit analysis (CBA)*** attaches a monetary value to health outcomes, for example, by asking the healthcare consumers (patients and general population) in general—what they would be willing to pay for the treatment or service that delivers a certain health benefit? The final measure for CBA is net monetary benefit and therefore allows comparison of interventions across healthcare specialities and between public sectors. For example, one could compare the monetary value of physiotherapy versus spinal fusion for scoliosis (between specialities) or levying taxes on sugary foods versus obesity education initiatives (between public sectors). However, measuring health outcomes in monetary terms remains a controversial subject due to several reasons.[8] Firstly, the ***willingness to pay*** for a treatment has been found to be directly proportional to the individual's income and ability to earn.[8,9,10,11] Further, CBA cannot be used in cases where a treatment or intervention results in a short-term outcome (e.g. pain relief) or causes psychosocial benefits only (e.g. increased self-efficacy). Lastly, process of care such as satisfaction with information provided by the healthcare provider and satisfaction with care and overall experience plays a huge role in the willingness to pay and hence, the monetary value of outcome.[11]

Cost-effectiveness Analysis

Cost-effectiveness analysis (CEA) is the most common type of economic evaluation found in the literature. CEA compares the costs and outcomes of two or more comparative interventions, in which outcomes are measured in natural, disease-specific units, such as cases successfully treated or the number of strokes averted.[5] An example would be the comparison of novel robotic-assisted thoracic surgery (treatment A) and existing video-assisted thoracic surgery (treatment B) with respect to tumor free margin (natural unit) and costs in patients with lung cancer. In this example, if treatment A is more expensive and less effective in obtaining tumor free margin, then treatment A is considered to be 'dominated' and not cost-effective as compared to treatment B. On the other hand, if treatment A is more effective and less expensive, it 'dominates' and is cost-effective.[12] However, realistically speaking, clinical decision making is often not as straightforward as the above example. Often comparative treatments are found to be more effective and more costly or less effective and less costly.

Under these circumstances, an ***incremental cost-effectiveness ratio (ICER)*** assists in quantifying the clinical and economic consequences of the treatment. An ICER is an estimate of the additional cost per unit of health outcome (mentioned below). When plotted in the form of a graph, with difference in cost between interventions (ΔC) on the Y-axis and difference in treatment effectiveness between interventions (ΔE) on the X-axis, it is called a ***cost-effectiveness plane***[13] (Fig. 12.2).

Incremental cost-effectiveness ratio (ICER)

$$\text{ICER} \frac{\text{Cost of new surgery S1} - \text{cost of prevalent surgery S2}}{\text{Effectiveness of new s0.05urgery S1} - \text{Effectiveness of prevalent surgery S2}} = \frac{\Delta C(\$)}{\Delta E}$$

$$\text{ICER} \frac{\$150,000 - \$100,000}{0.70 - 0.55} = \frac{\$50,000}{0.15} = 333,333.34$$

The above value is higher than the Canadian threshold of ICER ($100,000/unit of effectiveness) and hence, the decision is 'REJECT the new surgery'.

The X-axis shows the difference in effectiveness between the new treatment and the comparator and the Y- axis shows the difference in cost.

Traditionally, ICER was interpreted with the help of league tables of published ICER ratios.[5,14,15,16] However,

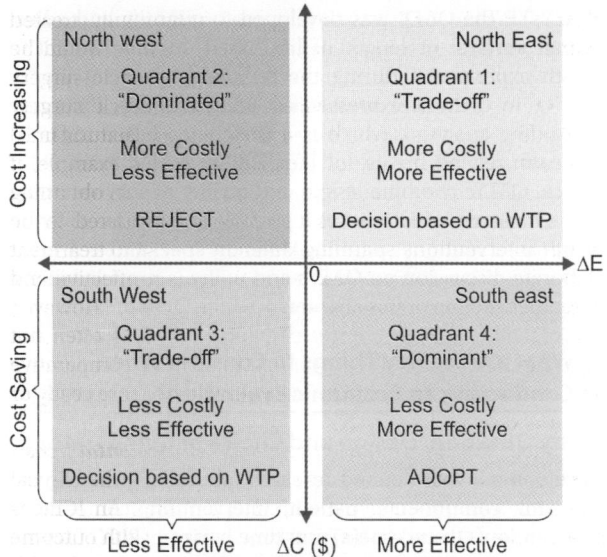

Fig. 12.2: Interpreting health economic evaluation results
Abbreviation: WTP—Willingness to pay

this approach was later disregarded as the ICER values for healthcare interventions in the league tables were derived using varying methods and due to the fact that the ICER for a given intervention varies depending on the comparative intervention.[14,15,16,17] Decision analysts often use an arbitrary cut-off or threshold, such as US $50,000 per amount of benefit (health outcome) to assess cost-effectiveness. Interventions with an ICER below the threshold, for instance, below US $50,000 per unit of health outcome are considered 'cost-effective' and deserving of funding. Country-specific ICER thresholds have also been established in the literature. In Canada, a threshold range of $20,000–$100,000 per amount of benefit (health outcome) is considered cost-effective.[18]

Cost-utility Analysis

Cost-utility analysis (CUA) is similar to CEA except that outcomes are measured in quality-adjusted life years

(QALYs).[19] The QALY was developed to quantify and adjust overall survival or length of life based on the amount of health experienced during the remaining years of life.[20,21] The 'Q' in QALY is expressed as 'utility' (hence, the name cost-utility analysis), which is a preference-based measure of health-related quality of life (HRQL) scaled from 0–1.[22] Hence, QALYs combine length and quality of survival into a single measure, which makes it possible to compare different health interventions spanning different specialities. A more elaborate discussion on QALYs and utility is provided in the outcomes section of this chapter.

What are the Key Things to Consider When Conducting an Economic Evaluation?

Study Question, Design and Choice of Comparator

Developing a well-defined research question, including the following components: patient, intervention, comparative intervention(s), outcome(s) and time horizon (PICOT) is the first step of an economic evaluation. The patient population and the intervention should be well defined. The choice of a comparative intervention should be aligned with the research question and the current clinical practice standards.[10] Whenever possible, efforts should be made to compare the new treatment with the standard of care. If the standard of care doesn't exist or cannot be established, the most prevalent or usual treatment(s) should be used. Nonetheless, the choice of the comparator(s) should be justified at the outset of the evaluation. Economic evaluations can also be conducted alongside a clinical trial or a prospective cohort study or via an economic model.

Trial and Model-based Economic Evaluation

There are two ways to conduct an economic evaluation: trial-based or model-based economic evaluation.

When an economic evaluation is conducted alongside a randomized controlled trial (RCT), they are referred to as a trial-based evaluation. The economic evaluation is often piggybacked onto phase 3 clinical trials, which are designed to assess the efficacy and adverse effects of the new drug or phase 4 trials, which examine the long term effectiveness following the approval of the drug by a regulatory body.[23] For example, CEA parallel to a RCT of two breast reduction techniques, namely vertical scar reduction and inverted-T shaped reduction was conducted and recently published.[24]

A trial-based economic evaluation has the advantage of the relative effectiveness of the intervention being directly derived from trial participants in a selection bias-free design.[25] They provide timely information with high internal validity. However, there are certain disadvantages of the trial-based economic evaluation.[25] Some of which are listed below:

- The number of comparative interventions and the follow-up duration (time horizon) in a RCT design is limited by the cost and practical issues associated with conducting a RCT
- The results of an economic evaluation based in a RCT are jurisdiction and context-specific and hence may have limited generalizability.
- Missing data in resource utilization and patient-reported outcomes is a significant limitation of a RCT design.
- The uncertainty estimates (variability) of a trial-based economic analysis are specific to that particular trial and hence, not sufficient for decision-making by themselves.

Model-based evaluation examines the expected costs and outcomes of the decision options by incorporating all relevant sources of evidence and applying mathematical techniques using computer software.[20,24] There are two types of models commonly used in health economic evaluation- decision tree and **Markov model**. Decision tree is the simplest form of decision-analytical modelling. It represents all potential diagnosis and treatment pathways of a specific health condition with their associated probabilities, costs and outcomes.[23] A Markov model, unlike decision tree, structures the health condition and its treatment process by means of mutually exclusive and exhaustive health states, with patients traversing from one health state to another based on transition probabilities.[23,26,27] The cost and outcomes are accumulated according to the nature of the health state and the duration of staying in that state.[27]

Model-based economic evaluation is an important supplement to the trial-based evaluation as it can: (1) compare all relevant alternatives; (2) transform the short- or mid-term endpoints to final consequences; (3) make conclusions relevant to the lifetime time horizon; and (4) enhance external validity of the results.[23,28]

Perspective

The ***perspective*** in an economic evaluation is the viewpoint from which the cost and consequences are recorded and evaluated.[29,30] The choice of perspective stems from the research question, influences the choice of outcomes and costs; hence, the perspective should be established before a study commences. An economic evaluation can be conducted from a number of different perspectives: patient, caregiver (direct/indirect), hospital, healthcare professional, industry, public/private payers or the society as a whole.[29,30] The Panel on cost-effectiveness in health and medicine[31] suggests using the societal approach for all economic evaluations due to the following reasons:

- ***Accounts for cost-transfer between and within sectors:*** The decisions on resource allocation in healthcare affect other sectors and vice versa. For example, the relationship between smoking and lung cancer is well known. When the government increases the cost of smoking by imposing higher taxes on the purchase of cigarettes, it results in reduced incidence of lung cancer resulting in saving of healthcare dollars, which can be allocated to other conditions or causes, resulting in a societal gain. A societal perspective assists in unmasking the cost transfer between unrelated sectors.
- ***Opportunity costs:*** As resources are finite, the decision to allocate resources to a particular healthcare service or health sector results in reduced resources to other service(s) or sector(s) such as education, housing and transportation. These are called ***opportunity costs***. Opportunity costs also occur when a novel surgery results in patients returning to work sooner than the alternative. Without accounting for these costs in an economic evaluation conducted from a

societal perspective, it is unlikely that the true value of an intervention can be determined.

- ***Study comparability:*** To assess the overall benefit of a particular healthcare intervention, especially for policy decision-making purposes, it is imperative that the results of studies be synthesized. However, such a meta-analysis is unfeasible when the studies include different perspectives. Hence, making the societal perspective the norm has been proposed in the literature.

Irrespective of the type of perspective selected for the study, the choice should be justified and the results must be presented separately for each study perspective.

Time Horizon

The time horizon is the length of time over which the cost and consequences of the comparative treatments are evaluated.[25] The choice of time horizon should be consistent with the research question and can vary from a few weeks to life time. It is recommended that the time horizon should be long enough to capture meaningful differences in cost and outcomes between the intervention and comparator(s)—for chronic diseases, a lifetime time horizon is recommended.[10] For example, a six-month time horizon may be suitable for assessing the cost-effectiveness of laparoscopic carpal tunnel release for carpal tunnel syndrome but may be ill suited for total knee replacement in patients with degenerative arthritis of the knee due to the potential risk for prosthetic fracture in the long term. It should be noted that long-term analysis does not necessitate that the primary data from patients be obtained over several years (or lifetime). Statistical techniques exist for extrapolating or modelling long-term patient-outcome data from short or intermediate term outcomes. A description of these techniques is beyond the scope of this book chapter.

Discounting

The cost and consequences of an intervention are worth more in the present than the future because: (1) patients/population consider the short-term outcome only; (2) the future is uncertain and (3) patients/population expect to obtain a compounded future in return for present investment.[32,33] **Discounting** allows for adjusting the cost and health benefit of an intervention to ***present values*** to reflect society's rate of ***time preference***. Canadian Agency for Drugs and Technologies in Health (CADTH) recommends a rate of 5% per year,[10] however, this rate is not universal and varies between different jurisdictions. The consensus is that ***discount rate*** should not be applied to evaluations less than one year, but a rate of 0% should still be mentioned in the report to avoid confusion.[10]

Outcomes

The measurement of health outcomes is a fundamental component of a full economic evaluation. As we already know, the type of health outcome measured determines the type of economic evaluation. Patient outcomes can be reported in natural units such as mortality, complications prevented HRQL in CEA, or weighted to produce a composite index of outcome, such as QALYs in CUA or converted to monetary value as in CBA.

- ***Health-related quality of life:*** 'As a construct, health related quality of life refers to the impact of the health aspects of a person's life on that person's overall wellbeing. Also used to refer to the value of a health state to an individual,[34] HRQL can be accessed via generic quality of life measures such as Short Form-36 (SF-36)[35] or condition-specific measures e.g. Disability of Arm, Shoulder and Hand Questionnaire (DASH)[36] or Oxford Hip Score (OHS).[37] The value of HRQL measures in an economic evaluation is limited but they are the most common measures used in RCTs or prospective cohort studies designed to assess cost-effectiveness of a surgical intervention.
- ***Quality adjusted life years:*** QALYs are calculated by multiplying the length of life years gained from an intervention with quality of life weights for the time duration (described later).[38,39] Quality of life weights need to be measured based on preference of relevant health states under certainty (often referred as 'value') or under

uncertainty (often referred as 'utility'). Throughout this chapter, utility is used to refer to preference-based quality of life weights in general. Utility is anchored at 0 for being equivalent to dead and 1 for being in full health, with negative for worse than dead. Figure 12.3 health state utilities can be obtained directly or indirectly.

- **Direct method**: Involves interviewing approaches that elicit preferences directly from the patient or general public. Standard gamble, time trade-off and visual analog scale are the most theoretically driven and empirically tested approaches in the literature.[40]
- **Indirect method**: Involves using generic (generic because they are derived from the general public) utility-based measures such as Health Utilities Index (HUI)[41], Short Form-6 (SF-6)[42] and EuroQoL-5D (EQ-5D).[43,44] More recently, condition-specific utility-based measures are also being used in the literature e.g. King's Health Questionnaire[45] and European Organization for Research and Treatment of Cancer Core Quality of Life Questionnaire (EORTC QLQ-C30).[46]

Quality Adjusted Life Years (QALY)
  QALY = Utility of health state × duration of health state
  E.g. let's say, palmar fasciectomy for Dupuytren's contracture results in 0.8 years in full health and a utility of 0.76, then
  QALY for palmar fasciectomy = 0.76 × 0.8
  = 0.608
  However, needle aponeurotomy for Dupuytren's contracture results in 1.4 years in full health and utility of 0.8, then
  QALY for needle aponeurotomy = 0.8 × 1.4
  = 1.12
  Hence, additional QALYs generated by needle aponeurotomy = 0.512

- **Monetary value for health outcomes:** These are collected using a **willingness to pay (WTP)** approach. The two most commonly cited methods used in WTP studies[10] are:
  - **Contingent valuation**: uses a hypothetical survey to assess an individual's maximum WTP for a service that cannot be assigned a market price.[47] For example, estimating WTP for prevention of motor vehicle

Fig. 12.3: Health state valuations

*Values between zero and minus 1 represent health states worse than death

accidents or introduction of a new drug to prevent a complication associated with surgery.
- ***Discrete Choice Experiment***: uses a comparison exercise for eliciting preferences and hence WTP where individuals choose between a set of two or more alternatives.[48]. This approach has been used in the evaluation of process effects and non-health outcomes.[49] For example, assessing healthcare attributes important for patient satisfaction for treatment.

Resource Use and Costing

The perspective of the study determines the resources to consider in an economic evaluation. An economic evaluation can be from the perspective of the society by considering all ***direct*** (e.g. healthcare related costs), ***indirect costs*** (non-healthcare-related costs) and productivity costs (time lost from work) or can be from the hospital perspective by considering only the direct costs. Figure 12.4 illustrates

> **Societal Costs**
> Productivity costs
> Time lost from work by patient
> Cost to employer to hire/train replacement for patient

> **Indirect costs**
> 1. Out of pocket expenses for over the counter drugs, gait aid, rehabilitation-related costs
> 2. Transportation costs (fuel, parking and bus fare)
> 3. Increased cost of health premium for private insurance
> 4. Cost to hire caregivers (baby sitters, house cleaners, etc.)

> **Direct costs**
> *Surgery-related costs*
> - Surgeon, anesthetist fee
> - Operating room nurse fee
> - Cost of medications, disposable costs (gloves, masks, instruments)
> - Radiology and pathology-related costs
> - Rehabilitation costs
>
> *Overhead costs*
> - Cost of OR, peri-operative room, cost of hospital stay
> - Cost of medications
> - Floor staff fee (nurse, PSW)

Fig. 12.4: Perspectives and relevant costs in surgical intervention(s)

an example to compare the different perspectives and the relevant costs to be included under each perspective. Two different approaches can be used to estimate costs:[50,51]

- ***Micro-costing (bottom-up approach):*** Each relevant item of resource use is identified and results in a precise context-specific estimate of resources for each patient. This approach is more accurate, but time-consuming.
- ***Macro-costing (top-down approach):*** Resource use at aggregate level is determined (i.e. at the level of diagnosis-related group) without collecting quantity and cost of individual resource utilization items. Studies that use a macro-costing approach have higher external validity and allow comparison across different health conditions, but at the expense of precision.

Uncertainty and Variability

Uncertainty refers to the degree of precision with which a quantity is measured, while variability refers to natural variation in some quantity. Irrespective of the type of economic evaluation or the methodology, i.e. trial-based or decision modelling, uncertainty and variability in the results are inevitable.[52] ***Sensitivity analyses*** are often used to assess uncertainty and variability by examining the degree of change in the results of economic evaluation when the estimates of the input variables vary. Two main types of sensitivity analysis are found in surgical literature:

- ***Deterministic sensitivity analysis:*** In this approach, predetermined values are assigned to variables and the impact of the change in results of economic evaluation is assessed. Either one (one-way deterministic sensitivity analysis) or multiple variables (multi-way deterministic sensitivity analysis) are varied at one time.[53,54]
- ***Probabilistic sensitivity analysis:*** A more sophisticated type of sensitivity analysis that varies the values of multiple variables according to pre-specified distributions for these variables. Probabilistic sensitivity analysis is widely used to deal with sampling/parameter uncertainty in economic evaluation. It provides a full picture of uncertainty of an economic evaluation.[23,55,56] The final result of the probabilistic sensitivity analysis can be plotted on a cost-effectiveness plane.

Critically Appraising a Published Economic Evaluation

Critical appraisal is a fundamental process in evidence based practice. The purpose of critical appraisal is to identify methodological shortcomings in the literature and provide the users of the research evidence the opportunity to make informed decisions about the quality of research evidence.

When conducting the critical appraisal of an economic evaluation, the methods must be scrutinized for the appropriateness of the choice of comparator, perspective, time horizon, type of methodology and the type of economic evaluation and outcomes. The type of statistical analyses conducted should be explicit and the results should be

described with transparency. Several guidelines on how to conduct and report economic evaluation have been published in the literature. A few that have been most widely accepted are given below:
- Good Research Practices for Cost-Effectiveness Analysis Alongside Clinical Trials: The ISPOR RCT-CEA Task Force Report[57]
- ISPOR Modelling Studies Task Force Report[26]
- Consolidated health economic evaluation reporting standards (CHEERS)[58]
- Drummond's checklist for economic evaluations[59]
- Philips's checklist for decision-analytic modelling[60]
- Ever's checklist for economic evaluation.[61]

Important Learning Points

- Economic evaluation is an important tool in maintaining the efficiency of healthcare systems, since they outline how to maximize health benefits with limited healthcare resources.
- Certain types of economic evaluation are more relevant in some contexts; thus, it is important to choose the right type of economic evaluation.
- The limitations of economic evaluation must be considered when its results are used to inform health policy decision making.
- Not all health economic evaluations are of the same quality. Perform a critical appraisal to determine the validity of a certain study.

Definitions

Benefit: Anything that results that is of value.
Clinical Effectiveness: The application of interventions which have been shown to be efficacious to appropriate patients in a timely fashion to improve patients' outcomes and value for the use of resources.
Cost: The economic definition of cost (also known as opportunity cost) is the value of opportunity forgone, strictly the best opportunity forgone, as a result of engaging resources in an activity. Note that there can be a cost without the exchange of money.

Cost benefit analysis (CBA): A form of health economic evaluation in which the benefits are expressed in monetary terms.

Cost-effectiveness analysis: A form of health economic evaluation where benefits are measured in terms of natural, disease-specific units such as cases successfully treated or the number of stroke averted.

Cost-minimization analysis: A form of health economic evaluation in which two comparative procedures with equivalent health outcomes are compared.

Cost-utility analysis: A form of cost-effectiveness analysis where benefits are measured in terms of a utility measure such as the QALY.

Decision-analysis: Explicit quantitative mathematical approach for prescribing conditions under conditions of uncertainty.

Demand: The quantity of a good buyers wish to purchase at each conceivable price.

Direct costs: All resources that are consumed in the provision of a health promotion program. These may be incurred by the health promotion service, community or clients.

Discount rate: The rate chosen to express the strength of preference over the timing of costs and benefits (see discounting and time preference).

Discounting: The most widely accepted method of incorporating time preference into the evaluation of a program when the costs and benefits do not occur at the same point in time.

Economic evaluation (economic appraisal): The comparison of alternative courses of action in terms of their costs and consequences, with a view to making a choice.

Effectiveness: The extent to which programs achieve their objectives, in real-life settings.

Efficiency: Maximizing the benefit to any resource expenditure or minimising the cost of any achieved benefit.

Health: A state of complete physical, mental and social well-being and not merely the absence of disease or infirmity.

Health economics: The study of how scarce resources are allocated among alternative uses for the care of sickness and the promotion, maintenance and improvement of health, including the study of how healthcare and health-related services, their costs and benefits and health itself are distributed among individuals and groups in society.

Health economists: Individuals who study health economics.

Incremental cost-effectiveness ratio: Obtained by dividing the difference between the costs of the two interventions by the difference in the outcomes, i.e., the extra cost per extra unit of effect.

Indirect costs: These relate to the losses to society incurred as a result of participating in the program, such as the impact on production, domestic responsibilities and social and leisure activities.

Markov model: A particular type of decision analysis that allows for the transfer between different health states over a period of time.

Micro-costing: An estimate is made for each element of resource use within the program and a unit cost is derived for each.

Opportunity cost: The cost of a unit of a resource is the benefit that would be derived from using it in its best alternative use.

Outcome: An indicator of health status that will be used to assess the difference between the treatment and/or control groups.

Perspective: The point of view from which an analysis is carried out. The social welfare perspective considers costs and benefits from the point of view of society.

Present values: The value today of future costs or benefits (after adjusting by discounting).

Quality adjusted life years (QALYs): Calculated by adjusting the estimated number of years of life of an individual is expected to gain from an intervention for the expected quality of life in those years. The quality of life score will range between 0 for death to 1 for perfect health, with negative scores being allowed for states considered worse than death.

Resources: Things that contribute to the production of output. Money gives a command over resources but is not a resource per se.

Scarcity: There will never be enough resources to satisfy human needs completely.

Sensitivity analysis: A process through which the robustness of an economic model is assessed by examining the changes in results of the analysis when key variables are varied over a specified range.

Time preference: Individuals are not indifferent to the timing of costs and benefits, preferring benefits sooner and costs later.

Utility: A measure of the 'satisfaction' (benefit) obtained from consuming goods and services.

Willingness to pay: This technique asks people to state explicitly the maximum amount they would be willing to pay to receive a particular benefit. It is based on the premise that the maximum amount of money an individual is willing to pay for a commodity is an indicator of the value to them of that commodity.

REFERENCES

1. Kernick D. Introduction to health economics for the medical practitioner. Postgrad Med J. 2003;79(929):147-50.
2. Mushkin SJ. Toward a definition of health economics. Public Health Rep. 1958;73(9):785-94.
3. Culyer, AJ., Newhouse JP. Introduction: the state and scope of health economics. Handbook of health economics 1 (2000): 1-8.
4. Drummond M. Economic analysis alongside control trials. London: Department of Health; 1994
5. Detsky AS, Naglie IG. A clinician's guide to cost-effectiveness analysis. Ann Intern Med. 1990;113(2):147-54.
6. Tan-Torres Edejer, T., Baltussen, R. M. P. M., Adam, T., Hutubessy, R., Acharya, A., Evans, D. B., & Murray, C. J. L. (2003). Making choices in health: WHO guide to cost-effectiveness analysis.
7. Robinson, Ray. "Economic evaluation and healthcare 2. Cost and Cost Minimization Analysis. British Medical Journal 307.6906 (1993): 726-728.
8. Cookson, R. Willingness to pay methods in healthcare: a sceptical view. Health Econ. 2003;12(11):891-4.
9. Russell S. Ability to pay for healthcare: concepts and evidence. Health Policy Plan. 1996;11(3):219-37.
10. Canadian Agency for Drugs and Technologies in Health. (2006). Guidelines for the economic evaluation of health technologies: Canada. In Guidelines for the economic evaluation of health technologies: Canada. CADTH.

11. Ryan M, Watson V, Amaya-Amaya M. Methodological issues in the monetary valuation of benefits in healthcare. Expert Rev Pharmacoecon Outcomes Res. 2003;3(6):717-27.
12. Haentjens P, Annemans L. Health economics and the orthopaedic surgeon. J Bone Joint Br. 2003;85(8):1093-9.
13. Black WC. The CE plane: a graphic representation of cost-effectiveness. Med Decis Making. 1990;10(3):212-4.
14. Drummond M, Torrance G, Mason J. Cost-effectiveness league tables: more harm than good? Soc Sci Med. 1993;37(1):33-40.
15. Birch S, Gafni A. Cost-effectiveness ratios: in a league of their own. Health Policy. 1994;28(2):133-41.
16. Mauskopf J, Rutten F, Schonfeld W. Cost-effectiveness league tables: valuable guidance for decision makers? Pharmacoeconomics. 2003;21(14), 991-1000.
17. Grosse SD. Assessing cost-effectiveness in healthcare: history of the $50,000 per QALY threshold. Expert Rev Pharmacoecon Outcomes Res. 2008;8(2):165-78.
18. Laupacis A, Feeny D, Detsky AS, et al. How attractive does a new technology have to be to warrant adoption and utilization? Tentative guidelines for using clinical and economic evaluations. CMAJ. 1992;146(4):473-81.
19. Robinson R. Cost-utility analysis. BMJ. 1993;307(6908):859-62.
20. Kaplan RM, Bush JW. Health-related quality of life measurement for evaluation research and policy analysis. Health psychology. 1982;1(1):61-80.
21. Weinstein MC, Stason WB. Foundations of cost-effectiveness analysis for health and medical practices. N Engl J Med. 1977;296(13):716-21.
22. Torrance GW. Utility approach to measuring health-related quality of life. J Chronic Dis. 1987;40(6):593-603.
23. Simoens S. Health economic assessment: a methodological primer. Int J Environ Res Public Health 2009;6(12):2950-66.
24. Thoma, A, Kaur MN, Tsoi B, et al. Cost-effectiveness analysis parallel to a randomized controlled trial comparing vertical scar reduction and inverted T–shaped reduction mammaplasty. Plast reconstr surg. 2014;134(6):1093-107.
25. Sculpher MJ, Claxton K, Drummond M, et al. Whither trial-based economic evaluation for healthcare decision making? Health Econ. 2006;15(7):677-87.
26. Weinstein MC, O'Brien B, Hornberger J, et al. Principles of good practice for decision analytic modeling in healthcare evaluation: report of the ISPOR Task Force on Good Research Practices—Modeling Studies. Value Health. 2003;6(1):9-17.
27. Petrou S, Gray A. Economic evaluation using decision analytical modelling: design, conduct, analysis, and reporting. BMJ. 2011;342:d1766.

28. Buxton MJ, Drummond MF, Van Hout BA, et al. Modelling in economic evaluation: an unavoidable fact of life. Health Econ. 1997;6(3):217-27.
29. Phelps CE. Perspectives in health economics. Health Econ. 1995;4(5):335-53.
30. Byford S, Raftery J. Economics notes: Perspectives in economic evaluation. BMJ. 1998;316(7143):1529-30.
31. Weinstein MC, Siegel JE, Gold MR, et al. Recommendations of the Panel on Cost-effectiveness in Health and Medicine. JAMA. 1996;276(15):1253-8.
32. Smith DH, Gravelle H. The practice of discounting in economic evaluations of healthcare interventions. Int J Technol Assess Health Care. 2001;17(2):236-43.
33. Gravelle H, Smith D. Discounting for health effects in cost-benefit and cost-effectiveness analysis. Health Econ. 2001;10(7):587-99.
34. Felce, D., & Perry, J. (1995). Quality of life: Its definition and measurement. Research in developmental disabilities, 16(1), 51-74.
35. Ware JE Jr, Sherbourne C D. The MOS 36-item short-form health survey (SF-36). I. Conceptual framework and item selection. Med Care. 1992;30(6):473-83.
36. Hudak PL, AmadioPC, Bombardier, C. Development of an upper extremity outcome measure: the DASH (disabilities of the arm, shoulder and hand) [corrected]. The Upper Extremity Collaborative Group (UECG). Am J Ind Med. 1996;29(6):602-8.
37. Dawson J, Fitzpatrick R, Carr A, et al. Questionnaire on the perceptions of patients about total hip replacement. J Bone Joint Surg Br. 1996;78(2):185-90.
38. Torrance GW, Feeny D. Utilities and quality-adjusted life years. Int J Technol Assess Health Care. 1989;5(4):559-75.
39. Williams A, Evans R, Drummond M. Quality-adjusted life-years. Lancet. 1987;329(8546):1372-3.
40. Bennett KJ, Torrance GW. Measuring health state preferences and utilities: rating scale, time trade-off and standard gamble techniques. Quality of life and pharmacoeconomics in clinical trials. 1996;2:253-65.
41. Horsman J, Furlong W, Feeny D, et al. The Health Utilities Index (HUI®): concepts, measurement properties and applications. Health Qual Life Outcomes. 2003;1:54.
42. Brazier J, Usherwood T, Harper R, et al. Deriving a preference-based single index from the UK SF-36 Health Survey. J Clin Epidemiol. 1998;51(11):1115-28.
43. Group E. EuroQol—a new facility for the measurement of health-related quality of life. Health Policy. 1990;16(3):199-208.

44. Brooks R, Group E. EuroQol: the current state of play. Health Policy. 1996;37(1):53-72.
45. Brazier J, Czoski-Murray C, Roberts J, et al. Estimation of a preference-based index from a condition specific measure: the King's Health Questionnaire. Med Decis Making. 2008;28(1):113-26.
46. Rowen D, Brazier J, Young T, et al. Deriving a preference-based measure for cancer using the EORTC QLQ-C30. Value Health. 2011;14(5):721-31.
47. Klose T. The contingent valuation method in healthcare. Health Policy. 1999;47(2):97-123.
48. Ryan M, Farrar S. Using conjoint analysis to elicit preferences for healthcare. BMJ. 2000;320(7248):1530-3.
49. de Bekker-Grob EW, Ryan M, Gerard K. Discrete choice experiments in health economics: a review of the literature. Health Econ. 2012;21(2):145-72.
50. Wolff, N. (1998). Measuring costs: what is counted and who is accountable? Estimation of incremental costs. Disease Management and Clinical Outcomes, 4(1), 114-128.
51. Lipscomb J, Yabroff KR, Brown ML, et al. Healthcare costing: data, methods, current applications. Medical Care. 2009;47(Suppl 1):S1-6.
52. Briggs A, Sculpher M, Buxton M. Uncertainty in the economic evaluation of healthcare technologies: the role of sensitivity analysis. Health Econ. 1994;3(2):95-104.
53. Richardson WS, Detsky AS. (1995). Users' guides to the medical literature: VII. How to use a clinical decision analysis. A. Are the results of the study valid? Evidence-Based Medicine Working Group. JAMA. 1995;273(16):1292-5.
54. Richardson WS, Detsky AS. Users' guides to the medical literature: VII. How to use a clinical decision analysis. B. What are the results and will they help me in caring for my patients? JAMA. 1995;273(20):1610-3.
55. Doubilet P, Begg CB, Weinstein MC, et al. Probabilistic sensitivity analysis using Monte Carlo simulation. A practical approach. Med Decis Making. 1985;5(2):157-77.
56. Sonnenberg FA, Beck JR. Markov models in medical decision making: a practical guide. Med Decis Making. 1993;13(4):322-38.
57. Ramsey S, Willke R, Briggs A, et al. Good research practices for cost-effectiveness analysis alongside clinical trials: the ISPOR RCT-CEA Task Force Report. Value Health. 2005;8(5):521-33.
58. Husereau D, Drummond M, Petrou S, et al. Consolidated Health Economic Evaluation Reporting Standards (CHEERS) statement. BMC Med. 2013;11(1):80.
59. Drummond MF, Jefferson TO. Guidelines for authors and peer reviewers of economic submissions to the BMJ. The BMJ Economic Evaluation Working Party. BMJ. 1996;313(7052):275-83.

60. Philips Z, Ginnelly L, Sculpher M, et al. Review of guidelines for good practice in decision-analytic modelling in health technology assessment. Health Technol Assess. 2004;8(36):iii-iv, ix-xi, 1-158.
61. Evers S, Goossens M, De Vet H, et al. Criteria list for assessment of methodological quality of economic evaluations: Consensus on Health Economic Criteria. Int J Technol Assess Health Care. 2005;21(02):240-5.
62. EBM Toolbox: A glossary of health economics terms. (2012, September 20). Retrieved June 21, 2015, from http://clinicalevidence.bmj.com/x/set/static/ebm/toolbox/678253.html

13. The Basics of a Diagnostic Test Study

Kathleen G Dobson,
Alonso Carrasco, Raman Mundi, Steve Rocha

Key Objectives

- Understand what a diagnostic test study consists of and its importance
- Learn about important considerations in the design of diagnostic test studies
- Understand the properties that define a diagnostic test
- Learn about how to interpret a likelihood ratio (LR) and receiver operating characteristic (ROC) curves
- Develop insight into the appraisal of studies of a diagnostic test.

What is a Diagnostic Test Study?

The reason to conduct a study of a diagnostic test is to determine if a test can accurately provide the correct diagnosis in a specific patient population. A diagnostic test is typically performed on patients with suggestive symptoms, but who present clinical uncertainty about having a specific disease. When performing a study of a diagnostic test, patients suspected of having a condition are assessed with both the test under investigation and a *reference standard*. The test under investigation is referred to as the *index test*. The index test may be of any method that provides information on the patient's health, including laboratory, function, clinical finding or imaging tests. The reference standard is regarded as the best available method for diagnosing the presence or absence of the target condition. Within diagnostic test studies, the results from the reference standard test should ideally be regarded as the truth about disease—whether it is present or absent. By comparing the outcomes of the index test directly to the outcomes of the reference standard, the diagnostic accuracy of the index test can be established and its properties expressed in several ways, as will be discussed below.[1]

Why do we Need to Conduct Studies of a Diagnostic Test?

As proper diagnosis is critical to ensure patient health and appropriate health services use, it is important to ensure that diagnostic tests can accurately and efficiently provide the correct diagnosis. The process of diagnosis can be broken down into successive steps. First, the clinician generates a differential diagnosis based on the patient's history and clinical presentation. The clinician will then assign each possible diagnosis a ***pre-test probability.***[2] These probabilities are based on disease prevalence in the patient population and on the physician's own experiences.[3] Secondly, once some diseases are discarded (low to very low pre-test probability), clinicians may still need to deal with several potential diagnoses to clarify further. It is under this residual uncertainty when diagnostic tests are most valuable. The right diagnostic test provides additional information to shift a clinician's uncertainty from an area where further testing is required to either an area of certainty in which treatment should be implemented (above treatment threshold) or an area in which no testing is warranted (below test threshold) (Fig. 13.1). This new information gathered through diagnostic testing changes the pre-test probability of the diagnosis to a new ***post-test probability.***[2]

Different diagnostic tests influence the probability of a patient's diagnosis. A diagnostic test when positive may increase the probability by a substantial amount and make a diagnosis highly likely (i.e. rule in the disease). Conversely, the same test when negative may only have minimal influence on probability and do little to exclude the diagnosis (rule out the disease).[3] The degree and direction in which a diagnostic test will influence probability is dependent on the properties of that test and these properties can only be established through studies of a diagnostic test in which the index test is compared to a reference standard.

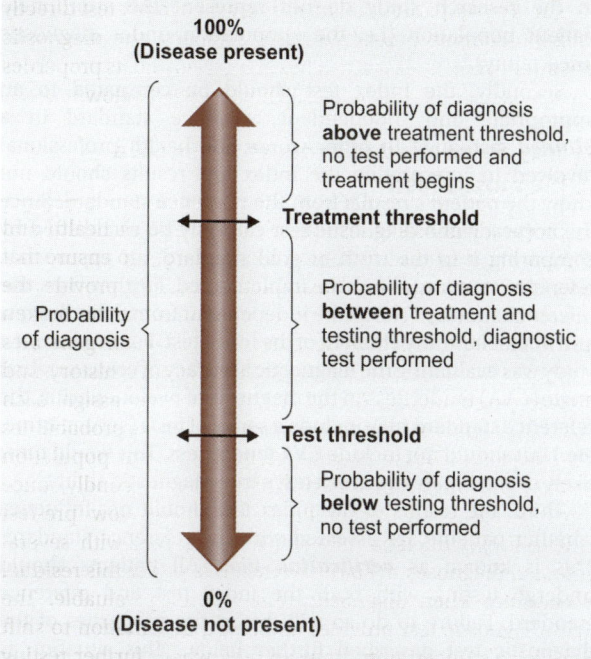

Fig. 13.1: Probability of diagnosis and diagnostic tests

What Should be Considered to Conduct an Ideal Study of a Diagnostic Test?

There are several steps that should be taken to increase methodological quality and minimize risk of bias when designing a diagnostic test study. First and foremost, patients enrolled in the study should face diagnostic uncertainty. Almost any test can differentiate between severely ill patient and healthy patient. To establish whether a diagnostic test will be useful in a clinical setting, the study must incorporate those patients that resemble the patient population of a clinical setting.[4] For example, if a new laboratory amniocentesis test to determine fetal chromosomal abnormalities wished to be tested, the study must be completed with a sample of pregnant women. ***Spectrum bias*** occurs when the patients in the research study do not represent the appropriate patient population (i.e. the population under diagnostic uncertainty).[5]

Secondly, the index test should be compared to an appropriate and independent reference standard in a **blinded** fashion.[2,4] In other words, the health professional involved in interpreting the index test results should not know the patient's results from the reference standard. Since the accuracy of a diagnostic test can only be established by comparing it to the truth or gold standard, an appropriate reference standard should be implemented. Furthermore, the reference standard should be independent from the index test and not include any element of the index test. For instance, if a study was evaluating the diagnostic accuracy of costovertebral angle (CVA) tenderness in the diagnosis of pyelonephritis, the reference standard may include a series of tests (serum, urine, etc.) but should not include CVA tenderness. This would most likely overestimate the index test's true diagnostic ability.

Third, the results of the index test should not influence whether patients are assessed with the reference standard. This is known as **verification bias**. All patients should undergo testing with both the index test and reference standard. Failure to do so will distort the properties of the diagnostic test described further below. This situation is particularly common when the reference standard requires invasive procedures for its verification.[6,7]

When reporting the results from the study, the manuscript should also report in detail all steps associated with performing the diagnostic test, including patient preparation, techniques and interpretation. The description should be have sufficient details to allow replication by readers.[6] A final tip is that when publishing a diagnostic test study, the title and abstract should clearly state that the study examines the accuracy of a diagnostic test. Including a MeSH heading of 'sensitivity and specificity' may also make it easier to retrieve your diagnostic study in electronic databases.[7]

What Results of the Diagnostic Test Study Should be Reported?

When reporting the results of a diagnostic study, there are five key properties of a diagnostic test that should be clearly

Table 13.1: Format of a 2 x 2 table

Index test	Reference standard	
	Condition present	Condition absent
Positive result	a	b
Negative result	c	d

presented: ***sensitivity, specificity, positive predictive value, negative predictive value*** and ***likelihood ratios (LR).***[6] To understand these parameters, it is useful to construct a 2 × 2 table that directly compares the index test and reference standard, as shown in Table 13.1. This table has 4 boxes: one for true positives (box a), one for false positives (box b), one for false negatives (box c) and one for true negatives (box d).[3]

To aid in understanding these concepts, we will present a hypothetical example. Let us suppose 100 patients are recruited in a study investigating the accuracy of the 'anterior drawer test' in diagnosing patients suspected of having full thickness anterior cruciate ligament (ACL) tears. The reference standard in this case is magnetic resonance imaging (MRI). The results of this trial are displayed in Table 13.2.

Sensitivity and Specificity

Sensitivity is defined as the proportion of patients with the target condition who have a positive test result (a/a + c).[3] As seen in the 2 × 2 table, only those patients with the condition (boxes a and c) are included in sensitivity calculation. If a diagnostic test has high sensitivity, it will be able to rule out a condition if the patient tests are negative. For example, if our anterior drawer test has a sensitivity of 100%, when the test is negative, it is very likely that the patient does not present

Table 13.2: Example 2 × 2 table—anterior drawer test for ACL tears

Anterior drawer test	MRI	
	ACL Tear	No Tear
Positive result	40 (a)	4 (b)
Negative result	20 (c)	36 (d)

with an ACL tear. However, even though a high sensitivity test will confidently detect those without the condition, a positive result may be indicative for other similar conditions, resulting in 'false' positives. Therefore, a sensitive test is most useful when a patient's diagnosis is negative. The mnemonic **SnNOut** (high **Sn**sitivity, **N**egative, rule **out**) is commonly used to remember this principle.[8]

Specificity is defined as the proportion of patients without the target condition who have a negative test result (d/ b + d).[3] As seen in the 2 × 2 table, only those patients **without** the condition (boxes b and d) are included in specificity calculation. A test that is highly 'specific' for a target condition will only be positive if that condition truly exists in the patient. Thus, tests with high specificity tend to rule in the diagnosis when positive. This concept can be remembered with the mnemonic **SpPIn** (high **Sp**ecificity, **P**ositive test, rule **in**).[8]

In our example trial comparing the anterior drawer test to MRI, among the 60 patients with an ACL tear, 40 were detected by the anterior drawer test. Among the 40 with no ACL tear, 36 had a negative anterior drawer test. Thus, in this example, the anterior drawer test has a sensitivity of 67% (40/60) and a specificity of 90% (36/40).

As mentioned, a sensitive test is important to rule out a certain condition (SnNOut), while a specific test is useful to rule in the condition of question (SpPIn). The main limitation of interpreting sensitivity and specificity values is that they cannot be used in predicting the probability of a condition in individual patients.[8] This is because sensitivity and specificity are based completely on the number of patients with or without disease in a study. Therefore, predictive values and LR are critical in determining the probability of an individual patient's disease after undergoing a diagnostic test.

Positive and Negative Predictive Values

Information from a diagnostic test shifts the pre-test probability to a new post-test probability—ultimately making the diagnosis more or less likely.[2,4] One method to establish the post-test probability is to calculate the **positive predictive value (PPV)** and **negative predictive value (NPV)** of the diagnostic test. The PPV is the proportion of patients with a positive test result that truly have the target condition (a/a + b). The NPV is the proportion of patients with a negative test result who truly do not have the target condition (d/c + d).

In our hypothetical ACL tear study, 44 patients had a positive anterior drawer test, of which only 40 truly had an ACL tear. Thus, the PPV of this test is 91% (40/44). In other words, if a patient suspected of having an ACL tear has a positive anterior drawer test, there is a 91% probability (post-test probability) that a tear does exist. Of the 56 patients with a negative test result, only 36 have no ACL tear. The NPV of the anterior drawer test is 64% (36/56). Hence, a negative test result indicates a 64% probability that the condition is absent or conversely, a 36% post-test probability of an ACL tear being present.

Likelihood Ratios

If a disease has a high prevalence in the appropriate patient population, the PPV will also be high, indicating that the baseline prevalence of the disease/condition is extremely important for determining post-test probability of disease. LR, the final and most important properties of a diagnostic test that should be present for is to take a disease's prevalence into account.[2,9,10] The LR is defined as the proportion of patients with the target condition who have a particular test result divided by the proportion of patients without the target condition who have the same test result.[3] Depending on the type of diagnostic test, the LR for a ***positive test*** (+) may be of interest. The LR+ is defined as:

LR+ = the probability of an individual ***with*** disease having a positive test/ the probability of an individual ***without*** disease having a positive test.

The numerator for the LR(+) equation is equal to the ***sensitivity*** of the test, while the denominator is equal to **1 − specificity** of the test.[5] Therefore, one can calculate the LR(+) as:

$$LR+ = sensitivity/ 1 - specificity; OR$$
$$LR+ = (a/a + c)/1 - (d/b + d) \text{ OR}$$
$$LR+ = (a/a + c)/(b/b + d)$$

Conversely, it may be more important to examine the LR for a ***negative test*** (−), which may be defined as:

LR− = the probability of an individual ***with*** disease having a negative test/ the probability of an individual ***without*** disease having a negative test.

The numerator for the LR(−) equation is equal to the converse of the sensitivity of the diagnostic test (1 − sensitivity), while the denominator is equal to the ***specificity*** of the test.[10] Therefore, one can calculate the LR(−) as:

$$LR- = 1 - \text{sensitivity}/\text{specificity; OR}$$
$$LR- = 1 - (a/a + c)/(d/b + d) \text{ OR}$$
$$LR- = (c/a+c)/(d/b + d)$$

In simple terms, the LR represents the ability of a test to move a clinician from a pre-test probability to a new post-test probability. The higher the impact of the index test on increasing or reducing the post-test probability, the more useful is the LR.

For the other concepts described in this section, we have only considered 'positive' and 'negative' test results in our 2×2 tables, but an important advantage of LR is that they are not restricted to such dichotomous outcomes. For instance, 3 separate LR could be calculated if a test categorized patients into high, intermediate and low categories. Furthermore, LR are simple to understand and allow for an easy conversion of pre-test probabilities to post-test probabilities.[2,3] This ratio can be determined for all test strata, whether dichotomous or not.

Referring back to our ACL tear study, the likelihood that a patient with an ACL tear will have a positive anterior drawer test is 67% (40/60, a/a + c) and the likelihood that a patient with no ACL tear will have a positive anterior drawer test is 10% (4/40, b/b + d). The LR for a positive anterior drawer test is thus 6.7 (0.67/0.10). That means a positive anterior drawer test is 6.7 times more likely to occur in a patient with an ACL tear than in a patient without a tear. The LR for a negative anterior drawer test can be calculated in the same way, which yields a value of 0.37. This means that a negative anterior drawer test is 0.37 times more likely in a patient with an ACL tear than a patient with no tear. Table 13.3 summarizes these key properties of a diagnostic test.

Table 13.3: Properties of a diagnostic test

Property	Explanation	2 × 2 table
Sensitivity	The proportion of patients with a given condition who have a positive test	a/a + c
Specificity	The proportion of patients truly free of a given condition who have a negative test	d/b+d
Positive predictive value	Proportion of patients with a positive test who have the condition	a/a + b
Negative predictive value	Proportion of patients with a negative test who truly do not have the condition	d/c + d
Likelihood ratio positive (LR+)	The relative likelihood that a given test would be positive in a patient with a condition of interest, as opposed to one without the condition	(a/a + c)/ 1 − (d/b + d)
Likelihood ratio negative (LR-)	The relative likelihood that a given test would be negative in a patient with a condition of interest, as opposed to one without the condition.	1 − (a/a + c) /(d/b + d)

How are LR of a Diagnostic Test Incorporated into Clinical Practice?

LR indicate by how much and in which direction the diagnostic test will change the pre-test probability.[10] A LR greater than 1 will raise the pre-test probability and the greater the value of this ratio, the higher the post-test probability will be. A LR of less than 1 will lower the pre-test probability and closer the value is to 0 the lower the post-test probability will be. A LR of 1 has no influence on the pre-test probability and the post-test probability will be equivalent to the pre-test probability.[4]

The LR can be used to determine the post-test probability in more than one way. Simple calculations can be done, in which the pre-test probability is converted to pre-test odds

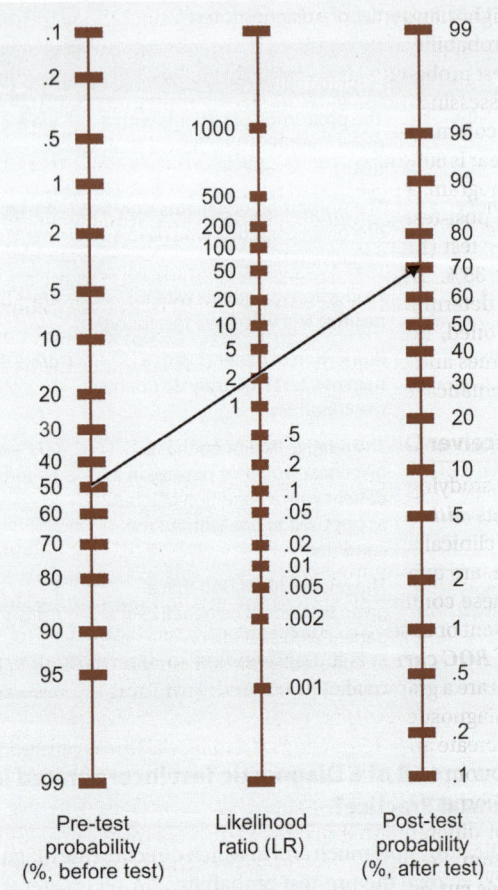

Fig. 13.2: Example of a nomogram (adapted from Fagan)[11]

and then multiply by the LR. This provides the post-test odds, which can be reconverted into a post-test probability. A different approach is to use a nomogram (Fig. 13.2).

A nomogram has three columns: (1) a left-hand column for pre-test probabilities, (2) a middle column of LR and

(3) a right-hand column with post-test probabilities.[11] The post-test probability is determined by anchoring a ruler at the given pre-test probability, running it through the corresponding LR and assessing the point at which the ruler intersects the right-hand column.[5] In our ACL study, the pre-test probability of an ACL tear is 60% (60 of the 100 patients have an ACL tear). Using a nomogram, a positive anterior drawer test (LR of 6.7) would give a post-test probability of about 90%. A negative anterior drawer test (LR of 0.37) would give a post-test probability of about 35%. These post-test probabilities are equivalent to those determined by calculating the PPN and NPV above. As mentioned, however, LR are not restricted to dichotomous outcomes and the use of a nomogram eliminates the need for mathematical calculations.

Receiver Operating Characteristic (ROC) Curves

When studying a clinical test, two patient groups are defined: patients ***with*** disease and patients ***without*** disease. However, many clinical tests, such as the measurement of blood hemoglobin, are quantitative and continuous in nature.[12] To translate these continuous measurements to determine if disease is present or absent, a clinical cut-off needs to be decided. The use of ***ROC curves*** is a common way to determine this. ROC curves are a graphical method for determining the best cut-off for a diagnostic test (Fig. 13.3).

To create an ROC curve, first a diagonal line is plotted from the bottom left hand corner at the origin and the top right hand corner (1,1); this line represents a diagnostic test that cannot differentiate a patient with a condition or without a condition. Secondly, the sensitivity (true positive rate) of all possible cut-points for the diagnostic test are plotted on the ***y axis***, with the false positive rate (1-specificity) plotted on the ***x axis***.[12] As it is nearly impossible to have a virtually-perfect test, the best-cut point for a diagnostic test will be the closest point to the top left corner.

Apart from helping to determine the best cut-off for a diagnostic test, ROC curves may be used to examine how accurate a diagnostic test is by looking at the ***area under the curve (AUC)*** on the graph.[13] An AUC value can fall between 0 and 1. A value closer to 1 represents a test with higher

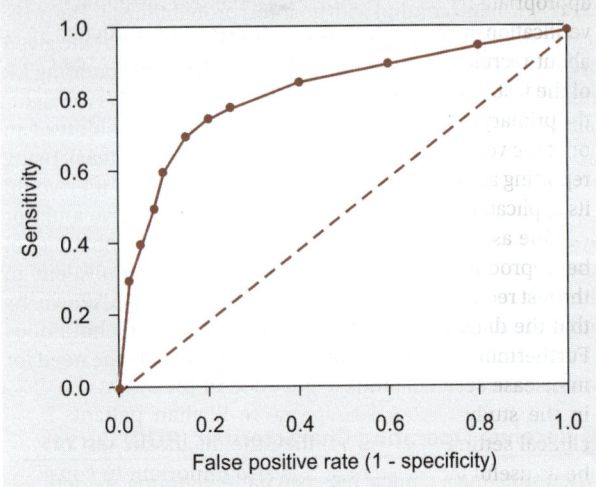

Fig. 13.3: Example of a ROC curve

diagnostic accuracy. In general, a diagnostic test with an AUC value greater than 0.9 has high diagnostic accuracy; a value between 0.7 and 0.9 indicates adequate accuracy; 0.5 and 0.7 indicates low accuracy; and 0.5 represents that the test cannot differentiate a patient with or without disease.[8] Lastly, a ROC curve may be used to compare the effectiveness of more than one diagnostic test by plotting multiple tests on the same graph.

How do you Appraise a Study of a Diagnostic Test?

Studies of a diagnostic test can be appraised for their methodological quality, their results and their applicability to the clinical setting.[14] The methodological features that minimize the risk of bias in these studies include a description of the enrollment process and characteristics of an appropriate sample of patients. For example, were patients recruited because they presented suspicious symptoms of disease, had a previous test result or have they undergone either the index or reference test?[7] As mentioned previously, the study should compare the index test to an independent and appropriate reference standard in a blinded fashion and avoid verification bias.[2,4,6,7] A study should provide sufficient detail about recruitment and testing procedures to allow replication of the test.[10] In appraising the results of a diagnostic test study, the primary concern is that LR for the diagnostic test be reported or at the very least, enough data be given to calculate them (i.e. reporting a 2 × 2 table).[6] Finally, the study must be appraised for its applicability to the clinical setting in question.

One aspect to consider is whether the diagnostic test can be 'reproduced' in the clinical setting. If resources differ or the test requires trained interpreters, then there is a possibility that the diagnostic test may not be successfully reproduced. Furthermore, patients in the clinical setting should be similar in disease severity to those included in the study. If patients in the study are on average more ill than patients in the clinical setting in question, then the diagnostic test may not be as useful in that setting. It is also important to consider if patients in the clinical setting will benefit from the test. If the diagnostic test itself is invasive and associated with adverse effects, its use may not be warranted. If the target condition has a poor prognosis but is highly responsive to treatment, then diagnostic testing will be more valuable in this case.[6]

Important Learning Points

- Studies of a diagnostic test directly compare an index test to a reference standard to determine the accuracy of the index test.
- It is important to include a sample of patients that face diagnostic uncertainty, to have an appropriate, blind reference standard and ensure all patients are assessed with both the index test and reference standard.
- Sensitivity, specificity, PPV and NPV indicate the discriminatory power of a diagnostic test and can be use to determine post-test probabilities.
- Due to the advantages over the other properties of a diagnostic test, LR have become the most valued measures of a diagnostic test in clinical practice. They provide a measure of how influential a diagnostic test will be in ruling in or ruling out a diagnosis.

- ROC curves may be used by plotting sensitivity and specificity to determine what the most appropriate dichotomous cut-point is for defining disease.
- A study of a diagnostic test should be appraised for the methods, the presentation of the results and the applicability of the study results to the clinical setting of interest.

Definitions

Area under the ROC curve: The area used for determining the accuracy of a diagnostic test.
Blinding: The index test and reference standard are assessed by interpreters who are unaware of the results of the other investigation.
Gold standard: A method having established or widely accepted accuracy for determining a diagnosis and providing a standard to which a new diagnostic test can be compared.
Index test: The test under evaluation in a study of a diagnostic test. It can include information gathering from the history, physical examination, function tests, laboratory tests, imaging tests and histopathology.
LR: The relative likelihood that a given test would be expected in a patient with a condition of interest, as opposed to one without the condition.
NPV: The proportion of patients with a negative test who truly do not have the condition (d/c+d).
PPV: The proportion of patients with a positive test who truly have the condition (a/a+b).
Post-test probability: The probability of having the target condition after the application of a diagnostic test.
Pre-test probability: The probability of having the target condition before the application of a diagnostic test.
ROC: A graphical method for determining the best cut-off for a diagnostic test.
Reference standard: The best available method for establishing the presence or absence of the condition of interest and serves as the 'truth' in a study of a diagnostic test. It can include laboratory tests, imaging tests, pathology and clinical follow-up.
Sensitivity: The proportion of patients with a given condition

who have a positive test (a/a+c).

Specificity: The proportion of patients truly free of a given condition who have a negative test (d/ b+d).

Spectrum bias: When the patients enrolled in the research study do not represent the appropriate patient population.

Verification bias: Bias caused by the results of the diagnostic test, which can influence whether patients are assessed with the reference standard.

REFERENCES

1. Bossuyt PM, Reitsma JB, Bruns DE, et al. Towards complete and accurate reporting of studies of diagnostic accuracy: the STARD initiative. Fam Pract. 2004;21(1):4-10.
2. Richardson WS, Wilson MC. Chapter 10: The process of diagnosis. In: Guyatt G, Rennie D, Meade MO, Cook DJ, editors. Users' Guide to the Medical Literature: Essentials of Evidence-Based Clinical Practice. 2nd ed. New York: McGraw-Hill Professional Publishing; 2008. p. 169-178.
3. McGee S. Evidence-based Physical Diagnosis, 3rd edition. Philadelphia: Elsevier Saunders; 2012.
4. Furukawa TA, Strauss S, Heiner BC, Guyatt, G. Chapter 12: Diagnostic tests. In: Guyatt G, Rennie D, Meade MO, Cook DJ, editors. Users' Guide to the Medical Literature: Essentials of Evidence-based Clinical Practice. 2nd ed. New York: McGraw-Hill Professional Publishing; 2008. p 195-222.
5. Newman TB, Browner WS, Cummings SR, Hulley SB. Chapter 12: Designing studies of medical tests. In: Hully SB, Cummings SR, Browner WS, Grady DG, & Newman TB, editors. Designing clinical research. 4th ed. Philadelphia: Lippincott Williams & Wilkins; 2013. p. 171–191.
6. Archibald S, Bhandari M, Thoma A. Users' guides to the surgical literature: how to use an article about a diagnostic test. Evidence-Based Surgery Working Group. Can J Surg. 2001;44(1):17-23.
7. Bossuyt PM, Reitsma JB, Bruns DE, et al. The STARD statement for reporting studies of diagnostic accuracy: explanation and elaboration. Ann Intern Med. 2003;138(1):W1–12.
8. Akobeng AK. Understanding diagnostic tests 1: sensitivity, specificity and predictive values. Acta Pediatr. 2007;96(3):338–41.
9. Greenhalgh T. How to read a paper. Papers that report diagnostic or screening tests. BMJ. 1997;315(7107):540-3.
10. Akobeng AK. Understanding diagnostic tests 2: likelihood ratios, pre- and post-test probabilities and their use in clinical practice. Acta Pediatr. 2007;96(4):487–91.

11. Fagan TJ. Letter: Nomogram for Bayes theorem. N Engl J Med. 1975;293:257.
12. Akobeng AK. Understanding diagnostic tests 3: Receiver operating characteristic curves. Acta Pediatr. 2007;96(5):644-7.
13. Mallett S, Halligan S, Thompson M, et al. Interpreting diagnostic accuracy studies for patient care. BMJ. 2012;345:e3999.
14. Sackett DL, Haynes RB. The architecture of diagnostic research. BMJ. 2002;324(7336):539-41.

14

The Basics of Reliability

Chloe Bedard, Anil jain

> **Key Objectives**
> - Understand the definition of reliability and be able to distinguish reliability from agreement and validity
> - Learn the different measures of reliability
> - Learn the different characteristics of a reliability study
> - Learn the important questions to ask when critically appraising a reliability study.

What is 'Reliability'?

The purpose of measurement is to quantify some characteristic or attribute that we view as unique to that subject or object.[1] That is, we want to record some information about an object that we believe may differ from other measured objects. Consider all of the 'Sample Characteristics' tables you have seen, we can easily agree they are composed of characteristics of the sample that are likely to differ among participants and do not contain information that is likely to be the same for each participant. As researchers, we are interested in characteristics that differ among people; the implication of this is that we need instruments of measurement that capture this variability. In other words, to be useful in measuring differences between participants, an instrument must be reliable.[2] The formal definition of reliability comes from ***Classical Test Theory (CTT)***, which starts with the conceptualization of a single subject's score as comprised of their 'true' score and the error of the measurement. The most reliable instrument would theoretically contain no error in its measurement and thus consistently represent the object of measurements 'true' score. 'True' in this sense does not technically represent the universal truth of the observation, but rather the average score that would be produced if the subject was measured an infinite number of times. Therefore, a person's 'true' score may be a biased score, however, it is *consistently* biased.[1] So we may define reliability as the consistency of a measurement; it is the extent to which an instrument provides the same measurement each time it is used under the same condition with the same subjects.[1,2]

The reliability coefficient is statistically defined as the ratio of between-subject variability to the total variability (*Equation 1*). Between-subject variability is the true difference between subjects. Total variability is the true difference between subjects in addition to *measurement error*. This can also be expressed in terms of variances, where σ^2_s is the variance due to true differences between subjects and σ^2_e is the variance due to error (*Equation 2*). The total variability will always be greater than the between-subject variability and so the reliability coefficient will always range from 0 to 1. A value of 0 indicates that all of the variation in the sample is due to error. A value of 1 indicates that all of the variation is due to true differences between subjects and represents perfect reliability.[1,2]

Equation 1: Definition of reliability
Reliability = True subject variability/(true subject variability + measurement error)

Equation 2: Reliability coefficient
Reliability = $\sigma^2_s / (\sigma^2_s + \sigma^2_e)$

There are two ways to increase the reliability coefficient: reduce the variance due to error or increase the between-subject variability. The first strategy is an example of what researchers are doing when they train observers or raters on how to administer a measurement instrument. To increase the between-subject variance, we may use a scale that allows more variability in subject responses, e.g. by using a 7-point Likert scale to measure an attribute, rather than a dichotomous scale. When subjects are able to make finer degradations of responses we capture more variability among them as compared to restricting their responses to one of two categories.[3] Between-subject variance can be artificially inflated when the instrument is applied to a heterogeneous sample of people. As stated above, a reliable instrument is one that is able to discriminate among subjects. Therefore, if subjects are inherently easy to discriminate between because we have recruited a sample of people who have contrasting characteristics, the instrument may *appear* to be highly reliable.[1] The alternative situation occurs when researchers apply an instrument to a relatively homogeneous sample in a clinical study yet report evidence of its reliability from a population that is more heterogeneous than the present study. The patients' test scores will no longer be reliable because the test cannot detect the small variability between patients and this will actually reduce statistical power.[4]

This highlights an important concept regarding reliability—it is not an inherent property of the instrument. The reliability coefficient is meaningless unless interpreted in the context of the measurement situation; that is, the sample, the raters, the administration methods, etc.[1] Therefore, it is more appropriate to speak about the reliability of the score produced by the measurement instrument in the context in which it was tested.[5]

Is Reliability the Same as Agreement?

Agreement is often confused with reliability. However, in some instances an instrument may produce highly agreeable but unreliable scores; this can occur when there are limited response options per item. For example, in the case of a checklist being applied to medical students to assess their competency, the response to each item is either yes, the student performed this action, or no, the student did not perform the action. In this example, we will have two raters per medical student so we can calculate inter-rater agreement and inter-rater reliability. Chances are high that the two raters will agree with each other for each student because there are only two responses for each item. However, we have much less information about each student and so the between-subject variability is restricted, thereby lowering the inter-rater reliability coefficient. This point may be further illustrated when thinking about the agreement and reliability of an instrument applied to a sample of participants who are all rated to have the *same* amount of the measure of interest. All raters should agree on the level of this attribute or characteristic but there will be no variability between participants, effectively bringing the reliability coefficient to zero. This is not to say that agreement and reliability are *always* inversely related, because we know that a highly reliable measurement tool is both consistent (i.e. agreeable) and able to discriminate between subjects.[1,2] As many researchers equate agreement with reliability it is important to make this distinction so readers can interpret results of reliability studies critically.

Is Reliability the Same as Validity?

Validity is the extent to which one can make accurate interpretations about the participant based upon the observations produced by the measurement tool.[6] To contrast this definition to reliability, we can recall our discussion of a 'true' score. This is the score that is consistently produced (i.e. contains minimal random error), however, may contain an aggregation of systematic biases the subject responds with. Regardless of the systematic biases present in every observation of this measurement, the scale may still be said to be reliable.[7] However for a scale to be valid, we must be certain that the observation produced by the measurement instrument does not contain systematic bias and is in fact only obtaining information about what it is supposed to be measuring.[6] Therefore, we can reason that reliability places an upper limit on validity such that a scale can only be as valid as it is reliable (***Equation 3:***).[6] The difference between reliability and validity is illustrated in Figs 14.1A to C. The bullseye in the middle of the target is the true value. Measurements can be both valid and reliable and are centered tightly around true value, as shown in A. On the other hand, measurements can be very reliable but not valid if they are systematically off the mark, as in B. Where only a few unreliable measurements are taken, these measurements also have low validity because they are likely to be off the true value by chance alone, as shown in C.

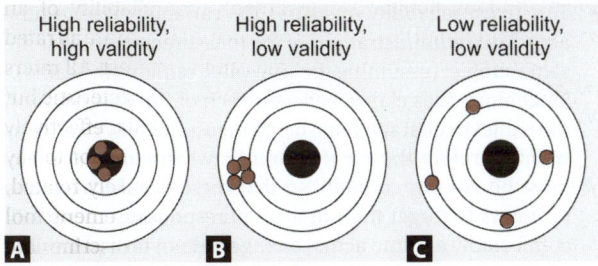

Figs 14.1A to C: Reliability versus validity[8]

Equation 3: Maximum validity

$$\text{Validity (max)} = \sqrt{\text{Reliability (of new test)} \times \text{Reliability (of the reference test)}}$$

What are the Different Measures of Reliability?

The most common measures of reliability include intra-rater, inter-rater, test-retest reliability and internal consistency. The first three measures of reliability assess the consistency across two or more test administrations, while internal consistency may be calculated after a single administration.

- Intra-rater reliability captures information about the variability within a single rater at two points in time to the same stimulus.[1,9] For example, the rating of a radiograph at one point in time by a rater is compared with the rating of the same radiograph at a different point in time by the same rater. Time is the only factor that varies between administrations. Intra-rater reliability will typically yield a higher reliability estimate than inter-rater reliability studies because it does not contain error due to other raters.
- Inter-rater reliability assesses the variability in scores across raters. Ideally different raters are using the exact same unbiased criteria to measure the subject and therefore we would expect raters to produce the same or very similar scores for the same subject.[1,10]

- Test-retest reliability measures the variability due to time across two administrations of the measurement tool for the same subject (assuming the true value remains the same).[1] Since time does elapse between each of the observations, the subject's characteristic being measured may change as well.[2] Therefore, the length of time between administrations must be chosen carefully so that there is sufficient time for raters to forget their first set of responses and yet still comfortably assume actual change did not take place. The appropriate time interval will depend on the measurement of interest and the instrument, however, the typical length of time between test administrations is between 2 and 14 days.[1] Low test-retest reliability coefficients should be interpreted cautiously as there are alternative explanations other than poor reliability of the tool, such as real change occurring between administrations.[1] Test-retest reliability is commonly calculated for scales that are self-administered because the rater is the subject.
- Internal consistency reflects the relationship between an individual's responses on each item within a single instrument and the overall score, suggesting whether or not the items appear to be measuring the same thing.[10] If each item on the scale is meant to measure a single attribute or characteristic, we would expect a high correlation between items and between each item and the total score. However, if the correlation between items is too high it may suggest that the items are redundant.[11] Another consideration of internal consistency is the number of items on the scale. The internal consistency will increase as the length of the scale increases, regardless of the actual relationship between items.[10] A third consideration of internal consistency arises in measurement tools with multiple subscales that would not be expected to correlate highly with each other; measures of internal consistency should be assessed within each subscale and not for the total scale.[11] It is important to remember that internal consistency does not include some types of measurement error, such as differences in times, observers and settings. Internal consistency is the weakest form of reliability and readers should interpret the results with caution.[2]

What are the Characteristics of a Reliability Study?

How do I Construct the Research Question?

In clinical research, it is important to first precisely construct an appropriate research question, defining the population, intervention, comparison, outcome and time. In a reliability study, investigators must determine which instrument they are testing, how this instrument will be used in clinical or research practice, to whom they will apply the measure and what type(s) of reliability they will measure in the study.[2] The research question should reflect the measurement situation in which the tool will be used. The intervention will be the instrument evaluated in the study. The comparison may be between raters, times or items. The outcome of a reliability study is the type of reliability being assessed. The time should be specified if it will be evaluated as a source of error (i.e. in test-retest reliability).

How do I Select the Patients/Subjects for a Reliability Study?

The reliability of an instrument should be evaluated in the sample it is intended to be applied to, because we cannot assume that the reliability of test scores in one sample is generalizable to other dissimilar samples. Therefore, it is important to select participants that are representative of the population for which the tool is intended.[1,12] For example, a study assessing a tool which measures shoulder range of motion in a physiotherapy clinic should include patients with all different ranges of motion. This diverse group of patients better represents actual practice than if only healthy patients with a large range of motion are included.

How do I Determine my Sample Size?

In a reliability study, there are two different samples that the researcher must determine the size of—the number of raters and the number of subjects. Karanicolas, et al.[2] recommends determining the number of raters based on generalizability and feasibility; i.e. how many raters will be used in a clinical or research setting and how many would be accessible for the research study. The sample size of the participants is more complex. There are several proposed sample size calculations that may be used and most require an estimation of the reliability, the minimum reliability that would be accepted, the level of certainty desired and the number of observations per subject. For specific formulas *see* Streiner, et al.[1] Increasing the sample size of the subjects will yield a more precise reliability estimate.

How do I Select Appropriate Raters?

Raters are a potential source of error and reliability tests can identify this variation. For instruments that are self-administered (e.g. quality of life questionnaires), the rater is the same as the subject. For other types of instruments, generally one or more raters apply the measure to multiple subjects. It is important to consider the expertize and practice setting of the raters selected for the reliability study. Raters who have a higher expertize level (i.e. due to a higher level of training) are more likely to assign a more reliable rating compared to raters with less experience; therefore, we must first identify the expertize of raters in actual practice. If raters of varying levels of expertize use the tool in practice then including raters with all potential levels of expertize will provide more informative results.[2]

How do I Assign Ratings?

All measurement tools should provide detailed instructions about the scoring or rating procedures that should be followed in clinical practice. The rating sessions in a reliability study should reflect the clinical practice environment and follow the exact scoring methods as outlined by the creators of the instrument.[2] Researchers should consider the additional information that is available to raters in actual practice, such as patient history. Raters should be supplied only with the information that would normally be made available in actual practice.[12] Lastly, in every reliability study it is important that each rater completes their evaluations in the same test settings. For example, if the study involves the review of radiographs, all raters should view the radiographs in the same format—either hard copy or computer image.[2]

How is the Data Analyzed?

Recall the statistical definition of reliability—the ratio of between-subject variance to total variance (***Equations 1 and 2***). These equations can be used to calculate an intraclass correlation coefficient (ICC); intraclass because it will be calculated within a single variable. The values used in this equation are derived from a repeated measures analysis of variance (ANOVA)[1]. The ICC formula may be manipulated to provide information about inter-rater, intra-rater and test-retest reliability, as well as internal consistency (*see* Weir, 2005[14] for more information). The ICC is typically used in measurement situations where the ratings are scored on a ***continuous scale***.[1] However, an ICC may be calculated for categorical ratings when the data is coded appropriately because the formulation is mathematically equivalent to a kappa (which will be discussed in the following paragraph).[15] The ICC is a very flexible and robust measure of reliability and can easily accommodate information across several raters, times and items.[1]

For ***categorical data***, the kappa statistic is typically used to measure reliability. The kappa statistic accounts for chance agreement by comparing the observed agreement with the possible agreement beyond chance.[16,17] Assessing agreement beyond chance is important especially in situations where there are skewed proportions of one category, because raters

Table 14.1: Strength of agreement categories for kappa statistic

Strength of agreement	Kappa statistic
Poor	<0.00
Slight	0.00–0.20
Fair	0.21–0.40
Moderate	0.41–0.60
Substantial	0.61–0.80
Almost perfect	0.81–1.00

will agree with each other more often than not.[1] The degree of agreement may be taken into account using a weighted kappa, so that large disagreements (i.e. differ by more than one category) are weighted more than partial disagreements (i.e. differ by only one category).[18] The weighted kappa statistic can be used to compare two or more observers, or two or more categories of responses.[2] The kappa statistic yields a minimum value of 0 indicating no agreement beyond chance and a maximum value of 1 indicating perfect agreement. Landis and Koch[16] have assigned labels to the corresponding ranges of kappa (Table 14.1).

How do I Interpret the Results?

The acceptable level of reliability depends on many variables, including the context and the purpose of the measurement. Often there are different standards of reliability depending on if the tool will be used in a clinical or research context. In a clinical setting, it is often the case that testing or treatment decisions will be made based upon the results of a single measurement;[1] in these contexts Nunnally[19] suggests that the instrument should have a reliability of at least 0.90. However, in a research setting, judgments are made based upon the mean value of a sample of participants and therefore we can afford a little unreliability. Nunnally[18] recommends a minimum coefficient of 0.70. A further consideration in a research setting is the sample size; results of studies with larger sample sizes may be less compromised by an unreliable instrument as compared to studies with smaller samples.[1]

Kirshner and Guyatt[19] argue that there are different requirements for reliability depending on the purpose of the measurement. Therefore, the results of a reliability study may be interpreted with a different lens depending on the purpose of the tool. If the instrument is used to ***discriminate*** between individuals, then the between-person variability should be large and the measurement error small; systematic differences between ***times*** will have little influence on the results. If the tool is used to ***evaluate*** a specific intervention, the between-subject variability is allowed to be small as long as the measurement error is small and consistent over time. For instruments that are used to ***predict*** an outcome, the between-subject variability should be large and measurement error small, as with discriminative tools, however systematic difference across administrations would be problematic.[19]

Finally, the results of a reliability study should always be interpreted in the context of their methods: it is important to consider whether the study subjects, raters and administration of the measure reflect the clinical or research setting where it will be in use. If the contexts are similar, then readers can reasonably expect similar reliability in their setting. However, if the settings are different, readers must interpret the results cautiously as they may not be able to generalize them to their own setting.[2] In the latter case, more research may be required to investigate the psychometric properties of the tool before it can be used in a particular setting.

What is an Example of a Reliability Study?

Kristensen, et al.[21] conducted a reliability study to assess the inter-rater reliability of the New Mobility Score in patients with acute hip fracture. Their research question would be, ***among patients with an acute orthopedic hip fracture, can different raters reliably assess pre-fracture functional level with the New Mobility Score instrument?*** The New Mobility Score evaluates the pre-fracture functional level with a score from 0 (i.e. patient is not able to walk at all) to 9 (i.e. the patient is fully independent). The patients included in the study were 48 consecutive patients with acute hip fracture at a median age of 84 years. All were admitted to an acute orthopedic hip fracture unit at a university hospital. The scores were assessed by two independent physiotherapists at the orthopedic ward. Reliability was evaluated using the ICC. The study found an inter-rater reliability of 0.98 (95% CI: 0.96-0.99) between the two physiotherapists.[10]

How do I Critically Appraise a Reliability Study?

Mokkink, et al.[22] have developed the Consensus-based Standards for the selection of health Measurement Instruments (COSMIN) reliability checklist which provides a framework to allow readers to critically appraise reliability studies. The reader should answer the following critical questions:

Design Requirements

- Was the percentage of missing items given?
- Was there a description of how missing items were handled?
- Was the sample size included in the analysis adequate?
- Were at least two measurements available?
- Were the administrations independent?
- Was the time interval stated?
- Were patients stable in the interim period on the construct to be measured?
- Was the time interval appropriate?
- Were the test conditions similar for both measurements? (E.g. type of administration environment, instructions)
- Were there any important flaws in the design or methods of the study?

Statistical Methods

- For continuous scores; was an intraclass correlation coefficient (ICC) calculated?
- For dichotomous/nominal/ordinal scores; was kappa calculated?
- For ordinal scores; was a weighted kappa calculated?
- For ordinal scores; was the weighting scheme described? (E.g. linear, quadratic)

Important Learning Points

- Reliability is the consistency of a measurement
- Reliability can be measured within an instrument, within a rater, between raters and across time
- It is important to construct an appropriate research question that reflects the measurement situation in which the tool will be used
- Interpretation of results is always context specific.

Definitions

Categorical data: Data values fall into unordered categories or classes.[22]

Continuous data: Data that represent measurable quantities but are not restricted to taking on certain specified values.[23]

Measurement error: The difference between the true value and the value obtained from a certain measurement.[1]

REFERENCES

1. Streiner DL, Norman GR, Cairney J. Reliability. In: Health measurement scales: a practical guide to their development and use. 5th edn. Oxford: Oxford university press; 2014. p. 159-199.
2. Karanicolas PJ, Bhandari M, Kreder H, et al. Evaluating agreement: conducting a reliability study. J Bone Joint Surg Am. 2009;91(Suppl 3):99-106.
3. Streiner DL, Norman GR, Cairney J. Scaling Responses. In: Health measurement scales: a practical guide to their development and use. 5th edn. Oxford: Oxford university press; 2014. p. 38-73.
4. Gronlund NE, Linn RL. 6th edn. Measurement and evaluation in teaching. New York: MacMillian; 1990.
5. Kraemer HC. Ramifications of a population model for k as a coefficient of reliability. Psychometrika; 1979;44(4):461-72
6. Streiner DL, Norman GR, Cairney J. Validity. In: Health measurement scales: a practical guide to their development and use. 5th edn. Oxford: Oxford university press; 2014. p. 227-253.
7. Stanley JC. Reliability. In: 2nd ed. Thorndike R, editor. Educational measurement. Washington: American Council on Education; 1971.
8. Fletcher RH, Fletcher SW. (2005) Clinical epidemiology: the essentials. 4th ed. Lippincott Williams & Wilkins, Baltimore.
9. Luiz RR, Szklo M. More than one statistical strategy to assess agreement of quantitative measurements may usefully be reported. J Clin Epidemiol. 2005;58(3):215-6.
10. Jordan K. Assessment of published reliability studies for cervical spine range-of-motion measurement tools. J Manipulative Physiol Ther. 2000;23(3):180-95.
11. Streiner DL, Norman GR, Cairney J. Selecting the Items. In: Health measurement scales: a practical guide to their development and use. 5th ed. Oxford: Oxford university press; 2014. p.74-99.
12. Boyle GJ. Does item homogeneity indicate internal consistency or item redundancy in psychometric scales? Personality and Individual Differences. 1991;12(3):286-289.
13. Irwig L, Macaskill P, Walter SD, et al. New methods give better estimates of changes in diagnostic accuracy when prior information is provided. J Clin Epidemiol. 2006;59(3):299-307.
14. Weir JP. Quantifying test-retest reliability using the intraclass correlation coefficient and the SEM. J Strength Cond Res. 2005;19(1):231-40.

15. Fleiss JL, Cohen J. The equivalence of weighted kappa and the intraclass correlation coefficient as measures of reliability. Educational and Psychological Measurement. 1973;33(3):613-619.
16. Landis JR, Koch GG. The measurement of observer agreement for categorical data. Biometrics. 1977;33(1):159-74.
17. Landis JR, Koch GG. An application of hierarchical kappa-type statistics in the assessment of majority agreement among multiple observers. Biometrics. 1977;33(2):363-74.
18. Cohen J. Weighted kappa: Nominal scale agreement with provision for scaled disagreement or partial credit. Psychol Bull. 1968;70(4):213-20.
19. Nunnally JC. Psychometric Theory. New York: McGraw-Hill; 1978.
20. Kirshner B, Guyatt G. A methodological framework for assessing health indices. J Chronic Dis. 1985;38(1):27-36.
21. Kristensen MT, Bandholm T, Foss NB, et al. High inter-tester reliability of the new mobility score in patients with hip fracture. J Rehabil Med. 2008;40(7):589-91.
22. Mokkink LB, Terwee CB, Patrick DL, et al. The COSMIN checklist for assessing the methodological quality of studies on measurement properties of health status measurement instruments: An international Delphi study. Quality of Life Research. 2010;19(4):539-49.
23. Pagano M, Gauvreau K. Principles of Biostatistics. 2nd edn. Pacific Grove: Duxbury Press; 2000.

15. Quick Guide to Assess Risk of Bias in Randomized Controlled Trials

Alonso Carrasco-Labra, Kathleen G Dobson

Key Objectives

- Acquire a better understanding of the features of randomized controlled trials (RCTs)
- Learn what bias is and how it may influence the results of a RCT
- Learn what is involved in conducting a RCT and what are the main methodological strategies implemented to avoid bias
- Be able to distinguish between low and high-risk of bias randomized trials using the cochrane risk of bias tool.

Bias in Randomized Controlled Trials

RCTs are recognized as the most reliable source of evidence in determining the efficacy and effectiveness of healthcare interventions. In this study design, participants are randomly allocated to one or more experimental and comparison arms with the objective of obtaining groups that are comparable with respect to both known and unknown prognostic factors. This ensures that the only difference between the study groups is that one of them receives the intervention under study; therefore, any benefit or harm measured can be reliably attributed to the intervention.[1] Nevertheless, this distinctive advantage of RCTs in determining causal inferences can be weakened by limitations and flaws in the planning, designing, implementing, analyzing and reporting, which can distort the effect of the intervention leading to an under or overestimation of the true treatment effect.[2]

Table 15.1: Summary of type of bias in randomized controlled trials

Types of bias	Definition
Selection bias	Systematic differences between baseline characteristics of participants which assigned to the intervention and comparison groups
Performance bias	Systematic differences between groups introduced by clinicians/researchers in the care provided to participants. These differences can also be introduced by participants in exposing themselves to factors other than the interventions of interest
Detection bias	Systematic differences between groups in how data is collected and how outcomes are assessed or adjudicated
Attrition bias	Systematic differences between groups due to the presence of participant withdrawals from the study
Reporting bias	Systematic differences between reported data in a publication of a trial and the initially planned but unreported findings.

What is Bias in the Context of Randomized Controlled Trials?

Bias, also referred to as systematic error, can be defined as 'any departure of results from the truth.'[3] In other words, bias is any factor or flaw in the process of conducting a study that deviates the results away from what they actually are (Table 15.1). There are several types of bias applicable to RCTs:

Selection Bias

In RCTs, ***selection bias*** is the presence of any systematic difference between baseline characteristics of participants allocated to the experimental and control groups. Empirical evidence shows that when researchers and/or clinicians are aware ahead of time as to which group (either experimental or control) their next eligible patient will be allocated to, they consciously or unconsciously may assign the patients with best prognosis or higher response to treatment into the experimental group.[4] It is also likely that the same phenomenon would happen if patients knew what study arm they were allocated to.[5] As a way to avoid the effect of this systematic difference between groups, researchers use ***random allocation***. Instead of clinicians or patients deciding which intervention to administer, it is the participant's chance making this decision for them. Each participant has a known and equal chance to be assigned to the intervention or comparison arm, with the key feature that the allocation to either group cannot be predicted.[5]

Some methods used to generate this randomization scheme are tables of random numbers or random number generator from computer software. Other methods such as allocating participants depending on the day of the week they consulted or the last digit from a patient's phone number are sometimes used by researchers, assuming that these methods are as reliable as the ones mentioned above. It is possible that patients enrolled on a Saturday night may differ from those enrolled on a Monday morning in many prognostic factors, creating imbalance between the groups and increasing the risk of selection bias. These methods are also problematic because of the openness of the allocation procedure. If it is known which arm the next patient will be allocated, it may also influence recruitment decisions, introducing additional bias to the results.[6]

To guarantee that study participants are assigned to the study arms in an unbiased manner, researchers should not only allocate them in a random fashion but also have to conceal that allocation. In other words, all the work done with creating an appropriate randomization scheme can be undone if such scheme is inappropriately implemented. ***Allocation concealment*** shields the research team and patients from knowing to what arm the next patient will be assigned. Without this key methodological strategy, other criteria rather than chance may be applied in the assignment process, resulting in study groups under comparison that are imbalanced in prognostic factors.[7] Empirical evidence suggests that failing to achieve a concealed allocation can overestimate the treatment effect upto 41%, as compared to studies implementing appropriate concealment methods.[8] Appropriate methods to achieve allocation concealment include sequentially numbered identical containers, pharmacy controlled lists and central randomization using phone or online contact. Methods like the sequentially numbered, opaque, sealed envelopes are more vulnerable and questionable compared to the other methods mentioned above.[3]

Allocation concealment should not be confused with blinding. It is primarily focused on avoiding selection bias and preserving the randomization scheme until allocation occurs. After the participants are assigned to the study arms (i.e. 'randomized'), researchers implement blinding in order to maintain the ***prognostic balance*** of background characteristics, which may influence the risk of the study outcome achieved by the randomization. Whereas allocation concealment can always be implemented, there are some situations where blinding is unfeasible (e.g. some surgical trials). Further information on blinding is described below.

Performance Bias

If randomization succeeded on creating prognostic balance between the intervention and comparison arm, this balance should be maintained while the trial is conducted. ***Blinding*** is the methodological strategy that ensures the participants that they do not know which study arm they have been assigned and allows researchers to achieve this goal.[9] ***Performance bias*** occurs when systematic differences are introduced to the intervention or control group in the clinical care that they receive or other factors that these groups may be exposed to, aside from the intervention under study.[10]

When participants are not blinded, knowing the nature of the intervention they are receiving may affect their response to that intervention and their judgment. For example, participants aware of being allocated to the arm receiving a new promissory drug under testing may provide more favorable results influenced by expectations rather than a real effect of such drug. In contrast, participants aware of being allocated to the control arm may feel undertreated or deprived from receiving an effective treatment; therefore, this may introduce deviations to the study protocol including issues of compliance and adherence to the study.[11]

Clinicians taking part in a trial should also be blinded. Knowing that a particular patient in the study was assigned to the control arm or is suffering from the adverse effects of the new drug, under study may influence clinicians' judgments, driving them to alter the way of healthcare which was initially planned or they may look more carefully for beneficial and harm outcomes. In other words, clinicians should be blinded to prevent *co-interventions* or differential administration of therapies that may affect the outcome of interest.[9]

The use of *placebo* in drug trials is the most important strategy to achieve blinding for patients, clinicians and other members of the research team. A placebo is defined as any 'biologically inert substance (typically a pill or a capsule) that is as similar as possible to the active intervention.'[12]

Detection Bias

Even if allocation concealment was appropriately implemented, clinicians and most of the researchers were effectively blinded, prognostic balance can still be endangered if those who are adjudicating or assessing the outcome are not blinded to which group the patient they are evaluating. If outcome adjudicators are blinded, this will help to avoid differential assessment of outcomes or *detection bias*. For example, an outcome adjudicator who knows the treatment allocation and has strong beliefs that the new treatment is better than the comparison may be more inclined to report more generous responses favoring the intervention under study.[13] Having data collectors and outcome assessors blinded is particularly relevant when blinding is unfeasible (e.g. surgical or complex educational interventions). One specific type of placebo applicable to non-pharmacological interventions is called a *sham procedure*. This type of procedures mimics the actual intervention in every way possible during the pre, peri and postoperative period; however, the key component responsible for the effect, is missing.[14] Data analysts can also be blinded to avoid bias in decisions while conducting the statistical analysis.[15,9]

Many studies report that the 'investigators' were blinded. This rather vague terminology does not allow one to really judge who was blinded. In addition, the use of the terms

Table 15.2: Groups in a RCT, the importance of blinding to avoid bias

Patients or participants	To avoid the effects of beliefs and other preconceptions (placebo effect)
Clinicians and healthcare providers	To avoid differential care or treatment administration (co-interventions) that could bias the assessment of outcomes
Data collectors and outcome adjudicators	To avoid bias during the process of collecting data and deciding whether the outcome of interest occurred in a patient
Data analysts	To avoid bias in decisions while conducting the analysis of the trial data.

'single' or 'double-blinded' to report who was actually blinded in a study has been slowly abandoned in favor of more explicit descriptions of all individuals that were unaware of treatment allocation.[13,16] Ideally, patients, clinicians, data collector, outcome adjudicators and data analysts should be blinded (Table 15.2). On average, it has been shown that non-blinded studies tend to overestimate treatment effects by almost 7%.[2]

Attrition Bias

In an ideal trial, all patients initially recruited and randomized receive the experimental or control intervention and are followed up prospectively to give time to the treatment to work and assess efficacy and safety outcomes. This means that, by the end of the trial, researchers will know exactly the status of each patient included in the study in relation to the measured outcomes. Unfortunately, most of the time, this is not the case. ***Missing participant data*** refers to outcome data for trial participants whose status on the outcome of interest is unknown. The main concern with patients lost to follow-up in a trial is that, usually, they have a different prognosis from those who remain enrolled in the study. For example, a patient in the experimental group suffers from a serious or unpleasant adverse event related to the intervention under testing, as a result the patient discontinues the treatment and never returns to subsequent follow-up visits.[9] The opposite situation can also occur; the participant is doing well and notices significant improvement in disease symptoms, so the participant sees no need to remain enrolled in the study. ***Attrition bias*** corresponds to 'systematic differences between groups in withdrawals from a study'.[10] Empirical evidence has shown that one in three trials showing statistically significant results to lose their significance when the analysis was repeated using plausible assumptions about the patients who were lost to follow-up.[17]

Picture a situation where a patient in a RCT who was not lost to follow-up, in other words, researchers are completely aware of the patient's status and are able to determine whether the outcome has occurred or not. This participant does not want to receive the intervention under study and declares himself as non-adherent. Where should this patient who did not receive the intervention he was initially allocated to be analyzed? As we have seen, maintaining the prognostic balance achieved with randomization is crucial and in order to maintain it, investigators follow a particular strategy called ***intention-to-treat analysis (ITT)***. When conducting ITT analysis all participants should be analyzed in the group to which they were initially allocated by the randomization scheme, irrespective of what intervention they actually received (i.e. either experimental or control intervention).[9] This allows researchers to maintain the prognostic balance gained with the randomization.

Reporting Bias

Selective outcome reporting corresponds to the selection of a subset of the original outcomes planned and recorded, on the basis of the results, for their inclusion in a publication of a RCT.[10] In other words, it refers to systematic differences between the findings that were reported compared to those that were omitted by the researchers. Empirical evidence suggests that outcomes that reach statistical significance are 2–5 times more likely to be appropriately and comprehensively reported, compared to those without statistical significance.[18] Some examples of selective outcome reporting are:[10]

- Selection of outcomes to report, based on the relevance of results.

- Selection of a specific data point to report amongst multiple repeated measures that were recorded.
- Selection of a different analysis for a particular outcome that deviates from the protocol to gain relevance or statistical significance.
- Selective under-reporting of data using expressions as 'non-significant results (p>0.05)' with no additional numerical data such as effect estimates (e.g. relative risks, odd ratios) and measures of precision (e.g. standard deviations, confidence intervals) to support the statement.

Assessing Risk of Bias in RCTs

Although there is evidence addressing the impact of different biases on the outcomes of RCTs, the assessment of a definitive presence of bias at an individual study level is not feasible. Therefore, a reader can only judge whether the study is at risk of bias and whether the issue is serious enough to warrant questioning the validity of the study findings. Hence, the Cochrane Collaboration has suggested to assessing the ***risk of bias***, defined as the extent to which the results reported from an individual study are affected by bias and consequently, should be practiced in the appraisal RCTs.

The Cochrane Risk of Bias Tool

To facilitate the assessment of risk of bias of RCTs, the Cochrane Collaboration has created the ***Cochrane Risk of Bias Tool***[10], which is composed of six bias domains: selection bias, performance bias, detection bias, attrition bias, reporting bias and other bias. The tool assesses 7 potential sources of bias:
1. Random sequence generation
2. Allocation concealment
3. Blinding of participants and personnel
4. Blinding of outcome assessment
5. Incomplete outcome data
6. Selective reporting
7. Other sources of bias.

When determining the risk of bias for an RCT, each potential source of bias assessed in the tool is judged as being either at low-risk of bias, high-risk of bias or unclear risk of bias. The use of the latter category, although not really informative, represents that there was not sufficient information reported in the manuscript of the RCT under assessment to reliably claim that the risk of bias was low or high. To ensure consistency and transparency, users of the tool are required to provide rationale for their decisions (support for judgment). Table 15.3 shows an example of an assessment conducted using the Risk of Bias Tool in a Cochrane systematic review[19] for an included RCT.[20]

Table 15.3: Example of the application of the Cochrane Risk of Bias Tool for RCTs (Example from the Cochrane systematic review: Ker K, Roberts I, Shakur H, et al. Antifibrinolytic drugs for acute traumatic injury. Cochrane Database of Syst Rev. 2015;5:CD004896. Conducted for the CRASH-2 trial*)

Domain	Judgment	Support for judgment
Random sequence generation (selection bias)	Low-risk	'Randomization was balanced by centre, with an allocation sequence based on a block size of eight, generated with a computer random number generator.' (p. 24)
Allocation concealment (selection bias)	Low-risk	'In hospitals in which telephone randomization was not practicable we used a local pack system that selected the lowest numbered treatment pack from a box containing eight numbered packs. Apart from the pack number, the treatment packs were identical. Hospitals with reliable telephone access used the University of Oxford Clinical Trial Service Unit (CTSU) telephone randomization service.' (p. 24)
Blinding of participants and personnel (performance bias)	Low-risk	'Both participants and study staff (site investigators and trial coordinating centre staff) were masked to treatment allocation.' (p. 24)

contd...

contd...

Domain	Judgment	Support for judgment
Blinding of outcome assessment (detection bias)	Low-risk	'Both participants and study staff (site investigators and trial coordinating center staff) were masked to treatment allocation.' (p. 24)
Incomplete outcome data (attrition bias)	Low-risk	'All analysis were undertaken on an intention-to-treat basis.' (p. 25) The data from four patients were removed from the trial because their consent was withdrawn after randomization.' (p. 25) The review authors judge that the proportion of missing outcomes compared with event risk is not enough to have a clinically relevant impact on the effect estimate.
Selective reporting (reporting bias)	Low-risk	Trial prospectively registered (ISRCTN86750102, NCT00375258, DOH-27-0607-1919 [p. 25]). Data on all prespecified outcomes presented in final report.

* Roberts I, Shakur H, Coats T, et al. The CRASH-2 trial: A randomized controlled trial and economic evaluation of the effects of tranexamic acid on death, vascular occlusive events and transfusion requirement in bleeding trauma patients. Health Technol Assess. 2013;17(10):1-79.

Important Learning Points

- The success of randomization depends on two factors: (1) generation of a random sequence to assign participants to the study arms and (2) allocation of participants in a concealed manner.
- Blinding of patients and researchers along with explicit descriptions of who was blinded in the study is crucial to avoid performance and detection bias.
- The larger the number of participants lost to follow-up, the more susceptible the study is to attrition bias.
- Selective outcome reporting occurs when decisions to report measured the outcomes are based on the results.

- The Cochrane Risk of Bias tool proposes a framework to assess the extent to which bias may have affected the results of a randomized controlled trial.

Definitions

Allocation concealment: Methodological strategy to make sure that the person who is enrolling participants in a randomized trial is unaware of to what study arm the next participant will be assigned to.

Attrition bias: Systematic differences between the groups under study due to participants' withdrawals.

Bias: Systematic deviation from the underlying truth because of a feature of the design or conduct of a research study.

Blinding: Condition of patients, clinicians and researchers participating in a study of being unaware of which participant were allocated to the intervention and control arm.

Co-interventions: Interventions other than the one under study that may affect the outcome of interest and when differentially applied, may introduce bias.

Detection bias: Intention to look more carefully for an outcome in one of the intervention groups.

Intention-to-treat analysis: Includes all randomized patients in the groups to which they were randomly assigned, regardless of their adherence with the entry criteria, regardless of the treatment they actually received and regardless of subsequent withdrawal from treatment or deviation from the protocol.

Missing participant data: Outcome data for trial participants whose status on the outcome of interest is unknown.

Performance bias: Systematic differences are introduced to the intervention or control group in the clinical care that they receive or other factors that these groups may be exposed to, aside from the intervention under study.

Placebo: Biologically inert substance that is as similar as possible to the active intervention. Placebo allows implementing blinding.

Prognostic balance: Balance achieved by randomizing participants to the study arms in relation to their biological, psychological and social characteristics, which confer increased or decreased risk of a favorable or unfavorable outcome. In addition, other unknown characteristics that may influence the outcome are also balanced by randomization.

Random allocation: Allocation of participants to groups under comparison by random chance.

Risk of bias: The potential of a study to have been adversely impacted by unintended or non-ideal circumstances.

Selection bias: Presence of any systematic difference between the baseline characteristics of participants allocated to the groups under study in a randomized controlled trial.

Selective outcome reporting: Inclination of authors to differentially report research results depending on their relevance rather than what it was actually measured.

REFERENCES

1. Higgins P, Altman DG, Gøtzsche PC, et al. The Cochrane Collaboration's tool for assessing risk of bias in randomized trials. BMJ. 2011;343:d5928.
2. Wood L, Egger M, Gluud LL, et al. Empirical evidence of bias in treatment effect estimates in controlled trials with different interventions and outcomes: meta-epidemiological study. BMJ. 2008;336(7644):601-5.
3. Lewis SC, Warlow CP. How to spot bias and other potential problems in randomized controlled trials. J Neurol Neurosurg Psychiatry. 2004;75(2):181-7.
4. Sackett DL. The tactics of performing therapeutic trials. In: Haynes RB, Sackett DL, Guyatt GH, Tugwell P, (eds). Clinical epidemiology: How to do clinical practice Research. 3rd edn. Philadelphia: Lippincott Williams & Wilkins; 2006. p. 66-172.
5. Altman DG, Bland JM. Statistics notes. Treatment allocation in controlled trials: why randomize? BMJ. 1999;318(7192):1209.
6. Altman DG. Randomization. BMJ. 1991;302(6791):1481-2.
7. Schulz KF. Assessing allocation concealment and blinding in randomized controlled trials: why bother? Evid Based Nurs. 2001;4(1):4-6.
8. Schulz KF, Chalmers I, Hayes RJ, et al. Empirical evidence of bias. Dimensions of methodological quality associated with estimates of treatment effects in controlled trials. JAMA. 1995;273(5):408-12.
9. Walsh M, Perkovic V, Manns B, Srinathan S, Meade MO, Devereaux PJ, et al. Therapy (Randomized Trials). In: Guyatt GH, Rennie D, Meade MO, Cook DJ, editors. Users' Guides to the Medical Literature: A Manual for Evidence-Based Clinical Practice. 3rd ed: McGraw Hill Education; 2015. p. 59-73.

10. Higgins JPT, Altman DG, Sterne JAC. Chapter 8: Assessing risk of bias in included studies. In: Higgins JPT, Green S, editors. Cochrane Handbook for Systematic Reviews of Interventions Version 510 (updated March 2011): The Cochrane Collaboration, 2011. Available from www.cochrane-handbook.org.; 2011.
11. Schulz KF, Chalmers I, Altman DG. The landscape and lexicon of blinding in randomized trials. Ann Intern Med. 2002;136(3):254-9.
12. Guyatt G, Meade MO, Rennie D, et al. Users' guide to the medical literature: A manual for evidence based clinical practice. 3rd edn. United States: McGraw Hill; 2015.
13. Schulz KF, Grimes DA. Blinding in randomized trials: hiding who got what. Lancet. 2002;359(9307):696-700.
14. Miller FG, Wendler D. The ethics of sham invasive intervention trials. Clin Trials. 2009;6(5):401-2.
15. Gøtzsche PC. Blinding during data analysis and writing of manuscripts. Control Clin Trials. 1996;17(4):285-90; 290-3.
16. Devereaux PJ, Manns BJ, Ghali WA, et al. Physician interpretations and textbook definitions of blinding terminology in randomized controlled trials. JAMA. 2001;285(15):2000-3.
17. Akl EA, Briel M, You JJ, et al. Potential impact on estimated treatment effects of information lost to follow-up in randomized controlled trials (LOST-IT): systematic review. BMJ. 2012;344:e2809.
18. Dwan K, Altman DG, Arnaiz JA, et al. Systematic review of the empirical evidence of study publication bias and outcome reporting bias. PLoS One. 2008;3(8):e3081.
19. Ker K, Roberts I, Shakur H, et al. Antifibrinolytic drugs for acute traumatic injury. Cochrane Database of Syst Rev. 2015;5:CD004896.
20. Roberts I, Shakur H, Coats T, et al. The CRASH-2 trial: A randomized controlled trial and economic evaluation of the effects of tranexamic acid on death, vascular occlusive events and transfusion requirement in bleeding trauma patients. Health Technol Assess. 2013;17(10):1-79.

16 GRADE—Understanding Grades of Healthcare Recommendations

Mark Phillips, S Rajasekaran

Key Objectives

- Gain a better understanding of the grading of recommendations assessment, development and evaluation (GRADE) approach
- Understand the importance of quality of evidence in recommendations with respect to study design, risk of bias, imprecision, inconsistency, indirectness and magnitude of effect
- Be able to understand and utilize the GRADE approach when developing clinical recommendations
- Be able to critically appraise clinical recommendations using the GRADE framework and determine the strength of the recommendation provided.

Overview of the GRADE Approach

The GRADE approach is a tool that is used to create and assess *clinical recommendations* in systematic reviews, clinical practice guidelines or health technology assessments. The GRADE approach rates both the quality of evidence, as well as the strength of the recommendations provided, through a structured and transparent methodology.[1]

The GRADE process begins with the development of a research question specific to the topic of interest, which is followed by the selection of all relevant outcomes to the research question. The quality of evidence is assessed for each individual outcome and categorized as either very low, low, moderate or high. GRADE assesses a number of factors that influence the quality of evidence in recommendations, including: *study design*, *risk of bias*,

imprecision**, **inconsistency**, **indirectness and ***magnitude of effect***.[1] Throughout this chapter we will outline how to utilize the GRADE approach to critically assess clinical recommendations, as well as how to use GRADE when developing clinical recommendations.

Research Questions and Determining Important Outcomes

The use of the GRADE approach to develop clinical recommendations begins with clearly defining an explicit research question. The most common tool for developing a strong research question is using the ***PICO*** method. PICO refers to patient/population, intervention, comparator and outcome. By determining and identifying each of the elements of PICO, the purpose and research question for the investigation can be clearly defined. It is important to consider how specific to define both the population and intervention, as being too narrow will limit the amount of evidence on the topic, but being too broad will include evidence that may not be easily comparable. This consideration should be carefully assessed when formulating a research question using the PICO method.[2]

The next step in GRADE is to determine all important outcomes to the research question of interest. These outcomes include efficacy measures, adverse events and safety measures, socioeconomic impacts (e.g. costs of treatments or burden on caregivers) and public health impacts (e.g. antibiotic resistance as a result of the treatment). It is important to not ignore an outcome due to a lack of reporting within the current evidence, but instead identify and describe the paucity of evidence on that particular outcome given in the literature available on the topic. After a complete list of outcomes has been identified, each outcome should be classified as critical, important but not critical or low importance.[2] These classifications will be useful later, when evidence is being evaluated and recommendations are being formulated.[2]

Rating Quality of Evidence Overview

Whether conducting a quality assessment within a systematic review or developing clinical recommendations, it is important to rate the quality of evidence associated with the identified outcomes.[1] GRADE quality assessment represents two different concepts depending on the context of its use. GRADE quality assessment within a systematic review represents the confidence behind outcome effect estimates, while GRADE quality assessments within clinical recommendation development represents the confidence in the outcome effect estimates to justify the corresponding recommendations made.[3]

The GRADE approach defines four levels of quality—high, moderate, low or very low. High level evidence provides the reviewer with confidence that 'the true effect lies close to that of the estimate of effect.'[3] Moderate level evidence indicates moderate confidence in the effect estimate, of which 'the true effect is likely to be close to the estimate of the effect, but there is a possibility that it is substantially different.'[3] Low level evidence is defined as evidence in which 'confidence in the effect estimate is limited—the true effect may be substantially different from the estimate of effect.'[3] Very low quality of evidence provides 'very little confidence in the effect estimate—the true effect is likely to be substantially different from the estimate of effect.'[3] A common misperception regarding quality of evidence is that it is directly indicative of the corresponding recommendations strength; however, this is not true. A weak recommendation may be based off of high quality evidence and conversely a strong recommendation may be based off of low quality evidence.[3]

Quality of evidence is rated initially by study design, with the highest quality rating given to randomized controlled trials (RCTs) and observational studies being low quality evidence. From this initial assessment based on the hierarchy of evidence, five criteria may possibly decrease the initial quality rating and three criteria may potentially increase the initial quality rating.[3] These eight criteria are fundamental in appropriately using the GRADE approach to rate the quality of evidence; therefore, they will be explained in detail in the subsequent sections.

Rating Study Limitations (Risk of Bias)

Whether a study is of high quality (RCT) or low quality (observational study), the quality of evidence can be downgraded due to potential risk of bias. Risk of bias should be determined for each individual outcome of interest. Risk of bias can be rated as:

- No serious limitations; in which case, the GRADE quality score does not change.
- The serious limitations; in which the quality is decreased by one level (e.g. a high quality study with serious limitations would be decreased to a moderate quality rating).
- Very serious limitations; in which the quality is decreased by two levels (e.g. a high quality study with very serious limitations would be decreased to a low quality rating).[4]

For the rating of risk of bias within RCTs, there are a number of potential study limitations, including: inappropriate sequence generation, inadequate allocation concealment, a lack of blinding, an incomplete account of all patients and outcome events (e.g. high loss to follow-up), selective reporting of outcomes, early study termination causing beneficial results, using non-validated outcome measures, carry-over effects within a crossover trial and recruitment bias within cluster-randomized trials. Each of these potential limitations should be considered and assessed for randomized trials. Potential limitations that should be assessed in observational studies to determine the overall risk of bias, include inappropriate eligibility criteria, flawed methodology in the measurement of the exposure and/or the outcome, a failure to address confounding variables such as prognostic factors and the reporting of incomplete follow-up data. The risk of bias assessments should be reported for all important outcomes and summarized within a table.[4]

Rating Publication Bias

Similar to study limitations, the quality of included studies can be rated down based on potential publication bias. Publication bias typically arises in bodies of evidence that include a large number of small studies, of which many are industry funded. It has been shown that studies without statistically significant results are less likely to be published. Consequently, systematic reviews performed on a small number of preliminary investigations may overestimate treatment effects and thus, should suspect publication bias.

Additionally, it has been suggested that industry sponsors may withhold negative results, so any body of evidence largely composed of commercially funded research suggests the suspicion of publication bias as well. The use of funnel plots to examine results patterns may aid in the discovery of publication bias, but should not be solely relied upon in the assessment of publication bias. The use of funnel plots should be used in addition to the aforementioned criteria of a body of evidence that contains many small or preliminary studies and a large volume of industry funded studies.[5]

Rating Imprecision

For dichotomous outcomes, there are two considerations that evidence may be rated down for imprecision. The first is if the total sample size is lower than the calculated *optimal information size* (OIS) and/or the total sample size is less than 400 (a threshold rule-of-thumb value).[6] The second is if the 95% confidence interval (CI) includes no effect and appreciable benefit/appreciable harm. GRADE suggests that the threshold for appreciable benefit or appreciable harm should be a relative risk reduction/relative risk increase of greater than 25%.[6] An exception for rating down due to imprecision is if event rates are very low, the 95% CI around the relative effect is very wide, but the CI around absolute effects is narrow. This situation does not call for a rating down of the quality of evidence.[6]

For continuous outcomes, the quality of evidence can be rated down for two reasons: (1) if the total sample size is less than the calculated OIS and/or the total sample size is less than 400 (a threshold rule-of-thumb value) and (2) the 95% CI includes no effect and the upper or lower confidence limit crosses the benefit or harm minimal important difference (MID).[6] If the MID is unknown or it was calculated using different outcome measures than the one in question, an effect size of 0.5 should be used to potentially downgrade the level of evidence.[6]

Rating down the quality of evidence due to imprecision is highly dependent on the difference in effect that the study aims to detect and the resulting OIS. The GRADE approach does not ensure agreement between all users of the recommendation; however, it does provide explicit criteria for the judgments being made regarding these values.[6]

Rating Inconsistency

Inconsistency refers to the variability of results within the body of evidence for the outcome of interest. Criteria for assessing inconsistency include similarity of point estimates, extent of overlap of CI, statistical test for heterogeneity and the I^2 statistic.[7] Rating down the quality of evidence for inconsistency should be considered when point estimates vary widely across studies, CI demonstrate little or no overlap, the statistical test for heterogeneity results in a low p-value and the I^2 statistic—a measure of the proportion of variation in estimates of effect due to differences within studies—is large. If inconsistency across these criteria is evident and unexplainable (e.g. cannot be explained by subgroup differences seen within the studies), the quality of evidence should be rated down by one level. Similar to the previously outlined criteria, it is not possible to rate up the quality of evidence for consistency; it is only possible to rate down if inconsistency is present.[7]

Rating Indirectness

Indirectness may be identified when a systematic review or clinical practice guideline's evidence includes studies with differences across their patient populations, interventions used or outcomes measured when compared to relevant studies on the topic. Patient differences may arise if a study has included a patient population that differs from the most relevant population outlined in the PICO statement derived at the beginning of the GRADE process.[8] Additionally, if the intervention or outcomes measured within a study differ from those determined in the PICO statement indirectness should be considered, as the results of this study may not be appropriately applicable to the specific research questions at hand. If the patient-important outcome that had been defined is replaced by a *surrogate outcome,* this suggests the presence of indirectness. A surrogate outcome may seem to correlate to the patient-important outcome of interest;

however, it is not appropriate to use this information in the interpretation of the outcome of interest. For example, the patient-important outcome for a study on osteoporosis is the number of fractures within the population, but an included study has instead provided measures of bone density, which is considered a surrogate outcome. Although bone density may potentially correspond to risk of fracture, this data should not be included in the assessment of evidence regarding the incidence of fracture occurrence.[8]

Finally, indirectness may be present and warrant a decrease in the quality of evidence rating if the interventions included have not been tested within head-to-head comparisons. A systematic review or clinical practice guideline may make comparisons between two treatment modalities that have never been compared head-to-head, but a comparison will still be made based on results of both modalities relative results versus placebo. This type of comparison should be considered too indirect to make inferences from and thus the quality of evidence for the clinical recommendation should be rated down by one level.[8]

Factors to Increase the Quality of Evidence Rating

The previously outlined factors are all potential ways in which the initial quality of evidence (determined from the study design) can be rated down to a lower quality of evidence. However, there are factors that should be considered that may potentially increase the quality of evidence rating for a given outcome. There are three ways in which the rating of quality of evidence may be rated up:
1. The presence of a large magnitude of effect
2. The presence of a ***dose-response gradient***
3. When all of the possible confounders or biases have been analyzed to report their correlation to the estimated effects.[9]

These factors are typically designed for rating up observational and nonrandomized studies. It may be appropriate to rate up the quality of evidence score of observational studies by one level if the magnitude of effect is large, while the score may be rated up two levels if the magnitude of effect is very large in a short period of time. If a dose-response gradient is demonstrated, the quality of evidence rating may also be rated up by one level. Finally, if an observational study provides in-depth analyses of prognostic factors and their effects on outcomes, the quality of evidence rating can be increased by one level.[9]

Resource Use and Rating Economic Evidence

The GRADE approach recommends, when providing a summary of findings, resource use associated with the intervention (e.g. days in hospital or clinician time), as well as economic evidence (e.g. cost data) be included for consideration by decision makers when developing recommendations.[10] This can be done by identifying differences in resource use and costs between alternate treatment modalities and comparing this information across all treatment options. The quality of evidence regarding resource use and cost should be appraised using the same criteria and process that has been discussed in previous sections to assess health outcomes.[10]

Making an Overall Rating of Confidence in Effect Estimates

Now that the quality of evidence for each important outcome has been assessed, a rating must be derived to represent the overall confidence in the estimates of effect provided by the evidence. Using the criteria that are used to rate down/up the quality of evidence, systematic review authors and guideline developers must create a single rating from these criteria for each individual outcome.[11]

Each rating for individual outcomes can now be combined to create an overall rating of the quality of evidence for the intervention in question. The guideline development group should create an overall rating of the evidence based on the ratings of individual outcomes that they feel are the most critical outcomes to their recommendation. The reasoning behind the decisions should be as transparent as possible so that all the judgments made are easily understood and clearly explained to the users of the clinical recommendation.[11]

Summary of Findings of Tables

A Summary of Findings (SoF) table should be constructed to present the quality of evidence ratings and the estimates of effect for each outcome. This table should include a measure of the burden or estimated risk of the corresponding outcome, a measure of the difference in risk between the intervention and control group, the relative magnitude of effect of the intervention, the number of patients and studies, the quality of evidence rating (including any explanations for why the quality of evidence has been rated down or rated up) and any additional comments for all of the included outcomes.[12] This table should not only include important health-related outcomes, but any resource use or cost related outcomes that have been assessed as well. Once the summary of findings table has been created, the guideline developers may now work to create a recommendation for or against the intervention in question.[13]

Formulating Recommendations from the Evidence

The group must consider what all (or at least most) informed clinicians would decide in light of the information provided in the SoF table. The recommendation can be categorized as either *strong* or *weak;* creating a scale of recommendations that range from *strong against, to weakly against,* to *weak for,* to *strong for* the use of the intervention in question.[14] If the benefits of the intervention drastically outweigh the drawbacks, the guideline developers should decide to make a strong recommendation for the use of the intervention. However, if the benefits are not obviously superior to the drawbacks or the drawbacks are potentially too significant to warrant the benefits, a weak recommendation for/against the intervention may be suggested accordingly. If the drawbacks of an intervention clearly outweigh the benefits, a strong recommendation against the intervention should be made.[14,15]

The development of the recommendation must carefully consider all available information, including the estimates of effect, the quality of evidence (confidence in the effect estimates), resource use and considerations of patient values and preferences. Decisions made and reasons behind recommendation decisions should be clearly and transparently reported in order to provide a detailed account of how and why the recommendation development group came to their recommendation decision.[15]

Important Learning Points

To recap the GRADE process:
- The GRADE approach should be used to critically assess or create clinical recommendations
- Formulate the research question, define a PICO statement and select all important outcomes
- Rate the evidence for each outcome from 'high', to 'moderate' to 'low' to 'very low'
- Evidence is initially rated based on study design using the hierarchy of evidence but this rating can rated down based on risk of bias, imprecision, inconsistency and indirectness or rated up based on magnitude of effect, the presence of a dose-response gradient or an in depth analysis of prognostic factors and confounders
- For each important outcome, provide a pooled estimate of effect and the quality rating of evidence behind that estimate of effect in a SoF table
- Guideline developers should consider which outcomes are crucial for their recommendation and weight the information regarding these outcomes heavily into their recommendation decision in terms of perceived benefits and drawbacks
- All reasoning placed behind the recommendation decision should be clearly and transparently reported.

Definitions

Clinical recommendations: Recommendations created by a development group that provide insight into the appropriateness and validity of any given intervention or treatment modality.

Dose-response gradient: The demonstration of an incremental increase in response to a given treatment modality as a result of incrementally increasing the dose.

Imprecision: Imprecision refers to the statistical assessment (typically CI) surrounding the measure of effect. If CI or other provided measures of variance are very large, the results may suffer from imprecision.

Inconsistency: Inconsistency refers to the heterogeneity of the estimated outcome effects from multiple studies. If results from multiple studies are variable even though they had the same research question, this may represent inconsistency.

Indirectness: Indirectness refers to the consistency across included study research questions/ PICO statements. Studies included in the same body of evidence should all address the same research question through a similar PICO statement (e.g. Studies should all include the same patient population, intervention, comparator/control and outcomes) and if there is variability between studies, indirectness should be considered.

Magnitude of effect: The extent of impact that the intervention has on the population.

Optimal Information Size: The number of patients required to develop an adequately powered randomized controlled trials.

PICO: Refers to patient/population, intervention, comparator and outcome. It is a tool used to identify the research question of a project.

Risk of bias: The potential of a study to have been adversely impacted by unintended or non-ideal circumstances.

Study design: The methodology behind a clinical study, which can be defined based on the characteristics of the study (randomization, control groups included, etc.)

Surrogate outcomes: An outcome that is closely related that is used to make inferences about the outcome in question.

References

1. Guyatt G, Oxman AD, Akl EA, et al. GRADE guidelines: 1. Introduction-GRADE evidence profiles and summary of findings tables. J Clin Epidemiol, 2011;64(4):383-94.
2. Guyatt GH, Oxman AD, Kunz R, et al. GRADE guidelines: 2. Framing the question and deciding on important outcomes. J Clin Epidemiol. 2011;64(4):395-400.
3. Balshem H, Helfand M, Schünemann HJ, et al. GRADE guidelines: 3. Rating the quality of evidence. J Clin Epidemiol. 2011;64(4):401-6.

4. Guyatt GH, Oxman AD, Vist G, et al. GRADE guidelines: 4. Rating the quality of evidence—study limitations (risk of bias). J Clin Epidemiol. 2011;64(4):407-15.
5. Guyatt GH, Oxman AD, Montori V, et al. GRADE guidelines: 5. Rating the quality of evidence–publication bias. J Clin Epidemiol. 2011;64(12):1277-82.
6. Guyatt GH, Oxman AD, Kunz R, et al. GRADE guidelines 6. Rating the quality of evidence—imprecision. J Clin Epidemiol. 2011. 64(12):1283-93.
7. Guyatt GH, Oxman AD, Kunz R, et al. GRADE guidelines: 7. Rating the quality of evidence—inconsistency. J Clin Epidemiol. 2011;64(12):1294-302.
8. Guyatt GH, Oxman AD, Kunz R, et al. GRADE guidelines: 8. Rating the quality of evidence—indirectness. J Clin Epidemiol. 2011;64(12):1303-10.
9. Guyatt GH, Oxman AD, Sultan S, et al. GRADE guidelines: 9. Rating up the quality of evidence. J Clin Epidemiol. 2011;64(12):1311-6.
10. Brunetti M, Shemilt I, Pregno S, et al. GRADE guidelines: 10. Considering resource use and rating the quality of economic evidence. J Clin Epidemiol. 2013;66(2):140-50.
11. Guyatt G, Oxman AD, Sultan S, et al. GRADE guidelines: 11. Making an overall rating of confidence in effect estimates for a single outcome and for all outcomes. J Clin Epidemiol. 2013;66(2):151-7.
12. Guyatt GH, Oxman AD, Santesso N, et al. GRADE guidelines: 12. Preparing summary of findings tables-binary outcomes. J Clin Epidemiol. 2013;66(2):158-72.
13. Guyatt GH, Thorlund K, Oxman AD, et al. GRADE guidelines: 13. Preparing summary of findings tables and evidence profiles-continuous outcomes. J Clin Epidemiol. 2013;66(2):173-83.
14. Andrews J, Guyatt G, Oxman AD, et al. GRADE guidelines: 14. Going from evidence to recommendations: the significance and presentation of recommendations. J Clin Epidemiol. 2013;66(7):719-25.
15. Andrews JC, Schünemann HJ, Oxman AD, et al. GRADE guidelines: 15. Going from evidence to recommendation-determinants of a recommendation's direction and strength. J Clin Epidemiol. 2013;66(7):726-35.

4. The Research Protocol

Section Outline

17. First Things First—The Research Proposal
18. Choosing the Outcome—A Primer
19. Common Quality of Life and Health Utility Outcome Tools
20. An Introduction to Sample Size
21. Estimating an Appropriate Sample Size—Advanced Concepts, Formulae and Examples
22. Planning Your Analysis—Keep it Simple
23. What are Subgroup Analyses and How Should You Interpret Them?

17

First Things First— The Research Proposal

Andrew Duong, Chuan Silvia Li

Key Objectives
- Understand the importance of a clinical research proposal
- Learn the basics of how to write a clinical research proposal
- Identify the sources of guidance and support.

What is a Clinical Research Proposal?

A research proposal is a formal document describing what is being studied and how the study will be conducted. Research proposals are written to submit to a ***funding agency*** to apply for funding for the study. From a research proposal, you can develop a formal study protocol to submit for ***ethics approval*** and to provide guidance to investigators on how to conduct study procedures. Ultimately, a research proposal should highlight the research question and its relevance to clinical practice.[1]

Why is this so Important?

A well-written research proposal is critical at the beginning of your study. Funding agencies will rely on the research proposal when deciding whether or not to award funding to a researcher for his or her study.[1-4] Also, ethics approval is required prior to beginning of any study. Without ethics approval you will not be able to start your study and to obtain ethics approval you need to have a proposal or a protocol.

Where do I Begin?

It is a good idea to begin your proposal by writing down your research question. Your research question is a brief summary of your population, intervention (if applicable), comparator and outcomes. Writing down the research question helps you to specify exactly what you want to study. An example of a research question is: 'Among patients of age 60 years and older, does total hip arthroplasty compared to hemiarthroplasty reduce revision surgery rates at two years post-surgery?'[5]

The population is 'patients of age 60 years and older'. The intervention is 'total hip arthroplasty'. The comparator is 'hemiarthroplasty'. The outcome is 'revision surgery rates at 2 years post-surgery'.

What Else do I Need to Know Before I Start Writing my Research Proposal?

The following is a list of questions that investigators should ask themselves:[1-3]
- Is the problem relevant?
- Is the study feasible?
- Is the question novel or has someone already answered the question?
- How much time do I need?
- How will I obtain the number of participants required for my study?
- Do I have adequate research staff available?
- How much will it cost?
- Can I implement the protocol in an ethical manner?

What Information do I need to Include in My Research Proposal?

The following outlines the typical sections you should include in your research proposal. Keep in mind that different funding agencies and ethics committees may want different sections, so make sure that you check with the organization that you are submitting your proposal or protocol to. It is common for funding agencies to require curriculum vitae (CVs) from investigators, letters of support from colleagues and institutional signatures.

Title

Your title should be concise and at the same time clearly state what your study is all about. You can be creative in order to draw the attention of your reader, but be careful because a grant application or manuscript can be rejected if the title is misleading.[2] Make it brief, clear and impactful.

Summary

The summary is the first thing a reader sees, so make sure you successfully and succinctly highlight the goals, design and rationale of your study.[2,3,4]

Introduction

The introduction should be relatively brief. This is where you introduce the subject matter and **study rationale**. The goal is to provide a brief overview of the topic, establish a framework for the research, explain why the topic is important and capture the attention of your readers.[1,4,6] It also puts the proposal in context. It is a good idea to start with a broad description of the problem and then move toward specifics.

Literature Review

Conducting a literature review will help you in many ways. You will be able to see what has already been done and discover ideas that may be applicable to your own study. You will also gain a deep understanding of the subject and gather the necessary information to support your argument. Exploration of other researchers' work can also identify additional study aims and potential issues that can be included to strengthen your own proposal. The best sources of relevant information are journal articles and conference proceedings. You can search online databases, such as Medline, to facilitate this process.[1,4,6] It is important that you are able to provide an integrated overview of your field of study. This means that you show awareness of the most important and relevant theories, models, studies and methodologies.

Importance of the Study

Describe the importance of the problem. Indicate how your research will refine, revise or extend existing knowledge in the area under investigation. How will it benefit the concerned stakeholders? State the larger implications and impact of your study.

Objectives

Clearly state the objectives of your study. You should choose a ***primary objective*** that will be used to answer your research question and you can have several related ***secondary objectives***.

Study Design

There are many research designs you can choose from including a randomized controlled trial, prospective cohort study, case-control study, case series and many other designs as outlined in Sections II and III of this book. Ensure that you are using the best design for your research question and justify why you are using that design.

Identify the Population

You must outline the ***eligibility criteria*** of your study population and explain how you are going to obtain your sample. An estimate of the number of participants that you will require and the ***sampling*** method that you choose to use should be included in your proposal as well.[1,4] It will be important to justify the need of your study population for your research and that you have attempted to minimize risks to participants, especially in vulnerable populations.

Describe the Setting

It is helpful to describe the environment in which your study will take place. Describing the setting will also allow other researchers to potentially replicate your study in the future or to decide if the results of your study can be applied to their patients.[1,2]

Outcomes

Clearly identify all outcomes that you are interested in, as well as exactly how and when these outcomes will be measured. Identify the type of information that you are interested in and how you will capture this data. For example, if your outcome of interest is quality of life, you can select from a multitude of questionnaires that measure quality of life such as the Short

Form-36 (SF-36). Make sure that your outcome makes sense in relation to your objective and that you are measuring the outcome in a valid and reliable manner.

Data Collection Plan

It is important to establish the procedures for data collection in order to prevent potential mistakes, inconsistencies and incomplete or missing data from occurring. A detailed data collection plan includes which information is collected at which time points and how it will be collected (e.g. patient questionnaires, imaging, laboratory tests, etc.). A clear plan minimizes the possibility of confusion, delays and errors. You should take the time to explain the plan to study participants and research personnel so that everyone involved is on the same page before participating.[1,2,4]

Data Analysis

The data that you collected needs to be analyzed and summarized in a way that answers your research questions. The description should include the plans for processing the data and the choice of the statistical method applied for each objective.[1,2,4] Fully describe your ***dependent variable(s)*** and ***independent variable(s)*** for the primary analysis and for any secondary analysis that you plan to conduct. You may also need a statistician's help for this part.

Study Limitations

A brief paragraph on the potential problems that your study may encounter is recommended. Try to think like a reviewer and ask yourself questions that he or she might ask you.[4] Highlighting potential challenges with a plan to address them strengthens your research proposal.

Budget and Timeline

In some cases, a budget and projected timeline may be required outlining the anticipated costs for running the study and how long will it take to complete your study. Expenses will include research personnel, supplies, equipments, travel expenses, participant compensation (if applicable) and administrative costs.[2,4]

Ethical Considerations

You should state your plan to minimize patient harm and maximize their benefit. For example, if you are testing a new drug, what are the possible side effects and how will you deal with them? How will you ensure confidentiality of study documents? You may also need to outline your plan for an independent data monitoring committee (DMC) or data and safety monitoring board (DSMB) to review your data periodically and to protect your study participants.

Knowledge Translation Plan

How do you propose to share the findings of your study with professional peers, practitioners, participants and the funding agency?

References

Make sure that you cite all publications used in your research proposal.[2]

What Else should I Keep in Mind?

- Writing research proposals takes longer than you think, so start early.[3,4,7]
- Include tables, figure and diagrams throughout your proposal if you feel they will enhance the document and make things more clear and concise.[4,6]
- Resist the temptation to put too many objectives or over-ambitious objectives that cannot be adequately achieved by the implementation of the protocol.
- Follow the guidelines. Different institutions/granting agencies have different instructions and requirements for research proposals.[2,3,4]
- Sell yourself. Show the reader that you are capable of carrying out the study and have access to the required resources.
- Help from your colleagues to write letters of support or act as collaborators can be very useful.[4]

- Read your research proposal over and over again to ensure that nothing is missing and it is scientifically sound. It may also be helpful to have some of your colleagues to proofread it for grammar and scientific merit once it is completed.[2,3,4,6]
- If your research proposal is rejected for the first time, make the necessary changes and submit it again. One of the best ways to learn is through trial and error.[4,7]

Who can I Go to for Help?

There are a number of individuals who can assist you in the preparation of a research proposal:
- In the literature review process, librarians can be very helpful in the database search.[5]
- You should talk to experts in the field to gain valuable knowledge and seek guidance in planning your study procedures.[3,6]
- Consider finding a mentor who has many years of research experience, especially in writing research proposals.[7]
- Contact the institutions whom you are submitting your proposal to, if you have any questions regarding their application process and requirements.[3,4]
- Statisticians can help with technical details of sample size and data analysis. It is a good idea to have a statistician as a co-investigator.

Important Learning Points

- A well-written research proposal is required before the start of any study. It is a document that allows a researcher to receive funding and approval to conduct his or her study.
- An investigator needs to consider numerous things before preparing a research proposal, such as time, costs, adequate research staff, the required number of participants and most importantly, whether or not the research question is clinically significant.
- There are many items that need to be addressed in a research proposal. Ensure that all relevant information is provided and explained in a clear and presentable manner.
- A research proposal should be read and revised numerous times before submitting.

- There are many resources available that offer guidance and support to anyone who is preparing a clinical research proposal.

Definitions

Dependent variable: The event being studied which is expected to change with changes in the independent variable.

Eligibility criteria: The characteristics that will include or exclude potential participants.

Ethics approval: Any study involving living participants requires the approval of an ethics committee.

Funding agency: Organizations that provide funding for research studies. An application must be completed, which is then reviewed by a committee that decides whether or not to award a researcher a grant.

Independent variable: The variable that is being manipulated that is expected to cause changes in the dependent variable.

Population of interest: The specific group of people that the researcher is interested in making inferences about from the study.

Primary outcome: The observation that is most clinically relevant in determining the effect of the intervention on key variables in the study; the outcome of greatest importance.

Sampling: The method employed by the researcher for selecting individuals for the study sample.

Secondary outcome: An outcome believed to be related to the primary outcome and is used in addition to the primary outcome.

Study rationale: A detailed explanation of the reasons why research on given topic is necessary.

REFERENCES

1. Saunderlin G. Writing a research proposal: the critical first step for successful clinical research. Gastroenterol Nurs.1994;17(2):48-56.
2. Bordage G, Dawson B. Experimental study design and grant writing in eight steps and 28 questions. Med Educ. 2003;37(4):376-85.
3. Paterson, B. (2002). Writing a successful research proposal. The Canadian nurse, 98(7), 16-17.

4. Chung KC, Shauver MJ. Fundamental principles of writing a successful grant proposal. J Hand Surg Am. 2008;33(4):566-72.
5. Bhandari M, Devereaux PJ, Einhorn TA, et al. Hip fracture evaluation with alternatives of total hip arthroplasty versus hemiarthroplasty (HEALTH): protocol for a multicentre randomized trial. BMJ Open. 2015;5(2):e006263.
6. Schmelzer M. How to start a research proposal. Gastroenterol Nurs. 2006;29(2):186-8.
7. Kreeger K. A winning proposal. Nature. 2003;426(6962):102-3.

18 Choosing the Outcome—A Primer

Alisha Garibaldi, Guruva Reddy

Key Objectives
- Understand the definitions of outcomes and measuring instruments in the context of clinical research and their importance in clinical research
- Learn how to select an appropriate outcome for a study
- Discover types of measuring instruments
- Gain knowledge of various recommended instruments.

What is an Outcome in a Clinical Study?

Major conclusions drawn from a clinical study are generally based on the ***outcome*** or end result that is measured in clinical studies. It is important to know how to evaluate the end result of a study and to understand what the evaluation will reveal about the intervention being tested.

Why is Choosing the Right Outcome Important in Clinical Research?

By choosing the right outcome and assessing it appropriately, the investigator can draw conclusions about the intervention and therefore make potentially important discoveries. Not taking time to thoroughly think about the outcomes and their assessment before the study begins may result in a waste of time and money for the sponsor, clinical sites and research staff. Although choosing a suboptimal outcome can still lead to a significant finding, it may not be clinically relevant. In addition, if the chosen outcome is not assessed properly, it could produce inconclusive or misleading results. It is therefore crucial to take time at the beginning of a study to carefully select an outcome and a method of assessing the outcome which will provide the most valid and reliable results.

How Many Outcomes can I Choose?

Studies often look at more than one outcomes. The ***primary outcome*** of a study is of greatest importance, in that it should be the most clinically relevant observation in determining the effect of the intervention. The ***secondary outcome*** is used in addition to the primary outcome and is defined as an ***outcome*** that is believed to be related to the ***primary outcome***. A benefit of having multiple outcomes is that if the finding of one outcome is inconclusive, the other outcomes could reveal an important finding. A disadvantage of having too many outcomes is that there is a risk of finding a significant result when actually there is none. This is also known as a false-positive or spurious result.[1] Additionally, including a surplus of outcomes can increase the burden on the research team and research participants which may result in missing data if research forms are time consuming to complete or add additional costs.

How do I Choose an Outcome for my Study?

When choosing an outcome, the first step is to think about the purpose of the study. The purpose of the study can be found by reviewing the research questions in the study protocol. These questions are to be used as a guide for finding an appropriate outcome. For example, if one of the research questions is 'Is soap solution more effective than saline solution in preventing infections in patients with open fracture wounds?', then a suitable outcome for this study would be the rate of infection. If the research questions are not as specific as this and only inquire about the overall effectiveness of an intervention, then the investigator must spend time reflecting on which outcome will best show the effectiveness of the intervention. For instance, if the purpose of the study is to test the effectiveness of a new surgical technique, how will you know if it is more effective than other similar techniques? Will the death rate show you this? Or return to function? It is important to consider all the possibilities.

What are Patient-important Outcomes?

In order to maximize the significance of study results, the outcome must be important to the patient as well as to the physician.[2] ***Patient-important outcomes*** are when the outcome is relevant and applicable to the patient in particular. For example, some orthopedic studies judge how effective an intervention is by assessing when the patient's fracture was healed radiographically. However, if a patient is healed by X-rays, but they are still not fully weight bearing and have not yet returned to their daily activities, then this outcome will not be as meaningful to them. A patient will be more willing to try an intervention when the outcome affects them positively. The more important the outcome is to patients, the easier it will be for the intervention to be accepted and used in regular clinical care.

What is a Measuring Instrument?

Once you have chosen an outcome, you will need to decide how you are going to measure your outcome. A ***measuring instrument*** is a means to measure the outcome of interest so it can be reported in a publication. A measuring instrument must be used in a clinical study in order to ensure consistent observations of the outcome as well as accuracy in measurement. Selecting the appropriate instrument is essential for outcome measures to be considered valid and clinically meaningful.[3] Common types of measuring instruments include questionnaires, imaging, laboratory tests, functional assessments and physical exams.

How do I Choose a Measuring Instrument for My Study?

When selecting a measuring instrument, it is strongly recommended to use an existing instrument that has been validated, as opposed to creating your own. Existing instruments may have been tested on various technical aspects including validity, reliability and generalizability. It is important to determine what has been tested for a particular instrument when deciding which instrument to use.[4] If a subjective outcome is necessary, ***adjudication*** may be required.

What if I Cannot Find the Perfect Measuring Instrument for my Study?

There will rarely be a measuring instrument that will fulfill all the needs of the investigator and the population that they are studying.[4] In choosing the appropriate measuring instrument for a study, there is usually a trade-off between the extent of evaluation versus its feasibility.[3,5] In other words, an instrument would ideally capture every aspect of the intervention's effect on subjects; however, using long and in-depth questionnaires or onerous laboratory testing procedures to collect this information is not always feasible. It is important to keep instruments as brief as possible while including the most important and relevant information so that it places minimal strain and inconvenience on the patients and research staff.[3] The validity, reliability, diagnostic accuracy and responsiveness of the outcome measure must not be compromised. To find the most suitable measuring instrument for your study, a balance can be found by taking into account the study design, study goals, cost and time constraints.[2] If an appropriate measuring instrument tool does not exist, you can create your own, but be aware that this takes a great deal of time, specific training and testing.

Important Learning Points

- Measuring outcomes appropriately allows investigators to draw accurate and significant conclusions about the intervention being tested.
- Patient important outcomes should be used to produce results relevant to patients and clinical practice.
- Measuring instruments are used to accurately assess the outcome and include questionnaires, imaging, laboratory tests, functional assessments and physical exams.

Definitions

Adjudication: When an outcome is determined by an independent person or group of individuals who are not involved in the study.[2]

Measuring instrument: An instrument that shows the extent or degree of something; ensures accuracy in measurement.

Outcome: An indicator of health status that will be used to assess the difference between the treatment and control groups.

Patient important outcome: An outcome that is valued by the patient as well as the physician.[2]

Primary outcome: The observation that is most clinically relevant in determining the effect of the intervention on key variables in the study. Hence, the outcome is of greatest importance.

Secondary outcome: An ***outcome*** believed to be related to the ***primary outcome*** and is used in addition to the ***primary outcome***.

REFERENCES

1. Bhandari M, Whang W, Kuo JC, et al. The risk of false-positive results in orthopedic surgical trials. Clin Orthop Relat Res. 2003;(413):63-9.
2. Bhandari M, Petrisor B, Schemitsch E. Outcome measurements in orthopedic. Indian J Orthop. 2007;41(1):32-36.
3. Fitzpatrick R, Fletcher A, Gore S, et al. Quality of life measures in health care. I: Applications and issues in assessment. BMJ. 1992;305(6861):1074-1077.
4. Patrick DL, Deyo RA. Generic and disease-specific measures in assessing health status and quality of life. Med Care. 1989;27(3 Suppl):S217-32.
5. Ware JE. Measuring patients' views: the optimum outcome measure. BMJ. 1993;306(6890):1429-30.

19

Common Quality of Life and Health Utility Outcome Tools

Rajeev Jetly, Ydo V Kleinlugtenbelt

Key Objectives

- Understand the definition of utility outcome tools and the importance of using them within the context of clinical research.
- Learn the major characteristics that dictate if a tool is of high quality or not
- Discover the differences between specific and general utility outcome tools
- Gain knowledge about the various outcome tools used in clinical research today.

What is a 'Life and Health Utility Outcome Tool'?

When assessing the quality of life of a patient, there is great importance behind evaluating the physical, mental and social wellbeing of one's health. Life and health utility outcome tools help to measure these aspects in a very comprehensive manner. These tools or tests encompass an extensive array of categories including those associated with daily life activities such as work, household undertakings and relationships with family or friends.[1] Many of these outcome tools come in the form of self-reported questionnaires, clinical assessments or interviews.[2] The most common of these is the self-report survey because it can collect the desired information in a practical manner that is both time and cost effective.[2] These tools help physicians and clinical researchers to understand the patient's perspective regarding gains and losses of regular function as a result of the treatment for a disease or injury. One can choose a suitable tool from many tools which are available. The decision to use one over the other lies in its ability and effectiveness in measuring the desired outcome.[1]

What Makes a Utility Outcome Tool Useful?

To be useful in the field of clinical research and medicine, both life and health utility outcome tools need to be reliable and valid. However, many tools do not contain both these properties. A test can be reliable but not necessarily valid, whereas a valid test is always reliable.[1] Therefore, understanding the distinction between the two is very significant.[1]

Reliability

Reliability is an indication of the inherent variability in the utility outcome tool in terms of measurement. Additionally, it estimates the degree to which the score for the same patients changes for recurring measurements under several explicit conditions:[3]

- Using different sets of items from the same measurement instrument (internal-consistency)
- Across time (test-retest)
- By different persons on the same occasion (inter-rater)
- By the same person (i.e. raters or responders) on different occasions (intra-rater).

This domain contains three measurement properties—measurement error, internal consistency and reliability.

1. ***Measurement error:*** This strictly addresses the amount of absolute measurement error within a utility outcome tool. The preferred value to express measurement error is the standard error of measurement (SEM). This represents the standard deviation of repeated measures of an individual.[3] Furthermore, another statistic directly related to SEM is the smallest detectable change (SDC). This is the minimal change that must be overcome to ensure a significant change has occurred.[3] Therefore, an observed change must be higher than the SDC threshold to confirm that a real change has occurred. When the measurement error is smaller than the minimal important change (MIC), the instrument is considered clinically worthwhile.[3] However,

when the measurement error is larger than the MIC, it is less useful. Therefore, the MIC and SDC can help to decide whether or not a real and clinically relevant change has occurred in a patient.[3] By understanding the extent of measurement error, users can better apply this tool when it is used for evaluative purposes such as assessing the effects of surgery or other treatments.[3]

2. ***Internal consistency:*** It is measured by estimating the degree of interrelatedness to which each individual test item measures the same construct.[3] As a result, this reliability estimate does not require repeated administration of the utility outcome tool. If items in a scale are summarized into a score, it should be known that the items are sufficiently correlated.[3] This correlation between a respondent's item-responses is established through internal consistency and suggests whether or not these items measure the same construct.[3] For example, suppose you wanted to give your patient a test of three items to measure their level of satisfaction after their treatment session. The first item is 'You are almost always satisfied after a session.' The second item is 'You almost always like your treatment session.' The third item is 'You almost never feel satisfied after a session.' If a patient agrees with the first two items and disagrees with the last, the test has a good internal consistency associated with it.

3. ***Reliability:*** This measurement property of the domain reliability can be broken down into ***test-retest reliability***, ***inter-rater reliability*** and ***intra-rater reliability***. The test-retest reliability evaluates the reliability of a test administrated at different times. On two different occasions, the measurement instrument must be given to a group of the same patients where the outcome is observed. This type of reliability is heavily dependent on the whether or not the outcome is stable to daily or weekly fluctuations.[3] The timing of the second occasion is extremely critical so that the time interval between occasions is long enough for the last score to not be affected by the recollection of the first.[3] If an interval is too short, this tends to result in an overestimated reliability. However, if the interval is too long, allowing the subject to change in-between occasions,

the reliability can be underestimated.[3] Generally, a typical interval is between 2 and 4 weeks. When looking at inter-rater reliability, an outcome tool uses judges or raters to allocate scores to patients. This reliability is represented by the degree of agreement between scores which is given to patients by two or more raters.[3] Inter-rater reliability can be estimated by having both raters administer the same patient. This is useful because if various raters do not agree amongst each other, the scale used for measurement may be ineffective or the raters need to be retrained.

Intra-rater reliability evaluates reliability across different times with respect to the rater.[3] This involves having one rater score the same instrument on two different occasions. Similar to inter-rater reliability, it is dependent primarily on good standardization and how well trained the raters are.[3]

Validity

It refers to the extent to which the utility outcome tool measures the construct(s) it proposes to measure.[3] This domain contains three measurement properties—content validity, construct validity and criterion validity.

1. ***Content validity:*** It expresses the extent to which the items of the measurement instrument adequately reflect the construct being measured.[3] Firstly, the aim of the measurement should be evidently clear with being predictive, evaluative or discriminative.[3] Secondly, the items in the instrument must be judged on comprehensiveness and relevance.[3] This is accomplished by several experts via a survey. Finally, the content of the measurement instrument should match the target population. There are many occasions where the instrument is used in a different population rather than the target population. For example, the disabilities of arm, shoulder and hand outcome tool contains items about doing household chores, participation in work and sexual activities. These items measure the physical function of an older, adult demographic. However, when this instrument is used upon children, these items may be less valid towards measuring their physical function.[3] Therefore, a tool that contains important items for this patients group such as playing games and attendance to school is needed.

2. ***Construct validity:*** This estimates the range of scores from the tool that are consistent with the hypothesis proposed before the test.[3] A hypothesis is usually based upon expected internal relationships, expected differences amongst relevant groups scores and the expected relationship of scores to other outcome tool results.[3] There is currently no agreement upon how many hypotheses should be tested or confirmed to verify if a tool is construct valid. However, it has been suggested that around 75% of hypothesis should be confirmed to ensure construct validity.[3] An example of construct validity is cross-culture validity. This estimates the degree to which the performance of the items on a translated or culturally adapted outcome instrument is an adequate reflection of the performance of the item of the original version of the outcome instruments.[3] Due to cultural differences and language, sometimes a translation is not sufficient. As a result, multiple translations by at least two translators should take place to ensure construct validity of the instrument.[3]

3. ***Criterion validity:*** It is the estimation of the extent to which the scores of a utility outcome tool are an adequate reflection of the 'gold standard'.[3] When choosing an instrument to compare to, it is extremely important that it is a 'gold standard'. This is usually the most difficult task to achieve simply because there are very few gold standard instruments available. Furthermore, the estimation of this validity depends on the type of data. When both the outcome and gold standard instruments have continuous scores, the preferred method is by presenting the correlation coefficient. This correlation is ideal when the score is above 0.70.[3] When the outcome instrument score is continuous and the gold standard has a dichotomous score, the preferred method is the area under the receiver-operated characteristic with a criterion of 0.70.[3] When both scores are dichotomous, the sensitivity and specificity are the selected methods to use.[3]

What are the Types of Life and Health Utility Outcome Tools?

There are two types of utility outcome tools. The first includes ***generic outcome tools*** that address health in a very comprehensive manner and can be applied in many situations. The second type includes *region/disease-specific outcome tools*. These tools are focused towards highly specific circumstances in life that relate to a specific function, problem or underlying disease process. Both of these utility outcome tools have their individual advantages and disadvantages. Understanding the difference between these two can help one in choosing which type of tool is best to capture the desired information. However, even though it is extremely important to think about this, many take the preferred approach of using standard generic instruments that are supplemented with region-disease specific qualities.[1] This usually proves to be more effective than using only one type of tool exclusively.[1]

1. *Generic outcome tools:* They measure an individual's general health status with respect to their physical symptoms, function and psychological status.[1] These generic instruments are very useful in that they cover a very broad scope of health-related quality of life concepts.[1] Along with this, they help provide a more complete overall view of an individual's health. Many generic outcome tools are administered in the form of questionnaires. A significant advantage associated with these tools is that it allows researchers to compare health status across different aspects including diseases, interventions, severities and different cultures.[1,2] However, generic tools also have their disadvantages. Sometimes these tools are not sensitive enough and lack the ability to detect small but significant changes of the patient being tested.[1,2] Along with this, generic outcome tools tend to be long and can result in poorer response rates.[1,2]

2. *Region/disease-specific outcome tools:* They are customized to inquire about the precise physical, mental and social aspects of health affected by a specific disease or condition in question.[1,2] These type of tools can be extremely helpful when trying to detect small changes over a short period of time.[1,6] However, disease-specific tools can be limiting since they are only used for precise conditions and within specific population groups.[1,2]

   It is important to note that even though it is called a region/disease-specific outcome tool, one should validate the use of these tools based upon each joint and pathology of concern. For example, the Disabilities of the Arm, Shoulder and Hand (DASH) is a test that is used to assess upper extremity. If given to a patient with a shoulder dislocation, the DASH can provide extremely useful information. However, if given to a patient with a fracture of the distal radius, even though the DASH can assess upper extremity regions, the results from the test may not be as helpful. Therefore, when deciding which utility outcome tool to use, one should ensure that the test chosen will result in the outcome of interest.

What are the Recommended Generic and Disease-Specific Outcome Tools?

When selecting a utility outcome tool, it is strongly advised that one uses an already existing tool rather than to develop another tool for the same construct.[2] Many outcome tools have existed for a great deal of time and undergone tests to verify technical aspects including reliability and validity. An overview of commonly used generic and region/disease-specific tools is given in Table 19.1

Short Form-36 (SF-36)

It is the most commonly used generic utility outcome tool. Being documented in almost 4000 publications over the years of 1988–2000, the SF-36 is a short 15-minute, multipurpose survey that is comprized of 36 questions.[1] The survey can be self-administered or interview-administered in a variety of languages. It has been proven to be extremely useful in the assessment of patient health status in both general and specific populations.[2] This test is capable of exhibiting

Table 19.1: Examples of commonly used measuring instruments

Generic instruments	Region/disease-specific instruments
• Short Form-36 (SF-36) • Short Form-12 (SF-12) • EQ-5D • Health utilities index (HUI)	• Disabilities of the Arm, Shoulder and Hand (DASH) • Western Ontario and McMaster Osteoarthritis Index (WOMAC) • Arthritis Impact Measurement Scales (AIMS)

beneficial results when comparing the relative burden of diseases in patients and in discriminating between health and cost benefits produced by different treatments.[1] On average, scores from the SF-36 tool tend to correlate with physicians' assessments of the severity of illness being questioned. However, the SF-36 can be limited due to its inability to take sleep into consideration and its low response rate to populations above 65 of age.[1]

The SF-36 is comprized of eight domains with each containing questions-associated to their section. These domains include general health, mental health, physical function, social functioning, role physical, role emotional, bodily pain and vitality.[1] Each domain is given a scaled score that is a weighted sum of all the questions within that domain.[1] All scales are transformed into a 0–100 scale based on the assumption that all questions are of the same weight. The lower the score the more disability; the higher the score the less disability.[1] In order to calculate these scores, special software is needed. The price of these heavily depends on the number of scores that need to be calculated. To summarize the results, the SF-36 tool is broken into a physical component summary and a mental component summary. With regards to both these areas, the validity and reliability of the SF-36 summaries range fairly high.[1]

Short Form-12 (SF-12)

The short form-12 questionnaire is essentially a shorter version of SF-36. This tool is self-administered and has only 12 questions that measure the health and quality of life of individuals.[2] Just like the SF-36, this outcome tool measures eight domains that are summarized in a physical and mental aspect. The summary of the test is represented in scaled scores ranging from 0 to 100. This test instrument has been extensively evaluated and has exhibited good construct validity, high test-retest reliability and high internal consistency.[1] Differences between SF–36 and SF–12 are given in Table 19.2

EQ-5D

The EQ-5D is a standardized generic utility outcome tool that measures the health status of patients to provide support for

Table 19.2: Differences between SF-36 and SF-12

Short form-36	Short form-12
• Provides more information about the nature of the differences in physical and mental results.	• Reproduces the SF-36 summary scales very well. Takes less time to complete.
• Less efficient and more expensive compared to SF-12.	• Less construct validity and sensitivity. That results in less precision for all eight scales.
• Used for studies with sample sizes less than 500 patients.	• Used for studies with sample sizes over 500 patients.

clinical and economic assessment.[1,4] This questionnaire is designed to be completed by one's self and can be applied to various health treatments and conditions. Being cognitively undemanding and taking only a few minutes to complete, the EQ-5D consists of five dimensions—self-care, usual activities, pain/discomfort, mobility and anxiety/depression.[4] Each of these dimensions has 3-5 levels that describe ones current health function. Patients are able to indicate their state of health by checking off boxes in each of the five dimensions that best describes their current status.[4]

Health Utilities Index (HUI)

The HUI is a family of generic utility outcome tools used for measuring the complete quality of life and health status of patients. The tool comes in the form of a self or interviewed administered survey that takes roughly 5-10 minutes to complete.[1] Along with this, the HUI is available in 35 different languages and can be written on paper or online. There are three versions of HUI known as HUI1, HUI2 and HUI3. However, although the HUI1 is still used, the HUI2 and HUI3 are much more frequently found in clinical and health population studies. The HUI2 describes 24,000 unique health status, whereas, the HUI3 describes 972,000 health status.[1] There has been multiple reliability and validity testing done on the HUI and has been proven to be comprehensive, reliable, responsible and valid.[1] This measurement tool itself provides descriptive evidence through multiple health categories including hearing, vision, speech, pain, self-care, emotion, cognition and mobility.[1] Every category has around 3–6 levels each with a description that allows patients to rank themselves accordingly.

Disabilities of the Arm, Shoulder and Hand (DASH)

The Disabilities of Arm, Shoulder and Hand utility outcome tool is a 30-item questionnaire that measures the physical function associated with people who have any of several musculoskeletal disorders of the upper limb.[1,2] This region-specific tool gives researchers and physicians the advantage of having a single, highly reliable and valid test to assess any joint in the upper extremity. The questionnaire is a self-report survey where patients rate the difficulty of function in daily life activities on a 5-point Likert scale.[1,2] The final score ranges from 0 to 100 with higher scores indicating severe upper limb disability. Along with this test, there is a shorter version available called QuickDASH containing only 11 items. However, this is only recommended for summary assessments since the full DASH has greater precision.[2] Both short and full DASH tests have high validity and reliability.

Western Ontario and McMaster Osteoarthritis Index (WOMAC)

The WOMAC Index is a disease-specific utility outcome tool that assesses and quantifies joint pain, stiffness and disability of patients who have knee and hip osteoarthritis.[3] It can be used to measure the progression of a disease or to determine a variety of effective treatments such as physiotherapy or surgery. Although, the WOMAC provides an excellent outlook on the patient's lower extremity functionality, it has been used for other conditions such as lower back pain, rheumatoid arthritis (RA), lupus and fibromyalgia.[3] Additionally, this outcome tool complements objective data from magnetic resonance imaging (MRIs), arthroscopy, radiographs and cartilage biopsies.[3] This 15 minute, self-administered questionnaire contains 24 questions that are divided amongst the categories of pain, stiffness and physical function. Being scored on a 5-point Likert scale, this test has a construct validity of 0.68–75 and a reliability ranging from 0.73 to 0.96.[3]

Patient-rated Wrist Evaluation (PRWE)

The PRWE is a joint-specific utility outcome tool that was developed to aid in the clinical assessment of specific wrist problems in patients. This questionnaire contains 15 items that are responsible for measuring wrist pain and determining the level of wrist disability during daily activities.[5] The items found in the PRWE are separated into two subscales where patients are able to rate their level of disability and pain from 0 to 10 for each item.[5] There are ten items in the function subscale divided into specific and usual activities whereas the alternate subscale gathers information regarding pain and contains 5 items. The maximum score in both sections is 50. Once both subscales are measured, the values are added to achieve a total score of a potential maximum of 100. A lower score in the PRWE is indicative of a better outcome. Some advantages of PRWE are that they are short, quick and reliable.[5]

Definitions

Construct validity: The range of scores from the tool that are consistent with the hypothesis proposed before the test.

Content validity: The extent to which the items of the measurement instrument adequately reflect the construct being measured.

Criterion validity: The extent to which the scores of a utility outcome tool are an adequate reflection of the 'gold standard'.

Internal consistency: The degree of interrelatedness to which each individual test item measures the same construct.

Inter-rater reliability: The degree of agreement between scores given to patients by two or more raters.

Intra-rater reliability: The degree of agreement across different times with respect to a single rater.

Measurement error: The difference between the true value and the value obtained from a certain measurement.

Reliability: The consistency of the data and its interpretation.

Test-retest reliability: The reliability of a test administrated at different times.

Validity: How well the data collected by the survey instrument reflects what the researcher set out to measure.

REFERENCES

1. Bellamy N. (2012). Western Ontario and McMaster Universities Osteoarthritis Index (WOMAC). Available from https://www.rheumatology.org/Practice/Clinical/Clinicianresearchers/Outcomes_Instrumentation/Western_Ontario_and_McMaster_Universities_Osteoarthritis_Index/
2. Bhandari M, Joensson A. Clinical research for surgeons. Stuttgart: Thieme. 2009;pp.101-15.
3. Bhandari M, Sancheti P. Understanding Outcomes Assessment. In: Clinical research made easy: A guide to publishing in medical literature. New Delhi: Jaypee Brothers Medical Publishers (P) Ltd; 2010.
4. Oemar M, Oppe M. (2013). EQ-5D-3L user guide: basic information on how to use the EQ-5D-3L instrument. Retrieved from http://www.euroqol.org/fileadmin/user_upload/Documenten/PDF/Folders_Flyers/EQ-5D-3L_UserGuide_2013_v5.0_October_2013.pdf
5. Navarro C, Ponzer S, Törnkvist H, et al. Measuring outcome after wrist injury: Translation and validation of the Swedish version of the patient-rated wrist evaluation (PRWE-Swe). BMC Musculoskelet Disord. 2011;12:171.
6. Scholtes VA, Terwee CB, Poolman RW. What makes a measurement instrument valid and reliable? Injury. 2011;42(3):236-40.
7. Ware J (2002). SF-36 Health Survey Update. Available from http://www.sf-36.org/tools/sf36.shtml#LIT.

20

An Introduction to Sample Size

Christopher Scott Smith, Ashok Shyam, Thuva Vanniyasingam

Key Objectives

- Understand the importance of sample size calculations in clinical research
- Identify the basic components required for calculating sample size
- Be aware of common pitfalls when calculating sample size
- Be able to report sample size calculations properly.

What is Sample Size and Why does It Matter?

Sample size is defined as the number of participants or experimental units included in a clinical study. This number is a key determinant of a study's statistical and clinical relevance and should not be determined arbitrarily, as issues can arise when a study is under or oversized.[1-3] When a study is undersized, its ability to detect significant differences between groups will be reduced, limiting the ability to detect meaningful differences between treatments. A study with an inadequate sample size and power can also result in misleading findings. This is demonstrated effectively in the study to prospectively evaluate reamed intramedullary nail in patients with tibial fractures (SPRINT) trial, a large clinical investigation evaluating operative treatments of tibial shaft fractures in over 1000 patients. A planned analysis of the first 35 patients provided findings that were the complete opposite of the final analysis conducted with 1226 patients. Interim analyses throughout the study indicated that only after 543 patients with closed fractures were enrolled did the results reflect the final advantage observed in the final analysis.[4] This example demonstrates the importance of having an adequate sample size to detect differences within the outcome and population of interest. Additionally, an oversized study can lead to a number of issues relating to unnecessary costs and ethical treatment of patients.

Calculating the sample size is an integral part of study planning and has become crucial when applying for both ethical approval and research funding. A well planned and detailed sample size calculation can demonstrate your competency as a researcher and help to determine if a study is feasible. This aspect of research planning should not be overlooked.

What should be Considered before Calculating Sample Size?

A researcher must first begin with a clearly defined research question. While determining the optimal sample size for a clinical study is a simple concept, it requires the investigator to understand a number of key assumptions that are influenced by components of the research question.[2] The investigator must identify the population of interest, the interventional and comparative treatments, the overall objective of the study and the time frame within which the study will run.

Defining these components of the research questions will allow the researcher to identify and review studies that incorporate a similar population of interest and primary outcome. These studies allow for the best estimate of the smallest effect size of interest between study groups and the variability (standard deviation) within the target population.[2,5,6]

All of these factors influence the underlying assumptions that are used to calculate a clinical study's sample size and should be well defined before moving forward with a sample size calculation or consulting with a statistician.[1]

What is Needed to Calculate Sample Size for a Clinical Trial?

There are a number of different methods that can be used to calculate sample size which vary by methodological design and objective of the study. While the first step in choosing the correct sample size calculation should be based upon the research question, study design and the study objectives. The basic components of sample size calculations remain constant. The investigator will need to determine the *type I (α) error*, *type II (β) error* or the statistical *power*, the *smallest effect size of interest* and the *variability* within the study population in order to calculate the sample size (Table 20.1).[1,2,5,7,8] These parameters have been defined below.

Type I (α) error: The chance of detecting a statistically significant difference between groups when there is no real difference is known as type I (α) error and leads the investigator to falsely reject the null hypothesis. This error is more commonly defined as a false positive. In clinical research the threshold p-value for significance, or alpha (α), is most commonly set to 0.05. This means that the investigator desires a less than 5% chance of drawing a false positive conclusion.[2]

Type II (β) error: In hypothesis testing, another type of error that can occur is type II (β) error. This type of error occurs when an investigator determines that there is no statistical difference between samples when in reality there is. This error is more commonly known as a false negative. Table 20.2 provides a summary of possible outcomes and errors that can occur during hypothesis testing.[2]

Table 20.1: Necessary components for sample size calculation

Necessary components for sample size calculations
• Type I (α) error
• Type II (β) error or Power
• Smallest effect size of interest
• Variability

Table 20.2: Possible outcomes in hypothesis testing

Reality	Sample	
	No difference	Difference
No Difference	True Negative	False Positive Type I (α) Error
Difference	False Negative Type II (β) Error	True Positive

Power: The power of a study reflects the ability to identify an effect that is present in a population based on a sample from that population. The statistical power of a study is the complement of the type II (β) error, which is defined as a false negative. To calculate the power of a study the investigator must subtract the (β) error from 1. Traditionally, the power of a study is set to 0.80 or an 80% chance of being able to identify a true effect, but sometimes more conservative values are used, like 0.90 (90%).[2]

The smallest effect size of interest: This is the smallest difference between study groups that the investigator determines to be of scientific and clinical interest. This difference is generally thought of as a minimal clinically important difference, which can be defined as a difference that would be considered meaningful and worthwhile by a patient and one that would make them consider repeating the treatment if it were their choice to make again.[2,6,9,10]

The variability: The variance is determined based on the standard deviation of an outcome of interest (primary outcome) for the population being included in the study. This is often estimated by the investigators using either a pilot study or information gained from previous research evaluating the same population and outcome of interest. This value is an estimate made by the investigator and should be based on the best information available.[3]

The parameters listed above are the key components in calculating sample size. An example of how these parameters can be combined to calculate sample size for a basic randomised control trial using continuous variables has been provided below. Note that formulas will differ based on trial design and objective. Sample size calculations and resources that can be used for calculation are covered in the next chapter.[1]

n = the sample size in each of the two groups

$\Delta\mu$ = the difference between population means of the two groups (minimal clinically important difference)

σ^2 = Population variance

a = alpha (usually 0.05)

b = power (usually 0.80)

$$n = \frac{2[(a+b)^2 \sigma^2]}{(\Delta\mu)^2}$$

Equation adapted from Noordzij et al.[2]

What are Some Common Pitfalls When Calculating Sample Size?

There are a number of issues that can arise when performing sample size calculations which may lead to inaccuracy in the final result. This can often arise from an inability to identify good estimates for the parameters used in sample size calculations.

The Effects of Selecting Alpha and Power

Traditionally, the alpha and power are set to 0.05 and 0.80, respectively.[1-3] While these values are adequate in most cases, other assumptions may be required depending on the topic of study. When the power of a study is increased or the alpha level is decreased the required sample size becomes larger. This relationship is depicted in Table 20.3.[5] Investigators should be aware of how changing these parameters can influence the sample size, and that sensitivity analyses are commonly performed by conducting sample size calculations

Table 20.3: Sample size and the relationship of effect size, power, and alpha level

Effect Size (%)	Power	Alpha	Sample size (per group)
10	0.80	0.05	384
5	0.80	0.05	1556
10	0.90	0.05	513
10	0.95	0.05	635
10	0.80	0.01	572
10	0.90	0.01	727
10	0.95	0.01	870
5	0.95	0.01	3531

using different values for the alpha, power and effect size. When in a situation of doubt the investigator should lean towards the larger sample size.[1]

Table 20.3. Illustrates the required sample size based upon effect size, power, and alpha assumptions. Table adapted from Devane et al.[5]

Estimating the Smallest Effect of Interest and the Variability

Selecting the smallest effect of interest and providing a good estimate of variability can be one of the most difficult tasks when preparing to calculate sample size. It is recommended that investigators use the minimal clinically important difference when selecting the smallest effect of interest. There are three methods that can be used to determine the minimal clinically important difference; distribution methods, the anchor based method, and the Delphi method. Distribution methods use statistical measures of spread, like standard deviation, to determine the minimal clinically important difference.[6,9,10] An example of this would be setting the minimal clinically important difference to one-half of an outcome score's standard deviation.[11-13] The anchor method compares changes in outcome scores to an 'anchor' or reference, like a baseline score. This method uses anchor questions to determine if the minimal change is where a patient feels they have improved compared to baseline due to the treatment.[11-13] The Delphi method relies upon experts, previous research, and the investigators experience to come to a consensus on setting the minimal clinically important difference.[11-13] It is important for the investigator to determine

---

Methods for Estimating the Smallest Effect of Interest

Distribution method: Uses statistical measures of spread to estimate the minimal clinically important difference.
Anchor based method: Uses a reference as an anchor to determine if changes in outcome are clinically important.
Delphi method: Relies on the opinion of a panel of experts to reach a consensus on the minimal clinically important difference based on the best available evidence.

which method will provide them with the best estimate for their sample population when determining the minimal clinically important difference.

The variance of the population of interest is another important assumption that the investigator must make in order to calculate sample size. This can be done by using previous research or a pilot study.[1,7] Investigators should be aware that pilot studies tend to be underpowered by definition and might not provide the best estimate of variance for this calculation.

Patient Withdrawal and Loss to Follow-up

Patients included in a study can withdraw their consent to take part in a study or be unable to complete the full study follow-up. The loss of study participants can affect a study's ability to detect differences between study groups, investigators should anticipate these potential issues and make adjustments to the calculated sample size accordingly. This means the sample size will need to be inflated, it is estimated that the calculated sample size is needed to be inflated by 5–15% to account for the potential loss of participants.[1]

Is There Anyone Who Can Help?

There are a number of people and resources that can help in the calculation of sample size. During the planning stage of a clinical trial, the investigator should consult with a biostatistician or an epidemiologist. These professionals can help guide the investigator to the appropriate sample size calculation for the study design and assist in conducting sensitivity analyses. Additionally, there are a number of resources that can be used to calculate sample sizes for some of the more common designs, a few examples of calculations and these resources have been provided in the next chapter.

How do I Report Sample Size Calculations?

Sample size calculations are an integral part of study design and should be properly reported in all applicable research publications. Commonly, sample sizes are reported using only the number of patients required, the alpha, and the power.[2] These statements are limited as they neglect to communicate the estimate of interest and the variability. Effectively communicating all of the assumptions that underlie the sample size calculation within a publication identifies the primary endpoint of the study for the reader and can alert them to potential problems relating to recruitment. When reporting the sample size calculation, the alpha, the power, the event rate in the control group, the treatment effect of interest, and, when applicable, the statistical software used to perform the calculation should be provided.[2,14] An example of a well reported sample size calculation has been taken from the SPRINT trial.[15]

'Our choice of sample size was based on the anticipated rate of the primary outcome (re-operation). All statistical hypotheses were two-sided. We chose alpha levels of 0.05 for the primary and 0.01 for the secondary outcomes. We evaluated 7 secondary outcomes, but because they were likely to be correlated the Bonferroni correction would have been excessively conservative we chose not to use this approach. The trial was designed to have a statistical power of 80% for the primary comparison. With our event rate of 13%, an additional 300 patients (total sample size=1200 patients) provided adequate study power (87%) for a treatment effect of at least 37%.'

Definitions

Anchor-based method: This method uses a reference as an anchor to determine if changes in outcome are clinically important.

Delphi method: This method relies on the opinion of a panel of experts to reach a consensus on the minimal clinically important difference based on the best available evidence.

Distribution method: This method uses statistical measures of spread to estimate the minimal clinically important difference.

Minimal clinically important difference: A difference that would be considered meaningful and worthwhile by a patient and one that would make them consider repeating the treatment if it were their choice to make again.

Pilot study: A small scale preliminary study conducted before the main research in order to check the feasibility or to improve the design of the research.

Power: The probability of rejecting a false null hypothesis. It is inversely proportional to Type II error (β).

Sample size: The number of participants or experimental units included in a clinical research study.

Smallest effect size of interest: The difference between study groups that the investigator determines to be of scientific and clinical interest.

Standard deviation: The standard deviation is the average difference between each value in the set and the cumulative mean.

Type I error: Incorrect rejection of the null hypothesis and concluding a relationship exists between two variables when in fact it does not. Also known as a spurious result.

Type II error: Incorrect acceptance of the null hypothesis and concluding no relationship exists between two variables when in fact it does.

Variability: The standard deviation of an outcome of interest within the study population.

REFERENCES

1. Bhandari M, Joensson A. Clinical Research for Surgeons. Thieme. 2008.
2. Noordzij M, Tripepi G, Dekker FW, et al. Sample size calculations: basic principles and common pitfalls. Nephrol Dial Transplant. 2010;25(5):1388-93.
3. Noordzij M, Dekker FW, Zoccali C, et al. Sample size calculations. Nephron Clin Pract. 2011;118(4):p.c319-23.
4. Bhandari M, Rampersad SA, Sprague S, et al. (Sample) size matters! An examination of sample size from the SPRINT trial study to prospectively evaluate reamed intramedullary nails in patients with tibial fractures. J Orthop Trauma. 2013;27(4):183-8.
5. Devane D, Begley CM, Clarke M. How many do I need? Basic principles of sample size estimation. J Adv Nurs. 2004;47(3):297-302.
6. Copay AG, Subach BR, Glassman SD, et al. Understanding the minimum clinically important difference: a review of concepts and methods. Spine J. 2007;7(5):541-6.

7. Zlowodzki M, Bhandari M. Outcome measures and implications for sample-size calculations. J Bone Joint Surg Am. 2009;91 Suppl 3:35-40.
8. Thoma A, Sprague S, Temple C, et al. The role of the randomized controlled trial in plastic surgery. Clin Plast Surg. 2008;35(2):275-84.
9. Carragee EJ, Cheng I. Minimum acceptable outcomes after lumbar spinal fusion. Spine J. 2010;10(4):313-20.
10. Jaeschke R, Singer J, Guyatt GH. Measurement of health status. Ascertaining the minimal clinically important difference. Control Clin Trials. 1989;10(4):407-15.
11. Bellamy N, Anastassiades TP, Buchanan WW, et al. Rheumatoid arthritis antirheumatic drug trials. III. Setting the delta for clinical trials of antirheumatic drugs—results of a consensus development (Delphi) exercise. J Rheumatol. 1991;18(12):1908-15.
12. Bellamy N, Buchanan WW, Esdaile JM, et al. Ankylosing spondylitis antirheumatic drug trials. III. Setting the delta for clinical trials of antirheumatic drugs—results of a consensus development (Delphi) exercise. J Rheumatol. 1991;18(11):1716-22.
13. Bellamy N, Carette S, Ford PM, et al. Osteoarthritis antirheumatic drug trials. III. Setting the delta for clinical trials—results of a consensus development (Delphi) exercise. J Rheumatol. 1992;19(3):451-7.
14. Gordis, Leon. Epidemiology. 4th ed. Philadelphia: Elsevier/Saunders, 2009. Print.
15. Bhandari M, Guyatt G, Tornetta P 3rd, et al. Study to prospectively evaluate reamed intramedually nails in patients with tibial fractures (S.P.R.I.N.T.): study rationale and design. BMC Musculoskelet Disord. 2008;9:91.

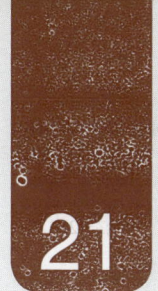

21

Estimating an Appropriate Sample Size—Advanced Concepts, Formulae and Examples

Thuva Vanniyasingam, Lawrence Mbuagbaw, Christopher Scott Smith

Key Objectives

- Learn the basic components and steps behind sample size estimation
- Understand the three types of comparisons in randomized controlled trials (RCTs)
- Learn sample size formulae for binary and continuous outcomes for two-arm parallel RCTs
- Become aware of programs available for estimating sample size
- Learn how to estimate and present a range of appropriate sample sizes.

What Basic Components are Needed for Sample Size Estimations?

As discussed in Chapter 20, information required for an appropriate sample size calculation includes:
- **Type I error** rate (α)
- **Power** of the study ($1-\beta$)
- **Smallest effect size of interest** (the effect in one group compared to the other)
- **Variability** (based on the standard deviation for each group in the population for continuous outcomes).

These factors are the backbone behind any sample size calculation and are particularly essential for a basic two-arm parallel group trial. They are briefly defined at the end of this chapter. Programs and formulae used to estimate the sample size will often require this input. Additional components may be needed for other designs like cluster trials or factorial design trials. The effect size is often informed by a clinically important difference between groups, an expected difference, or an affordable difference. Holding all other factors constant, a larger sample size is required to detect a smaller effect size.

What are the Basic Steps for Sample Size Estimation?

The following steps are needed for any sample size estimation:
- Specify your null and alternative hypotheses.
- Set your desired type I error rate (e.g. $\alpha=0.05$) and power (e.g. $1-\beta=0.80$).
- Define your study population and collect information relevant to the parameters of interest (such as means and standard deviations of each group or proportion with the outcome of interest in your control group).
- Define your minimal clinically important difference.
- Calculate sample size over a range of reasonable parameters.
- Select the sample size for use.

What are the three Types of Comparisons Made in Randomized Controlled Trials?

The most popular type of RCT design is the parallel trial where subjects are randomly placed into two or more arms, treated with different interventions and followed up at the same time.[1] Comparisons between groups differ based on what they are trying to demonstrate—clinical superiority, equivalence and non-inferiority.
- Superiority trials are the most popular RCTs and are suitable when an investigator is interested in knowing whether or not one treatment is more clinically efficacious than another treatment. This is performed in one of two ways: an investigator will either test if (a) a significant difference exists between two groups; a traditional comparison or (b) test if one treatment is better than the other treatment.
    - *Example (a):* A protocol for a multicentre RCT describes a plan to assess whether there is a significant difference on the impact of total hip arthroplasty, in comparison to hemiarthroplasty, on rates of unplanned secondary procedures within 2 years among individuals with displaced femoral neck fractures.[1]

- **Example (b):** Trial investigators are interested in whether fibrin pad is more safe and effectively hemostatic, in comparison to the standard of care, for managing severe soft-tissue bleeding encountered by patients receiving intra-abdominal and thoracic surgical procedures.
- Non-inferiority trials are used to determine whether one treatment is no worse (by a specific margin) than the other.
  - **Example:** Trial investigators want to determine whether intravenous tranexamic acid (a hemostatic agent) is non-inferior to topical application of tranexamic acid for postoperative blood transfusion rate among patients who have undergone total knee arthroplasty.[3]
- Equivalence trials are appropriate among studies where the interest is in testing if a treatment is as good as a comparator. If the observable difference between them lies within a predetermined interval, then the two therapies are considered to be equivalent.[2]
  - **Example:** A randomized controlled equivalence trial was conducted to determine whether hand-rubbing (with an aqueous alcoholic solution) was as effective as surgical hand-scrubbing in preventing 30-day surgical site infections for consecutive patients who experienced clean and clean-contaminated surgery. The authors set an 'equivalence interval' which specifies the degree of difference that the investigators would accept to conclude that the treatments are equivalent.[4]

Why is Hypothesis Testing Important in RCTs?

The initial step to a scientific process is the generation of a hypothesis. This is then critically tested through experiments and observational studies. Generally, the null hypothesis suggests that there is no association between the main predictor of interest (e.g. a treatment) and the outcome (e.g. mortality), while the alternative hypothesis proposes that they are associated. The alternative hypothesis can have a single direction of association between the main variable and outcome (one-sided, i.e. treatment will reduce mortality) or have both directions (two-sided, i.e. treatment may reduce or increase mortality). Table 21.1 further outlines the null (H_0) and alternative (H_1) hypotheses for each type of trial along with an

Table 21.1: Null and alternative hypothesis of clinical superiority, non-inferiority and equivalence trials

Trial	Hypothesis	Interpretation
Superiority a. when d=0 *Traditional comparison	$H_0: \Delta = 0$ $H_1: \Delta \neq 0$	H_0: There is no difference between the two treatments. H_1: The two treatments are different.
b. when d>0	$H_0: \Delta \leq d$ $H_1: \Delta > d$	H_0: One treatment is not superior to the other. H_1: One treatment is superior to the other by a minimum difference of d.
Non-inferiority	$H_0: \Delta \geq d$ $H_1: \Delta < d$	H_0: A given treatment is inferior to the other. H_1: A given treatment is non-inferior to the other.
Equivalence	$H_0: \Delta \leq d_1$ or $\Delta > d_2$ $H_1: d_1 < \Delta < d_2$	H_0: The treatment differences do not lie within an interval (d_1, d_2) that indicates clinical equivalence. H_1: The differences between two treatments lie within an interval (d_1, d_2).

*The traditional comparison for a superiority trial is the most popular type. A superiority trial where d > 0 implies that there is enough evidence to ensure that the difference between two treatments will not go in the opposite direction.

interpretation. The difference between two groups is the factor of interest, where Δ represents the true difference between groups and d is the minimum clinically important difference.

- For continuous outcomes, Δ is the true difference of the means between two groups ($\Delta = \mu_1 - \mu_2$).
- For binary outcomes, Δ is the difference of the true proportions between two groups ($\Delta = p_1 - p_2$).

How do I Manually Estimate Sample Size?

Sample size calculation formula for RCTs vary based on design. A variety of software and websites are available to perform calculations for each type of unique study. The two most commonly used sample size estimations are tailored for parallel two-arm trials and are presented below:

1. **_Binary outcomes_**[5]

   $H_0: p_1 - p_2 = 0$

   $H_1: p_1 - p_2 \neq 0$

   $$n = \frac{\left(z_{1-\alpha/2}\sqrt{2\overline{p}(1-\overline{p})} + z_{1-\beta}\sqrt{p_1(1-p_1) + p_2(1-p_2)}\right)^2}{d^2}$$

   where,

   p_1 = Proportion of individuals who experience the outcome in group 1

   p_2 = Proportion of individuals who experience the outcome in group 2

   $\overline{p}$ = $(p_1 + p_2)/2$

   d = Minimum clinically meaningful difference between the two proportions

   Z_x = Standard normal deviate of x

   α = Type I error

   β = Type II error.

   This is for continuous outcomes that follow a normal distribution and incorporate groups with different variances (or standard deviations).

2. **_Continuous outcomes or Common values for Zx_**[6]

   $H_0: \mu_1 - \mu_2 = 0$

   $H_1: \mu_1 - \mu_2 \neq 0$

   $$n = (\sigma_1^2 + \sigma_2^2) \times \left(\frac{z_{1-\alpha}/2 + z_{1-\beta}}{d}\right)^2$$

   where,

   α_1 = True standard deviation of the population in group 1

   σ_2 = True standard deviation of the population in group 2

   d = Minimum clinically meaningful difference between the two means

   Z_x = Standard normal deviate of x

   α = Type I error

   β = Type II error

Common values for Z_x:

For $\alpha = 0.10$, $z_{1-\alpha/2} = 1.64$
For $\alpha = 0.05$, $z_{1-\alpha/2} = 1.96$
For $\alpha = 0.01$, $z_{1-\alpha/2} = 2.58$

For power = 80%, $z_{1-\beta} = 0.84$
For power = 90%, $z_{1-\beta} = 1.28$

Application for Continuous Outcome RCTs

Example 1: Estimating the difference between two means in a clinical superiority trial:

Suppose an investigator is interested in conducting a two-arm parallel trial to compare a new treatment versus a standard (control) treatment with a continuous response variable of systolic blood pressure (SBP). The treatment is expected to reduce blood pressure and a trial was set up to test whether the mean SBP for the treatment group was less than the mean treatment of the control group. The parameter of interest is the difference between the two. A minimum clinically relevant difference of 30 mmHg is expected between groups. A power of 90% and significance level of α=0.05 is specified. Variability can differ between groups and previous studies have demonstrated the data to be approximately normally distributed with the standard deviation (SD) of 20 mm Hg in the treatment arm and 40 mm Hg in the control arm.

What is an appropriate sample size estimate?

Information Provided:

Expected difference: $d = 30$
An acceptable level of significance: $\alpha = 0.05$
Power of the study: $1-\beta = 0.90$
SD in control group: $\sigma_2 = 40$
SD in treatment group: $\sigma_1 = 20$

Calculation by formula:

$Z_{1-\alpha/2} = 1.96$

$Z_{1-\beta} = 1.28$

$$n = (\sigma_1^2 + \sigma_2^2) \times \left(\frac{Z_{1-\alpha/2} + Z_{1-\beta}}{d}\right)^2$$

$$= \frac{(20^2 + 40^2) \times (1.96 + 1.28)^2}{30^2} = 23.33$$

$\approx$ 24 individuals per group

Total sample size = 2n = 48 individuals.

Determine a range of sample sizes: In order to determine an optimal sample size that is clinically relevant, cost efficient, feasible and sufficiently powered, it is important to consider a range of sample sizes under varying conditions. Table 21.2 presents sample sizes appropriate for various clinically meaningful mean differences between treatment and control arms based on example 1. Sample sizes are presented for experiments with a power of 70%, 80% and 90%. The standard deviation is 20 mmHg in the treatment group and 40 mmHg in the control group, $\alpha = 0.05$. The effects of power and mean difference on sample size are shown in Figure 21.1.

Figure 21.1 displays the relationship between power and mean difference (effect size) with sample size estimates. As the minimal clinically important difference increases, the required

Table 21.2: Sample size calculations for varying clinically meaningful differences and power

Details	Mean Difference	Total Sample Size (Power =70%)	Total Sample Size (Power =80%)	Total Sample Size (Power =90%)
SD in control group = 40 SD in treatment group = 20 An acceptable level of significance α = 0.05 Power = 70, 80%, 90% Range in mean differences = 10–50	50	14	16	20
	40	18	22	30
	30	30	38	50
	20	64	82	108
	15	112	142	190
	10	250	316	424

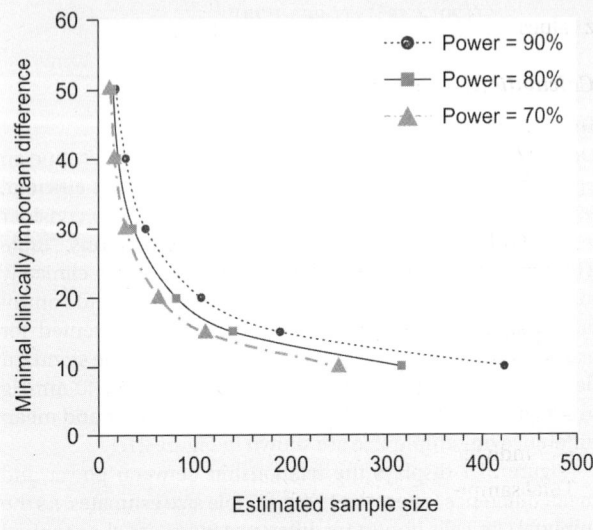

Fig. 21.1: Sample size estimations for varying clinically meaningful differences and power

sample size decreases. In contrast as power increases, sample size increases.

Application for Binary Outcome RCTs

Example 1: Calculating the difference between two proportions in a clinical superiority trial:

Suppose a 50% event rate is expected in the control group of an experiment and we are interested in an experiment with a clinically important difference of 25% reduction with the new treatment using a significance level of 0.05 and power of 0.90.

Information needed:

Expected difference:	$p_2 - p_1$	= 0.25
Level of significance:	α	= 0.05
Power of the study:	$1-\beta$	= 0.90
Proportion (control):	p_2	= 0.50
Proportion (treatment):	p_1	= 0.25
Average of expected rates:	$\bar{p}$	= $(0.5 + 0.25)/2$

z values:
$$= 0.375$$
$$z_{1-\alpha/2} = 1.96$$
$$z_{1-\beta} = 1.28$$

Calculation by Formula:

$$n = \frac{\left(z_{1-\alpha/2}\sqrt{2\overline{p}(1-\overline{p})}+z_{1-\beta}\sqrt{p_1(1-p_1)+p_2(1-p_2)}\right)^2}{d^2}$$

$$= \frac{\left(1.96\sqrt{2(0.375)(1-0.375)}+1.28\sqrt{0.25(0.75)+0.5(0.5)}\right)^2}{(0.25)^2}$$

$$= \frac{\left(1.96\sqrt{0.469}+1.28\sqrt{0.391}\right)^2}{(0.25)^2}$$

$$= 76.6$$

≈ 77 individuals per arm

Total sample size $= 2n = 2 \times 74 = 148$

Determine a range of sample sizes: Table 21.3 and Figure 21.2 present a range of sample sizes under varying conditions for the investigator to choose from. Sample sizes are presented for experiments with a power of 70%, 80% and 90% and a range in differences from 0.1 to 0.4. The effects of these variations on

Table 21.3: Sample size estimations for varying clinically meaningful differences in proportions and power

Details	Difference	Total Sample Size (Power =70%)	Total Sample Size (Power =80%)	Total Sample Size (Power =90%)
Proportion in control group=0.5 α=0.05 Power=70, 80%, 90% Range in differences = 0.1–0.4	0.4	32	40	52
	0.3	62	78	104
	0.25	92	116	154
	0.2	148	186	248
	0.1	610	776	1038

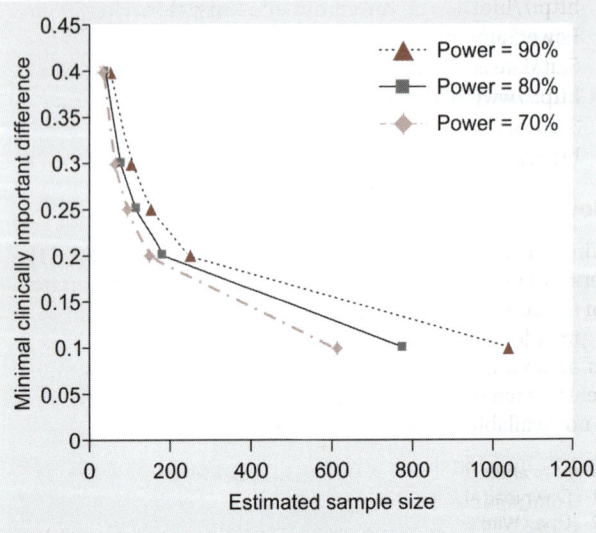

Fig. 21.2: Sample size estimations for varying clinically meaningful differences and power

Figure 21.2 depicts the influence of power and minimal clinically important difference in proportions on sample size estimations. As the minimum clinically important difference increases, the required sample size will reduce. As the power of a study increases, more subjects are required.

What Programs are Available for Sample Size Estimation?

Several computer programs and websites now exist to assist in sample size calculations, below is a list of other software available. Calculations between programs may vary slightly depending on the resource used due to rounding, formulas and continuity corrections embedded within formulas.

- WinPepi is available for free at:
  http://www.brixtonhealth.com/pepi4windows.html
- PS: Power and Sample Size Calculation software is available for free download at:

http://biostat.mc.vanderbilt.edu/twiki/bin/view/Main/PowerSampleSize
- StatMate is available for purchase at:
http://www.graphpad.com/scientific-software/statmate/
- StudySize is available for purchase at:
http://www.studysize.com/index.html

How do I Estimate Sample Size with WinPepi?

WinPepi is a free program available for downloading, with a series of user-friendly functions. The method and references for the derivations used to estimate sample sizes are provided. It provides details of its methods along with references in its manual if an investigator is interested in the derivations behind each sample size calculation. Please note that WinPepi is not available for Mac operating systems.

Steps to enter the sample size window in WinPepi:
1. Download and install WinPepi.
2. Open WinPepi and select the option **COMPARE2** under **OPEN A WinPepi PROGRAM**. The window will change.
3. Select **Sample size** in the menu bar.
4. Select the most suitable type of comparison for your study, enter the requested values and hit **Run** at the bottom.

For binary outcomes:
1. Open the sample size window in WinPepi.
2. Under the **Sample Size** tab of **COMPARE2**, select **Proportions (comparison)**.
3. Enter values for α and 1-β as a percent under **Significance level %** and **Power %** (e.g. Enter 5 for α=0.05 and 90 for 1-β=90%, respectively).
4. Enter 1 for **ratio of sample sizes B:A.**
5. Enter the proportion in A (new treatment) and B (standard treatment) (e.g. 0.25 and 0.2 respectively).
6. Note the other options also available to enhance the estimation.

For continuous outcomes:
1. Open the sample size window in WinPepi.
2. Under the **Sample Size** tab of **COMPARE2**, select **Means (comparison)**.
3. Enter values for α and 1-β as a percent under **Significance level %** and **Power %** (e.g. Enter 5 for α=0.05 and 90 for 1-β=90%, respectively).

Contd...

Contd...

4. Enter 1 for ***ratio of sample sizes B:A.***
5. Enter the standard deviation in ***A*** (new treatment) and ***B*** (standard treatment) under ***SD in A*** (e.g. 20) and ***SD in B*** (e.g. 20), respectively.
6. Enter the anticipated difference between the two under difference (e.g. 30)
7. Note the other options also available to enhance the estimation.

Other Considerations

Continuity Correction

For some software, a continuity correction factor is used to adjust the sample size estimations of dichotomous outcomes. For some software where the binomial distribution is approximated with a normal distribution, a sample size value is provided along with a continuity corrected sample size estimation. For software where the continuity factor is not used, the sample size can be expected to be smaller. Slight variations in sample size estimates can be expected between software. Consulting with a statistician will provide further clarity in what sample size estimate should be used.

Correction for Attrition

Sample size estimations are performed to determine the appropriate number of individuals required to maintain a level of significance and power when conducting analyses. Investigators who anticipate participant dropout to occur in the study must estimate this proportion to ensure they have an adequate number of individuals for their study. This proportion of subjects who do not complete the study can be accounted for in the sample size estimations using the following formula:

$$\text{Sample size adjusted for attrition} = (\text{sample size}) \times \frac{1}{1-(\text{proportion of dropouts})}$$

Categorical Outcomes

Multileveled categorical outcomes are often converted to dichotomous outcomes or assumed to be continuous for sample size estimations. To produce a dichotomous outcome, levels of the ordinal variable are grouped together based on either the skewed distribution of the variable or clinical rationale. To produce a continuous outcome, levels of the ordinal outcome are assumed to be values of a continuous variable. This is typically performed when outcomes have six or more levels or when averaging the values among each level makes sense.

Clustered Samples

Designs where individuals are sampled in groups and are often performed to improve the efficiency and cost-effectiveness of a study. Cluster RCTs are often used because the unit occurs naturally (e.g. children in a classroom, people in a village, both eyes on the same head, etc). The pitfall to clustered samples is the strong correlation of data from units within each cluster. This needs to be accounted for sample size estimations. For example, suppose RCTs enrolled patients from hospitals of five different countries, randomly allocating half of the patients to an intervention group and the other half to a standard therapy group. Patients from each country may share similar characteristics that result in responding to the treatment/service in a similar manner. The sample size depends on the correlation of the effect of the intervention among individuals within these clusters, often referred to as the intraclass correlation coefficient (ICC). Estimating this value can be based on previous studies or determined from a pilot study. It also depends on the number of clusters and the number of units within each cluster. There are many techniques when determining a sample size for a study that contains clustered samples; seeking assistance from a statistician is advised.[7]

Definitions

Power: The probability of rejecting a false null hypothesis. It is inversely proportional to Type II error (β).

Smallest effect size of interest: The difference between study groups that the investigator determines to be of scientific and clinical interest.

Type I error: Incorrect rejection of the null hypothesis and concluding that a relationship exists between two variables when in fact it does not. It is also known as a spurious result.

Type II error: Incorrect acceptance of the null hypothesis and concluding that no relationship exists between two variables when in fact it does.

Variability: The standard deviation of an outcome of interest within the study population.

REFERENCES

1. Bhandari M, Devereaux PJ, Einhorn TA, et al. Hip fracture evaluation with alternatives of total hip arthroplasty versus hemiarthroplasty (HEALTH): protocol for a multicentre randomized trial. BMJ Open. 2015;5(2):e006263.
2. Koea J, Baldwin P, Shen J, et al. Safety and Hemostatic Effectiveness of the Fibrin Pad for Severe Soft-Tissue Bleeding During Abdominal, Retroperitoneal, Pelvic and Thoracic (non-cardiac) Surgery: A Randomized, Controlled, Superiority Trial. World J Surg. 2015;39(11):2663-9.
3. Gomez-Barrena E, Ortega-Andreu M, Padilla-Eguiluz NG, et al. Topical intra-articular compared with intravenous tranexamic acid to reduce blood loss in primary total knee replacement: a double-blind, randomized, controlled, noninferiority clinical trial. J Bone Joint Surg Am. 2014;96(23):1937-44.
4. Parienti JJ, Thibon P, Heller R, et al. Hand-rubbing with an aqueous alcoholic solution vs traditional surgical hand-scrubbing and 30-day surgical site infection rates: A randomized equivalence study. JAMA. 2002;288(6):722-7.
5. Wittes J. Sample size calculations for randomized controlled trials. Epidemiol Rev. 2002;24(1):39-53.
6. Moore AD, Joseph L. Sample size considerations for superiority trials in systemic lupus erythematosus (SLE). Lupus. 1999;8(8):612-9.
7. Hulley SB, Cummings SR, Browner WS, Grady DG, Newman TB: Designing clinical research (Fourth Edition). Philadelphia, USA: Lippincott Williams & Wilkins; 2013.

Planning your Analysis— Keep it Simple

Kerry Tai, Kim Madden, Ashok Rajgopalan

Key Objectives

- Learn about different types of data and how to appropriately summarize this data with numbers and graphs
- Why, when and how to conduct different statistical tests with collected data
- Gain knowledge of hypothesis testing
- Recognize the difference between statistical significance vs clinical significance.

Types of Data

Data is the primary component of a statistical analysis. In order to properly describe relationship between sets of data, one must understand the basic characteristics of data. Understanding the type of data you are collecting is necessary in order to choose the correct type of data analysis to interpret your results. A set of data can be used to describe various characteristics of an observation and it comes in two general forms: categorical or continuous.[1] These types of data are described below:

Categorical Data

This is a type of data that consists of two or more categories. For example:
- Yes/No
- Male/Female
- Blunt/Penetrating/Burn
- Blood type A/B/AB/O

- Cancer stage I/II/III/IV.

Categorical data can be further divided into binary, nominal or ordinal data. **Binary data** is the simplest form of categorical data and is limited to only two categories, for example yes/no or male/female. **Nominal data** are observations that fit into categories with no inherent scale, for example blunt/penetrating/burn or blood type A/B/AB/O are two examples of data that lack a natural ordering or progression from one to the next category. **Ordinal data** are categories that have some meaningful order, but have no definitive amount, for example cancer stages I/II/III/IV have an obvious ordering and progression of categories.[1]

Continuous Data

This type of data, as implied by its name, can be obtained from a continuum or a continuous scale and can take on any value and can be reported to as many decimal places as the measuring device will allow.[1] For example:

- Age
- Temperature
- Height
- Weight.

Continuous data can be further divided into interval or ratio data. **Interval data** are similar to ordinal data where there is an inherent order, but the differences between values on the scale are consistent. There is also no true zero with interval data. For example, the difference between 25°C and 20°C is 5°C, as is the same between 10°C and 5°C. While we do have 0°C in temperature measurements, there is no clear definition of zero as 0°C and it does not mean that there is 'no temperature/no heat'.

Ratio data have an order, consistent values between the units and a true zero. For example, an individual can be 0 to 100+ years old and each number is separated by the same proportion, a year. Age is considered to be ratio data as person can truly have an age of 0.[1]

Descriptive Statistics

To make the message more meaningful and clear which can be easily understood by readers, it is essential to condense the information in a large dataset. Descriptive statistics can be used to describe and summarize the information collected in a meaningful way. This is an important way to present data to allow simple interpretation. Descriptive statistics can only be used to describe data, it does not allow us to make conclusions regarding any hypothesis that may have been made.[2]

Common ways to describe the data include providing information on the magnitude and variability of the data. Continuous data are typically described with ***measures of central tendency***, while categorical data are usually expressed ***as percentages or proportions***.[2]

The most common and well known measure of central tendency is the ***mean*** which is mathematical average of all data. The mean is equal to the sum of all the values in the dataset divided by the number of values in the set. Another common measure of central tendency is the ***median*** which is the middle value for the set that has been arranged in the order of magnitude, whereby half the data lies below and half the data lies above. Lastly, the ***mode*** is the most frequent value encountered in the dataset.[2] For example, using the dataset 8, 2, 5, 1, 6, 4, 3, 5, 3, 3, 15. The mean is 5, the median is 4 and the mode is 3.

Variability for continuous data can be reported using the ***standard deviation*** to describe the variation or spread of data within the dataset. The standard deviation is the average difference between each value in the set and the cumulative mean. If the data points are very close to the mean, the standard deviation will be close to 0, whereas if the data points are spread out over a wide range of values, the standard deviation will be higher. Using the standard deviation, one can tell if the data distribution is normal or bell curved. If the distribution is normal or bell curved we can assume what percentage of data points lie between each standard deviation. Following this distribution, approximately 68% of values are between ±1 standard deviation, 95% between ±2 standard deviations and 99.7% between ±3 standard deviations (Fig. 22.1).[2]

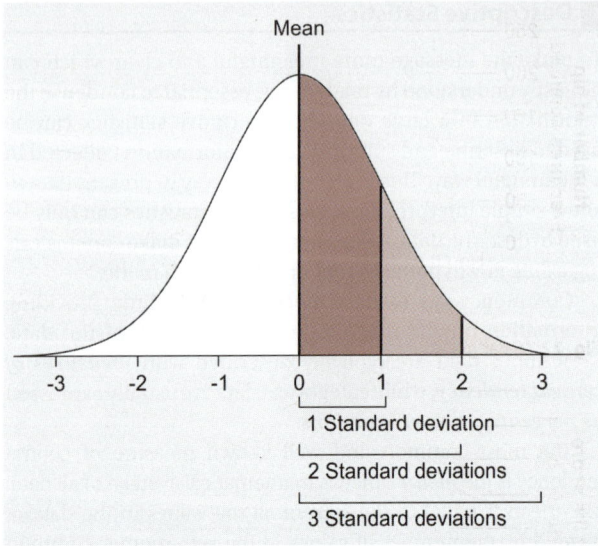

Fig. 22.1: A normal distribution showing mean and standard deviations

Presenting Your Data

We can describe data quantitatively, as described above, but we can also aim to provide a graphical summary of the data. Depending on the type of data and message one is trying to communicate, different types of graphs can be used. When you have a continuous dependent variable and a categorical independent variable such as the number of hip fractures admitted (continuous) to four different hospitals (categorical), a bar graph or column graph would work best as you can visualize the different categories easily. (Fig. 22.2) When you have a continuous dependent variable and a continuous independent variable such as health related quality of life (continuous) or over time (continuous), a line graph would work best to present the data (Fig. 22.3). To show several groups with proportions or percentages that add to 100% such as proportion of surgeons preferring different irrigating solutions for open fractures,[3] you can use a pie graph (Fig. 22.4)[1].

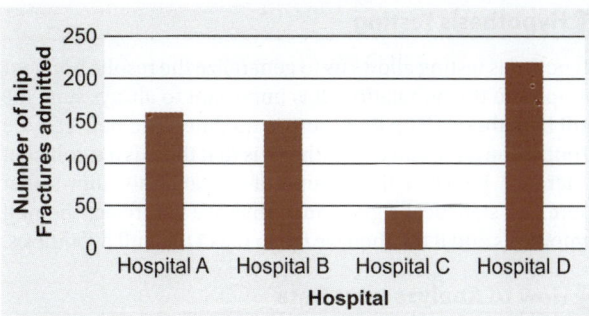

Fig. 22.2: Bar graph

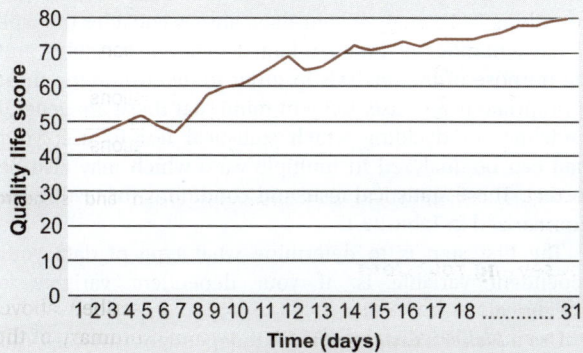

Fig. 22.3: Line graph

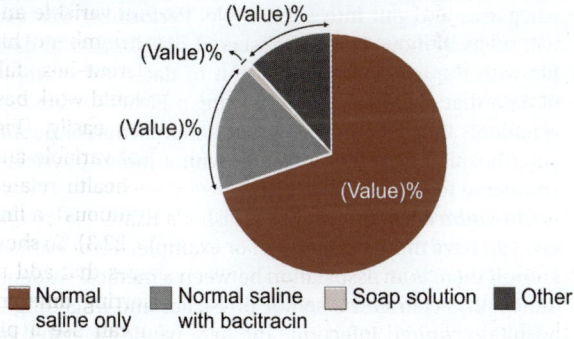

Fig. 22.4: Pie graph

Hypothesis Testing

Hypothesis testing allows us to generalize the results from our samples to the population. It is important to always state the null hypothesis (H0); that there is no difference between the groups. The alternative hypothesis is that there is a significant difference between the groups. If the analysis shows that there is a statistical significance then we can reject the null hypothesis and if not then we fail to reject the null hypothesis.

How to Analyze your Data

To find differences between groups or to determine associations one needs to analyze the data beyond just describing it. To analyze your data, always consider the type of data, number of independent/dependent variables and the purpose of the analysis in order to determine the most appropriate test to use. Keep in mind that these are general guidelines in deciding which statistical test to use; your data can be analyzed in multiple ways which may also be correct. These statistical tests and conditions for testing are summarized in Table 22.1.

The first step is to determine what type of data your dependent variable is. If your dependent variable is categorical.

- Use a ***Fisher's exact*** test if the independent variables and dependent variables are both binary. In order to perform this test, the data must be counted and divided into categories and put into a 2x2 table. Performing this test will measure how well the observed distribution of data fits with the expected distribution of data.[4] An example of data that could be analyzed using a Fisher's exact test is patients that get a hospital-acquired infection or do not get a hospital-acquired infection with a junior physician compared to a senior physician.
- A ***Chi-square*** test is a lot like a Fisher's Exact test except you can have more categories. For example, if you want to know if there is an association between a medical student, junior physician and a senior physician and in getting a hospital-acquired infection. The data would be stated in 2x3 table and cannot be done with a Fisher's Exact test.

Planning your Analysis—Keep it Simple

Table 22.1: Common statistical tests and conditions for testing

If Your dependent variable(s) (DV) is...	And your independent variable(s) (IV) is/are...	Then perform this statistical test
Binary	1 categorical IV with 2 categories	Fisher's Exact*
	Multiple IVs of any data type	Logistic Regression**
Categorical with 2 or more categories	1 categorical IV with 2 or more categories	Chi-square
Continuous and normally distributed	1 categorical IV with 2 categories	Independent t-Test
	1 categorical IV with 2 categories and paired data	Paired t-Test (or dependent t-Test)
	1 categorical IV with more than 2 categories	Analysis of variance (ANOVA)
	2 categorical IVs with multiple levels	Two-way ANOVA
	1 continuous IV	Correlation
	Multiple IVs of any data type	Linear regression
Continuous but not normally distributed	1 categorical IV with 2 categories	Mann-Whitney U
	1 categorical IV with 2 categories and paired data	Wilcoxon Matched Pairs
Continuous time-to-event	Multiple IVs of any data type	Survival analysis

*Fisher's exact test is also used when 2x2 chi-square analysis have too few expected events in one or more cells.
**There are more complex types of logistic regression for non-binary categorical DVs.

- ***Logistic regression*** can be used when you have more than one independent variable. Regression analysis adjust other variables that you are interested in. For example, if you want to determine if there is a significant association between getting a hospital-acquired infection with a junior or senior physician and you also want to take into account the patient's age, gender and other comorbidities.

If your dependent variable is continuous

- You can use the *t-Test* to determine whether or not there is a significant difference between the means of the two different groups.[4] For example, comparing the mean amount of time for a fracture to completely heal in an inpatient setting vs outpatient setting. If your dependent variable is not normally distributed, use a Mann-Whitney U test. If you have paired data you should use the **Paired t-Test**. For example, if you want to see if there is a difference in the mean test scores of the same group of surgical residents before course and after a course. If your data is paired and the dependent variable is not normally distributed, use Wilcoxon matched pairs instead.
- If your independent variable is categorical (three or more groups) and your dependent variable is continuous, you can use analysis of variance (ANOVA) to determine whether or not there is a significant difference between the means of the three or more independent groups. The ANOVA test can tell us if at least two groups were different from each other, but it cannot tell us which specific groups were different.[4] For example, comparing mean operations times between three different surgical techniques in a cohort of patients with a fractured hip–internal fixation, hemiarthroplasty and total hip arthroplasty. Additionally, if your groups have been split in two independent factors, you can perform a two-way ANOVA to determine if there is an interaction between the two factors and the dependent variable.[4] For example, we can compare the mean operations times of the three different surgical techniques (internal fixation, hemiarthroplasty, and total hip arthroplasty), but between surgical residents and surgical fellows.
- When dealing with two continuous variables, you can use a ***correlation analysis***. Usually the value that is calculated is called the ***R-squared value*** and can be used

to determine if a correlation exists or not. An R-squared value can range from 0 to 1 with a value of 0 meaning no correlation and 1 meaning that the two variables are completely correlated. A positive correlation indicates that the variables increase and decrease in parallel. A negative correlation indicates that when one variable increases the other variable will decrease.[2] For example, you can determine if there is a correlation between length of a surgical procedure and amount of patient-controlled analgesia used postoperatively.
- ***Linear regression*** is like logistic regression but is usually used when the dependent variable is continuous. For example, you can look at the association between amount of patient-controlled analgesia used post-operatively and length of a surgical procedure while taking into account the patient's age, gender and comorbidities.
- *Survival analysis* like Cox proportional hazards regression, is a more complicated type of regression analysis when your dependent variable is a time to a particular event. You need to know whether the patient had the event of interest and how long after baseline that the event occurred. For example, you can use survival analysis to analyze the death time in patients with metastatic bone disease while taking into account the type of treatment they received.

Statistical Significance vs Clinical Significance

It is important to note that even if the results of a statistical test indicate that the findings are statistically significant, it may not necessarily indicate that the results are also clinically significant or meaningful. The ***effect size*** can be very small even if the results are statistically significant, especially if a study has a large sample size. ***Cohen's d*** is a common measure of effect size that can be calculated with the following formula:

$$d = \frac{\text{sample mean 1} - \text{sample mean 2}}{\text{Pooled standard deviation}}[5]$$

It is always important to use clinical judgment as well as sound statistical knowledge when recommending a change in practice based on study results.

Definitions

Analysis of variance (ANOVA): A statistical test to determine if there are any differences between the means of three or more groups.

Binary data: Data which can only be classified as two categories like yes/no.

Cohen's d: A common measure of effect size that is the difference between two means divided by the standard deviation.

Correlation: The degree by which two continuous variables vary together.

Effect size: The magnitude of strength of an association.

Fisher's exact test and ***Chi-square (χ^2) test:*** Statistical tests that determine how expected proportions compare to observed proportions.

Interval data: Interval data is classified into categories where there is order, the exact differences are known, but there is no true zero.

Linear regression: A statistical analysis to predict a continuous dependent variable based on one or more independent variables.

Logistic regression: A statistical analysis to predict a binary dependent variable based on one or more independent variables.

Mean: The sum of values divided by the number of values in the dataset.

Measure of central tendency: Measure that describes the central position of the data set using a single value.

Median: Is the number in a data set that falls in the middle so that half of the values lie above and half below this number.

Mode: The value that occurs most frequently in a dataset.

Nominal data: Nominal data is classified into categories, but does not have an inherent order or scale.

Ordinal data: Ordinal data is classified into categories and has an inherent order.

Paired t-Test: A statistical test to determine if there is a difference between two means using paired data.

Ratio data: Ratio data is continuous data that has order, a meaningful scale and there is a true zero.

Standard deviation: The standard deviation is the average difference between each value in the set and the cumulative mean.

Survival analysis: A statistical analysis to predict the time to an event based on one or more independent variables.

t-Test: A statistical test to determine if there is a difference between two means.

REFERNCES

1. Bhandari M, Joensson A. Clinical Research for Surgeons. Stuttgart: Thieme, New York. 2009.
2. Bhandari M, Sancheti P. Clinical Research Made Easy–A guide to publishing in medical literature. Jaypee Brothers Medical Publishers (P) Ltd. Indian J Orthop. 2010;44(3):356.
3. Petrisor B, Jeray K, Schemitsch E, et al. FLOW Investigators. Fluid lavage in patients with open fracture wounds (FLOW): an international survey of 984 surgeons. BMC Musculoskelet Disord. 2008;9:7.
4. Norman GR, Streiner DL. Biostatistics: The Bare Essentials. 2008, B.C. Decker, Hamilton.
5. Cohen J. Statistical Power Analysis for the Behavioral Sciences (second ed.). (1988). Lawrence Erlbaum Associates.

What are Subgroup Analyses and How should You Interpret Them?

Erika Arseneau, Jean-Eric Tarride

Key Objectives

- Understand what subgroup analysis is and when it is used
- Be able to recognize characteristics of a well-designed subgroup analysis
- Learn how to interpret and apply results of subgroup analyses.

What is a Subgroup Analyses?

Once a clinical trial has been performed and the effect of a certain intervention has been discerned, it may be of interest to determine whether the intervention is more or less effective in certain subsets of the population. To investigate this, a ***subgroup analysis*** can be performed.

S***ubgroups*** are populations within the study sample that can be categorized by some sort of differential quality—ideally a baseline characteristic (e.g. sex, age, severity of disease, time of drug administration, etc.).[1] Subgroup analyses estimate treatment effects within specified subgroups to identify any differences. If conducted appropriately, the results of a subgroup analysis can guide clinical decision making and improve patient care by identifying which patients will benefit most or be harmed most from a particular treatment.[2] Unfortunately many of these analyses are not performed according to recommended guidelines and have a reputation for creating falsely positive results.[3]

What does a Well-designed Subgroup Analysis Consist of?

A Sound Rationale

The goal of a subgroup analysis should be in keeping with the intentions of the trial at hand and have a sound clinical basis.[4] A strong rationale considers the clinical applicability and practical utility of the subgroup analysis.[4] Can the results be applied to common patient populations (i.e. various demographics or comorbidities)? If the intervention is of rare use or the populations to which it is applied are very small, a subgroup analysis will lack practical utility.[3]

The justification for a subgroup analysis is greatly strengthened by the use of external evidence. This evidence may be the result of a past clinical trial indicating a possible difference in treatment effect between subgroups or may be guided by clinical experience.[5]

A Priori Hypothesis(es)

The hypothesis(es) generated and wanting to be tested in subgroup analysis should be stated at the beginning of the study (*a priori*).

Details of the hypothesis should also be given at the beginning of the study and included in the study protocol. This includes a clear definition of the characteristics that will define the subgroups, the direction of the expected subgroup effect and an estimated size of the subgroup effect.[4] Unfortunately many studies often fail to report some or all of these data.[6] In fact it was reported by a large research consortium known as DISCO, that as few as 6.7% of 252 articles published between 2000 and 2003 provided an *a priori hypothesis* for their subgroup analysis.[2]

A Small Number of a Priori Hypotheses

Many investigators will look for differences in large numbers of subgroups.[7] However, subgroup analysis should only be used to answer a minimal number of questions. Increasing the number of tests performed within a subgroup analysis inherently increases the chance of finding a falsely positive result.[4] The presence of a false positive is also known as a ***Type I error.***[8]

Sufficient Power to Discern Between Group Effects

Clinical trials are often designed to be just large enough to find an overall treatment effect, typically with ~80% ***power.***[4] Subgroups of trial populations are thus inherently much smaller in sample size and are frequently underpowered to detect between group effects.[1] This increases the probability of concluding that there are no subgroups differences when in fact there may be some differences, also known as a ***Type II error.***[8] Considering possible subgroup analysis prior to the beginning of a trial, will help in sample size calculations which can account for possible between group effects and power the trial appropriately. Of course, increasing trial size is not done without an associated cost.

Subgroups are Defined Based on Pretrial Characteristics

Subgroups should never be defined on a variable that is affected by the treatment.[4] They should only be defined based on disease characteristics obtained before randomization or individual patient characteristics such as age or sex. Subgroups that are defined based on outcome driven data can result in biased or invalid conclusions.[5]

Why do Subgroup Analyses have Such a Bad Reputation?

Subgroup analyses are often criticized for their use of ***post-hoc analysis*** and their tendency to create ***spurious results***.

What is Post-hoc Analysis and why is it Criticized?

Post-hoc analysis occurs when a hypothesis is generated after study completion. These hypotheses are generally seen as unreliable and biased because they are generated from data rather than being tested by the data. Sometimes you will hear this being referred to as '***data-dredging***'.[9] In addition, subgrouping the population after study completion runs the risk of having unbalanced treatment assignments between groups, which would completely invalidate the process of ***randomization***.[4] Similarly, categorizing patients based on factors that have emerged after treatment may show statistically significant differences, that only occur because one subgroup had a better prognosis than the other, rather than because the intervention actually had an effect.[5]

Consider for instance that you are interested in investigating whether compliance is a predictive factor for effectiveness of a given treatment. To investigate this, you categorize patients into two groups (<80% compliance and ≥80% compliance) and assess the effect of the treatment on both groups. The analysis shows that the ≥80% compliance subgroup benefits from the intervention more than the <80% compliance subgroup. Upon closer examination you realize that patients who were very compliant with their medication were also younger, had fewer baseline symptoms and were of a higher income bracket. Now the question arises, did the compliant group benefit from the intervention more because of the treatment or because they had a better prognosis?

To circumvent some of these issues, a technique can be considered during trial design known as ***stratified randomization***. This technique consists of stratifying the population by the variable of interest and then performing randomization. Stratified randomization would ensure that baseline characteristics are consistent across the treatment groups and that the treatment allocation is balanced between subgroups.[8]

Are all Post-hoc Subgroup Analyses Bad?

No. Although alone they can be considered unreliable, post-hoc subgroup analysis can often give rise to new questions that can be answered in future clinical trials. If numerous other studies have consistently reported similar subgroup effects, this may provide enough evidence to guide some clinical decision making.[10]

What is a Spurious Result and why are they so Common Among Subgroup Analyses?

A spurious result occurs when a relationship is reported to be significant when in fact it is not. This is otherwise known as a false positive or Type I error.[8] These can occur when researchers try to make multiple comparisons simultaneously, which is the case with many subgroup analyses. This phenomenon is statistically known as the problem of ***multiplicity*** or multiple testing. It is based on the fact that if you perform multiple tests at the same time, you inherently increase the probability that you will eventually find a statistically significant result, even if there are none to be found.[4]

Consider the following:

Testing 1 hypothesis:

p(at least 1 significant result) = 1−p (no significant results)
$$= 1-(1-0.05)$$
$$= 0.05$$

Therefore there is a 5% chance of observing a significant result even if there are none.

This is called the Type I error rate.

Testing 20 hypotheses:

p(at least 1 significant result) = 1−p (no significant results)^{20}
$$= 1-(1-0.05)^{20}$$
$$= 0.64$$

Therefore there is a 64% chance of observing a significant result even if there are none. The Type I error rate is 59% higher when testing 20 hypotheses than it would be if you were testing just one.

There are various statistical corrections that can be made to accommodate multiple testing but in practice they are rarely used.[5] Statistical corrections lower the critical p-value to neutralize the risk of Type I error. The most common type is known as the ***Bonferroni correction.***[4] Using the Bonferonni correction, the p-value is adjusted to α/n; where α is the critical value and n is the number of hypothesis being tested. Using the example above, statistical significance would be granted to test results with p<0.0025 (0.05/20).

A Classic Example of Subgroup Analysis Gone Wrong

To demonstrate the pitfalls of a poorly executed subgroup analysis, researchers from the International Study of Infarct Survival 2 (ISIS-2) categorized the study population by their astrological sign. They found that aspirin had a beneficial effect on mortality overall but it had a slightly adverse effect for the astrological signs Gemini and Libra.[11] Clearly this conclusion lacks any credible biological reasoning (or *biological plausibility)*. In fact it was meant to highlight that testing 12 different zodiac signs results in an increase in Type I error and is meant to be a warning for researchers to avoid the consequences of multiple testing.

This warning is not without merit. Many examples have been found throughout the literature on subgroup analysis that have been proven false. For instance the conclusions that antihypertensive treatment for primary prevention is ineffective in women or that thrombolysis is ineffective >6 hours after acute myocardial infarction have both been consistently refuted.[3]

How are Subgroup Analyses Performed?

To determine if a subgroup effect exists, it is not important to test whether the treatment is efficacious in each subgroup separately (which can be done using methods similar to the main analysis, e.g. t-test, Chi-square, etc.) rather it is imperative to test and see whether the treatment effect differs between subgroups.[4] Statistically this is known as a test for *interaction*. Usually this procedure is performed using a statistical test known as *regression*. If an interaction effect exists, this indicates that the efficacy of the treatment differs between subgroups.[3]

Subgroup effects can either be considered a *quantitative* or a *qualitative interaction.* A quantitative interaction occurs when the intervention is beneficial or harmful to all subgroups but the magnitude of the effect varies between subgroups (e.g. intervention has greater benefit in women than men). A qualitative interaction occurs when the intervention is beneficial for some subgroups and harmful to others (e.g. intervention results in a 3 years increase of survival for men and 1 year increase in mortality for women).[1] Quantitative interactions are known to be more common than qualitative interactions.

How are Subgroup Analyses Reported?

In addition to providing details on study design, studies should indicate details of how and why subgroups were selected along with the number and type of post-hoc/a priori hypotheses.[9] Multiplicity should be addressed and any statistical corrections made to compensate for this multiple testing should be described. Studies should also report whether any prognostic factor imbalances are present, even if they used the stratified randomization approach.[3]

Subgroup effects should be reported as a ***relative risk*** measure rather than an ***absolute risk*** measure.[4,5] Absolute risk is the difference in overall risk for being on the intervention versus off. Relative risk is an estimate of the proportion of risk that is removed by the treatment and is a relative measure between subgroups.[8] In general relative risks usually remain consistent across subgroups, whereas absolute risk does not. Therefore, to identify a true subgroup effect relative risk is the preferred measure.[5]

Finally, the findings that should be emphasized during reporting of a clinical trial is the overall treatment effect not the subgroup analysis results. Subgroup analysis findings should be reported and indicated, especially if it is a new finding, that the results need to be replicated or investigated in future studies.

Guidelines for Interpretation and Application of Subgroup Analysis

When evaluating subgroup analysis for clinical use, you should first examine the design of the study. Does the subgroup analysis contain the characteristics of a methodologically sound subgroup analysis? For instance, does the study include a statement of the rationale for the subgroup analysis, provide a small number of a priori hypotheses and perform the analysis based on pretrial characteristics?

Second you should consider the magnitude of the subgroup effect. If the magnitude of the difference is high, there is an increase in the likelihood that the finding is true and not a spurious result.[3]

Claims of a subgroup effect are more credible if pretrial biological studies or similar interventions support the findings.[5] This is why it is also especially important that results of subgroup analysis be considered in the context of biological plausibility.[6] Is the result consistent with our current understanding of biology?

Along similar lines it is important to consider whether the results have been repeated by other studies. If so, this may add credibility to the findings.[3]

Lastly, it is important to consider how the results of the subgroup analysis apply to the patients you are treating. Clinical trials almost always vary in their design, population, intervention and outcome. They also have very strict inclusion and exclusion criteria so it may be unlikely that the patients included in the study are comparable to your own.[3]

Below are a set of questions you should ask yourself when interpreting and applying the results of a subgroup analysis:[3]
- Can chance explain the subgroup effect?
- Is the subgroup effect consistent across studies?
- Was the subgroup hypothesis one of a small number of hypothesis developed a priori with a direction specified?
- Was the magnitude of the subgroup effect large?
- Is there strong pre-existing biological support for the subgroup effect?
- Are the characteristics of the subgroup population similar to that of my patient?

Can you Compare Results of Subgroup Analyses from Different Studies?

That depends. If you are using the results of subgroup analysis from various studies to guide future research, a qualitative evaluation can be used to examine trends found across studies. If however, you are using the results of multiple studies to guide patient care you have to be very careful when examining their applicability.[9] A common aid in this process is known as a ***meta-analysis*** which summarizes the results of many studies and pools them to provide an overall estimate of the effect.[5]

Definitions

Absolute risk: The overall risk difference between receiving an intervention versus not.

A priori hypothesis: A hypothesis generated before the research study takes place.

Biological plausibility: The proposal of a causal relationship that is consistent with existing biological and medical knowledge.

Bonferroni correction: A statistical method used to correct the consequences of multiple testing or multiplicity.

Data-dredging: The use of data mining to identify statistically significant results within a dataset that only occur by chance.

Interaction: A statistical test used to determine whether treatment effects differ across subgroups.

Meta-analysis: Statistically combining quantitative data from several studies to yield a single pooled summary estimate.

Multiplicity: The act of testing multiple hypothesis simultaneously. Also referred to as multiple testing.

Post-hoc analysis: The act of creating and testing hypothesis after the research study has been conducted.

Power (1-β): The probability of rejecting a false null hypothesis. It is inversely proportional to Type II error (β).

Qualitative interaction: The treatment effect is beneficial to one subgroup and harmful to another.

Quantitative interaction: The treatment effect is beneficial or harmful to all subgroups but the magnitude of the effect is different across subgroups.

Randomization: Allocation of participants to groups under comparison by random chance.

Regression: A statistical method used to determine whether relationships exist between specified variables.

Relative risk: The ratio of the risk of disease in exposed individuals to the risk of disease in non-exposed individuals.

Spurious result: A wrongful inference suggesting two events or variables have a causal relationship, when in fact they do not.

Stratified randomization: The act of subgrouping a patient population based on a certain variable prior to randomly allocating them to a treatment group.

Subgroup: A population within the study sample that can be categorized by some sort of differential quality—ideally a baseline characteristic.

Subgroup analysis: Act of comparing treatment effects between subgroups to identify any differences.

Type I error: Incorrect rejection of the null hypothesis and concluding a relationship exists between two variables when in fact it does not.

Type II error: Incorrect acceptance of the null hypothesis and concluding no relationship exists between two variables when in fact it does.

REFERENCES

1. Yusuf S, Wittes J, Probstfield J, et al. Analysis and interpretation of treatment effects in subgroups of patients in randomized clinical trials. JAMA. 1991;266(1):93-8.
2. Group DS. Subgroup analyses in randomized controlled trials: cohort study on trial protocols and journal publications. BMJ. 2014;349:g4539.
3. Bhandari M, Robioneck B. Advanced Concepts in Surgical Research (First). New York: Thieme.2012
4. Dijkman, B. (2009). How to Work with Subgroup Analysis: Users' Guide To the Surgical Literature, 52(6), 515–522.
5. Sun X, Ioannidis JP, Agoritsas T, et al. How to use a subgroup analysis:users' guide to the medical literature. JAMA. 2014;311(4):405-11.
6. Wang R, Lagakos SW, Ware JH, et al. Statistics in medicine—reporting of subgroup analyses in clinical trials. N Engl J Med. 2007;357(21):2189-94.
7. Guyatt G, Drummond R, Maureen M, et al. Users' guides to the medical literature: a manual for evidence-based medicine (Second). McGraw Hill. 2002.

8. Gordis L (2009). Epidemiology (Fourth). Philidelphia, PA: Saunders Elsevier.
9. Oxman AD, Guyatt GH. A consumer's guide to subgroup analyses. Ann Intern Med. 1992;116(1):78-84.
10. Rothwell PM. Treating individuals 2. Subgroup analysis in randomized controlled trials: importance, indications and interpretation. Lancet. 2005;365(9454):176-86.
11. Randomized trial of intravenous streptokinase, oral aspirin, both, or neither among 17, 187 cases of suspected acute myocardial infarction: ISIS-2. ISIS-2 (Second International Study of Infarct Survival) Collaborative Group. Lancet. 1988;2(8607):349-60.

5

Doing Research

Section Outline

24. Study Roles—Who does What?
25. Research Ethics Approval—A Must Before any Clinical Trial
26. Why do we Need Patient Consent? Designing a Good Consent Form
27. Collecting Data—it all Begins with a Good Data Form

24. Study Roles— Who does What?

Mark Gichuru, M Borate

Key Objectives

- Understand the roles of a principal investigator
- Understand the delegation of responsibilities of a principal investigator
- Understand the roles of a research coordinator
- Understand the roles of a clinical research associate
- Understand the roles of a clinical research nurse
- Understand what education and experiences are required for each role.

What are the Roles of a Principal Investigator?

The *principal investigator (PI)*, also known as the clinical investigator, is ultimately responsible for the conduct of a *clinical trial*, ensuring that the research is fair, sound and equitable to study participants.[1] The PI is responsible for overseeing the design of the study *protocol* (if the PI is the sponsor), deciding which clinical trials to conduct, the ongoing performance of the study and any conclusions drawn upon the completion of the trial.[1] If the PI is conducting clinical research with an investigational agent (drug or biologic), it is their responsibility to comply with all applicable rules and regulations according to the local regulatory agency.

The PI is also responsible for drug accountability, which includes supervising the proper handling, administration, storage and destruction of investigational agents.[1] Drug accountability ensures the safe and proper use of investigational products and thus, are a significant components of audits conducted by either the local regulatory agency or any sponsor.[1] Principal investigator should continuously be involved in this aspect of conducting their clinical trials, if responsibilities are delegated to another study member. The PI is also responsible for the monitoring and reporting of *adverse events (AEs)*.[1] If drug accountability is delegated to other study personnel, the PI should remain aware of AEs because they may trigger the need for a dose adjustment or medical device review. Data collection and documentation of all study-related matters should be assigned to a qualified individual and should communicate with the PI.

How does the Principal Investigator Delegate their Responsibilities in a Clinical Trial?

The PI and any co-investigators are the lead in the clinical research team (Flowchart 24.1). The PI delegates specific tasks to study personnel to assist in running the clinical trials effectively. One way to ensure effective communication between PI and staff is to generate a delegation log, which is a signed record of which study-related tasks have been assigned to which individual.

According to FDA regulation 21 Code of Federal Regulations 312.3:[4] 'In the event an investigation is conducted by a team of individuals, the investigator is the

Flowchart 24.1: Members within a clinical research team

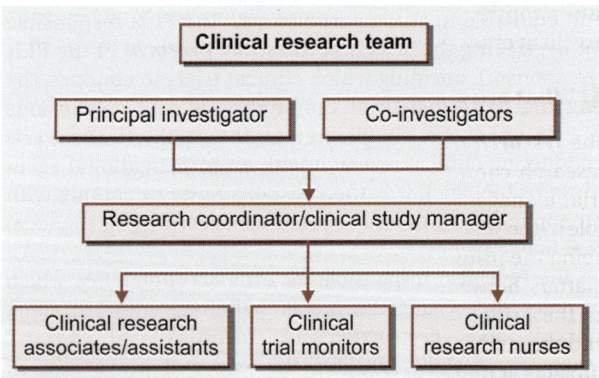

responsible leader of the team. 'Sub-investigator' includes any other member of that team.'

The FDA goes further to clarify that sub-investigator includes any individual that make direct/significant contributions to the data or perform study-related procedures.[4] In general, if an individual is directly involved in the performance of procedures required by the protocol and the collection of data, that person should be included on the delegation log.

In this way, the PI delegates some of their responsibilities onto other members that the PI determines capable of ensuring running of the clinical trial efficiently. However, the PI remains ultimately responsible for all study-related activities conducted by the study personnel.

What do I Need to Become a Principal Investigator?

A PI is typically a physician with a medical degree or a dentist in case of dental studies. Someone with a doctor of pharmacy (Pharm D) or a doctor of philosophy (PhD) may be a PI if the study is non-interventional or if the intervention is not a medical act or if a physician is a co-investigator. This individual has substantial expertise in their field that is related to the project and protocol and a strong research background (5–10 years of experience). This individual will have strong leadership skills and ability to work independently and supervise people in order to manage multiple projects and priorities. They must also be highly self-motived, have excellent organization oral and written communication skills.

What are the Roles of the Research Coordinator?

The *research coordinator (RC)* also known as the clinical research coordinator, clinical trial coordinator or clinical trial manager, is often considered having the most crucial role in the successful execution of a clinical trial.[5] Along with being the primary contact for the majority of study-related matters between several different audiences, the RC acts as the bridge between sponsor/pharmaceutical company and the study subjects.[6] The RC may interact with the study subjects acting as primary contact during the course of the

Flowchart 24.2: Responsibilities of the research coordinator

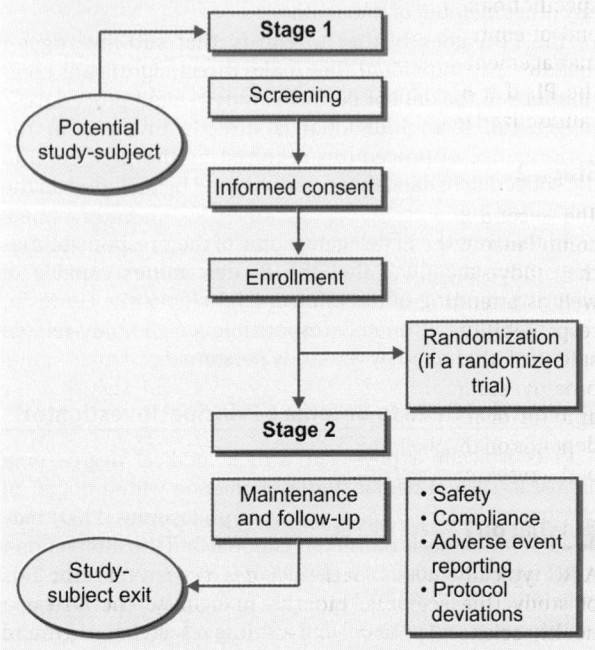

study and relay study-specific information to the clinical research team, PI and/or sponsors.[7] The RC's responsibilities are split into two distinct stages—screening/enrolling and maintenance (Flowchart 24.2).

Stage 1

The first stage includes recruiting, screening and enrolling patient-subjects into a clinical trial, along with the management of all applicable regulatory documents such as ***Research Ethics Board (REB)***, ***Institutional Review Board (IRB) or Ethics Committee (EC)*** submissions and regulatory applications.[5] During these processes, the RC visits the study-subjects and discusses the clinical study, walking them through the ***Informed Consent Form (ICF)*** and answering any study-related questions.[5] Depending on the clinical trial, the RC may be responsible for overseeing specific financial aspects of the study, including the financial end of contract negotiation and fee collection.[5] Financial management of the clinical trial is the responsibility of the PI. If it is a randomized study, the patients are then randomized to their intervention group.[5]

Stage 2

The second stage of a RC's role is maintaining patient compliance within the study. This involves ensuring that the study-subjects are taking the study intervention as well as attending all scheduled follow-up visits.[5] It is the responsibility of the RC to follow protocol and ensure the safety of the study-subjects. Although these two stages broadly summarize the responsibilities of the RC, the amount of responsibility the RC has on the trial largely depends on the responsibilities of the PI and other members of the research team.

What do I Need to Become a Research Coordinator?

A RC typically holds a bachelor's degree in a relevant field of study (life sciences, biology, pharmacy, chemistry or health sciences), along with at least 2 years of related work experience in the pharmaceutical industry/CRO environment or a research setting. A master's degree is often preferred or a certification in clinical research coordination. A RC must have exceptional time management skills, oral and written communication skills and a sound knowledge of clinical research and applicable regulatory guidelines.

What are the Roles of the Clinical Trial Monitor?

A ***clinical trial monitor (CTM)*** is involved in all stages of a clinical trial. A CTM may work directly for a pharmaceutical company, a ***contract research organization (CRO)***, in academia or freelance their skills independently.[8] Clinical trial monitors work is either full-time or part time and in the field (home-based) or at the office of their employment/at the investigational site. They are accountable for numerous responsibilities, such as study start-up activities, site monitoring and study close-out activities. More specifically, these roles/responsibilities may include:[8]

- Investigator identification and selection
- Clinical trial site selection
- Protocol and case report form (CRF) development
- Ensure trials abide by ***International Conference on Harmonization of Good Clinical Practice (ICH-GCP)***
- Guidelines for the safety of human participants
- Collect and process necessary regulatory documents from investigational sites
- Train site staff on the trial specific and industry standards
- Coordinate investigator meetings
- Prepare presentations and manuscripts for publication.

A CTM will often work with a sponsor for approximately 1-2 years on a small number of clinical trials.

What do I Need to Become a Clinical Research Associate/Assistant?

Similar to the RC, most clinical research associate (CRA) positions require a minimum a bachelor's degree in life sciences, biology, pharmacy, chemistry, health sciences or a related scientific field. A nursing degree or qualification may be required depending on the clinical trial/investigational product. Some employers may require a certification in clinical research. Most pharmaceutical companies/CROs require a minimum of 1-2 years of monitoring experience or regulatory experience in a related field. Clinical Research associates must demonstrate knowledge of ICH-GCP and local regulations, project management skills and the ability to work independently and within a team, strong attention to detail and possess excellent verbal and written communication skills.

What are the Roles of the Clinical Research Nurse?

The ***clinical research nurse (CRN)*** shares similar responsibilities to the RC and CRA, although focuses more on the care of research participants.[9] CRNs work primarily as a team in hospitals and other medical facilities with medical

professionals who deal with clinical research studies. CRN responsibilities include but are not limited to:[9]
- Identifying and screening patients
- Reviewing eligibility criteria
- Randomization of participants
- Scheduling visits and tests as per the study protocol
- Ensuring investigator product compliance
- Monitoring patient safety and wellbeing.

In addition, the CRNs may be responsible for reporting AEs to the RC and IRB and completing CRFs.[9] The CRN should be involved in protocol development and have working knowledge of how data will be collected and interpreted to ensure the trial is successful.

What do I Need to Become a Clinical Research Nurse?

To become a clinical research nurse (CRN), a bachelor's degree in nursing (BSN or BScN) is required. Nurses must have official licensing in most countries by writing an entry-to-practice exam. Additional certification is required to work in certain areas of specialization (oncology, virology, etc.) and several years of work experience as a nurse is often essential to the role (minimum of 2 years as a nurse or research experience). To excel in this position, a CRN requires strong judgement and decision-making skills, critical thinking skills, time management skills and strong oral and written communication skills.

Important Learning Points

- The PI is ultimately responsible for the conduct of a clinical trial and the safety and wellbeing of all participants.
- The PI may delegate their responsibilities to other study personnel but still remains ultimately responsible for all aspects of a clinical trial.
- The RC acts as the 'hub' of the clinical trial, liaising between sponsor/pharmaceutical company and the patient-subjects.
- The CRA is responsible for several activities in a clinical trial, including study start-up, monitoring and study close-out.

- The CRN shares the same responsibilities as the CRA in addition to the care of research participants.
- Many similarities and differences exist between the education and experience requirements for each role (Table 24.1).

Definitions

Adverse event: Any unfavorable or unintended sign, symptom or disease associated with the use of a medical intervention under investigation.

Case report form: A questionnaire used to collect data from each participant in a clinical trial.

Clinical trial monitor: Research professionals responsible for numerous activities in all phases of a clinical trial.

Clinical research nurse: Research professionals that focus on the care of patient participants; typically work in a hospital or medical facility setting.

Clinical trial: A method of research designed to test an investigational product/device on human participants.

Contract research organization (CRO): A person or organization (commercial, academic, etc.) contracted by the sponsor to perform one or more of a sponsor's trial related duties and functions.

Informed consent form: A form signed and dated by a subject who voluntarily confirms his or her willingness to participate in a clinical trial. This form is signed and dated after the patient is informed of all aspects of the trial that are relevant to the subject's decision to participate.

International conference on harmonization of good clinical practice (ICH-GCP): The ICH-GCP guideline was developed to provide a unified standard for the European Union, Japan and United States, as well as those of Australia, Canada, the Nordic countries and the World Health Organization (WHO). Good clinical practice (GCP) is a standard for the design, conduct, performance, monitoring, auditing, recording, analyzes and reporting of clinical trials that provides assurance that the data and reported results are credible and accurate and that the rights, integrity and confidentiality of trial subjects are protected.

Table 24.1: Education and experiences required for each role in the clinical research team

Position	Principal investigator	Research coordinator	Clinical trial monitor	Clinical research nurse
Education	• Physician (MD) or (co-investigator physician) • PharmD • PhD	• BSc (life sciences, biology, pharmacy, chemistry or health sciences) • Master's degree preferred	• BSc (life sciences, biology, pharmacy, chemistry or health sciences) • BSN • Certification in clinical research with experience	• BSN • Licensing • Additional certification for specific areas (oncology, virology, etc.)
Experience	• 5–10 years research experience • Expertise in field of research	• 2 or more years related work experience • 1–2 years research experience	• 1–2 years of monitoring experience • 1–2 years regulatory experience	• 2 or more years of nursing experience • 1–2 years research experience

Principal investigator (PI): The person that assumes responsibility for the conduct of a clinical trial.

Protocol: A document describing the purpose, background, design, methods and organization of a clinical trial.

Research coordinator: The 'hub' of the clinical trial; liaises between principal investigator, clinical research team, sponsor, sites and study-subjects.

Research ethics board (REB) or institutional review board (IRB) or ethics committee (EC): A committee that formally monitors all research projects to make sure that they meet ethical and scientific standards.

REFERENCES

1. Baer AR, Devine S, Beardmore CD, Catalano R. Clinical investigator responsibilities. J Oncol Pract. 2011;(2):124-8.

2. Food and Drug Administration Guidance for Industry: Investigator Responsibilities—Protecting the Rights, Safety and Welfare of Study Subjects. Retrieved 2015 from: http://www.fda.gov/downloads/Drugs/.../Guidances/UCM187772.pdf
3. Health Canada (2013). Guidance for Records Related to Clinical Trials. Retrieved 2015 from: http://www.hc-sc.gc.ca/dhp-mps/compli conform/clini-pract-prat/docs/gui_68_tc-tm-eng.php
4. Food and Drug Administration (2014) Investigational New Drug Application, Code of Federal Regulations, 21CFR312.3. Retrieved April 2015 from: http://www.accessdata.fda.gov/scripts/cdrh/cfdocs/cfcfr/CFRSearch.cfm? 312.3
5. Fisher JA. Co-ordinating 'ethical' clinical trials: The role of research coordinators in the contract research industry. Sociol Health Illn. 2006;28(6):678-94.
6. Mueller MR. From delegation to specialization: Nurses and clinical trial co-ordination. Nurs Inq. 2001;8(3):182-90.
7. Fisher JA, Kalbaugh CA. Altruism in clinical research: Coordinators' orientation to their professional roles. Nurs Outlook. 2012;60(3):143-8.
8. Stonier PD. Careers with the pharmaceutical industry. In: G Hayes (ed). The Clinical Research Associate; 2nd edition. England, UK: John Wiley and Sons Ltd; 2007; p. 67-76.
9. Gallin JI, Ognibene FP. Principles and Practice of Clinical Research. In: Diane St Germain, (ed). Data management in clinical trial; 3rd edition. London, UK: Elsevier; 2012; p. 92.

25

Research Ethics Approval— A must Before any Clinical Trial

Zenon Sirko, S Rajasekaran

Key Objectives

- Be able to define research ethics as well as appreciate its importance
- Understand from where research ethics originated
- Understand the main roles of the research ethics board (REB)
- Understand the basic model of research ethics
- Be able to understand what classifies an action as 'research misconduct'.

What is 'Research Ethics' and Why is it Important?

Research is a vital part of the scientific world; without it there would be no new information, no progress. It is key to the discovery and development of new procedures, drugs, machines and so much more. However, when conducting research, especially research that requires the use of human subjects, it is very important that rules and guidelines must be followed. These guidelines are necessary to ensure the protection of the subject from any physical, emotional or psychological harm and can be classified under the umbrella of research ethics. **Research ethics** is defined as rules for researchers to follow the separate acceptable and unacceptable behavior when conducting research.[1]

The National Institutes of Health (NIH) stresses that research ethics is imperative as it holds the researcher accountable to the public and protects the research subject from unwarranted risk and harm. Research ethics increases support from the public substantially. This is extremely significant due to the fact that the majority of research is publically funded, therefore unethical treatment of research subjects would likely lead to the loss of funding for a research study. Also, research ethics promotes the honesty in collaborative work, ensuring that researchers are given credit for their respective contributions as well as protecting their intellectual property.[1]

What are the Origins of Research Ethics?

It is believed that the beginning of research ethics dates back to 1947 with the creation of the ***Nuremburg Code***. This code consists of 10 basic principles for research ethics, which were created in the wake of the horrendous acts and experiments performed by Nazi doctors and scientists on Jewish prisoners during World War II.[2] These acts led to the painful and inhumane deaths of thousands. The Nuremburg Code consists of the 10 following guidelines:[6]

1. The human subject must voluntarily consent.
2. The goal of the research must be beneficial to society.
3. Research must be based on prior animal testing, with reasonable expected results.
4. Any and all unnecessary harm to the subject must be avoided.
5. There should never be a risk of serious injury or death of the subject.
6. The amount of risk to the subject should never be more than the potential benefit of the study.
7. All necessary resources for the safety of the subject must be present in order for the study to be carried out.
8. The researcher conducting the experiment must be qualified scientifically.
9. At any point during the experiment, the subject has the right to remove themselves with no negative consequences.
10. At any point during the experiment, the researcher must terminate the experiment if they believe that continuing the study will lead to the harm or death of the subject.

These 10 rules effectively shaped the guidelines and regulations of research ethics to this day, in the hope that the atrocities committed in the name of research during World War II are never repeated.

How is Research Conduct Monitored/What is the Research Ethics Board?

A key aspect of research ethics is the presence of an independent third party, which has the role of reviewing and monitoring the research study. These parties ensure that all proper ethical protocols are followed in the creation and execution of a research study. Before a researcher is allowed to conduct an experiment, they must propose their study to the independent party. If it is approved, then the researcher may begin the study. If not, the researcher must revise the study until it receives approval.[7]

Most commonly, this third party is known as the ***Research Ethics Board (REB), Institutional Review Board (IRB), or Ethics Committee (EC).*** The Canadian Government describes the REB as the following:[7]

- A board established by an institution that reviews all research conducted under its jurisdiction. This board must be appointed by the highest acting power of the institution and a working relationship must be maintained between the two of them. This working relationship should consist of communication, funding and the availability of resources. The REB acts on behalf of the institution.
- REB must consist of a minimum of five members, with men and women both being accounted for. When considering the minimum size of the REB, the breakdown of their respective expertise is as follows:
  - Minimum of two members with a background and expertise in research.
  - Minimum of one member with a background and expertise in ethics.
  - Minimum of one member that has a good working knowledge of the law, but is separate from the acting institution's legal counsel or adviser.
  - Minimum of one member that is strictly a member of the community, with no affiliation whatsoever with the institution.

The size of the REB for an institution should have a relative correlation to the size of the institution.

- As stated previously, researchers must propose their research study to the REB before they are permitted to have human subjects participate. However, the researcher is not required to receive permission from the REB before the exploratory phase of the study. As could be presumed, the higher the potential risk to the subject, the higher the 'level of scrutiny' will be from the REB. The potential risk will also determine the frequency of status reports required by the REB, with a minimum of one status report a year as well as a status report summarizing the study once it has concluded.
- Researchers have the responsibility to report any problems that may arise during the study to the REB, as well as submit a request to the REB if they would like to change their study protocol from the one previously approved. The researcher must await approval by the REB before they may implement these changes. Also, as stated previously, if a researcher does not receive approval from the REB originally, they have the right to have their proposal reconsidered. This is contingent on the fact that they make changes that the REB deem sufficient to ensure the study is carried out ethically.

What are the Main Pillars of Research Ethics?

The National Institutes of Health (NIH) Clinical Center has published 7 basic ideologies of research ethics.[4] They are as follows:

1. ***Social and clinical value:*** Essentially, there must be a justifiable reason for conducting the research. The subject will likely experience some inconvenience or risk attributed to the study, so as a researcher you must make it worth the possible sacrifice by the subject.
2. ***Scientific validity:*** The researcher must answer the questions being asked. If he/she does not, then it is a waste of time and money, as well as puts the subject at unnecessary risk. To avoid this, make sure the research questions are realistic and has an attainable goal.
3. ***Fair subject selection:*** All people should have equal opportunity to become a subject in a study, considering

they meet the legitimate scientific criteria that make them eligible for it. Therefore, researchers must have a genuine reason for excluding a patient from a study, e.g. increased risk due to an external factor.

4. ***Favorable risk/benefit ratio:*** It is imperative that the perceived benefits of research study outweigh the risks for the subject. There are many potential risks for a research subject and the researcher should take every precaution possible to minimize those risks. It is clearly unethical and impractical for the risks associated with a study to be greater than the potential benefits.

5. ***Independent review:*** It is a key that a third party, usually an independent review panel such as the REB, review the proposed study before it begins. They must also monitor the study while it is in progress. This is to ensure that all the previous criteria for an ethical research study have been met. For example, ensuring there is no bias in the proposed method of selecting subjects.

6. ***Informed consent:*** The vast majority of the time, informed consent is necessary in order to enroll a subject into a study. Informed consent is ensuring that the patient has a full understanding of the proposed study and how it will affect them specifically. Also, under no circumstance should the patient ever be forced to enroll in a study, they must always be enrolled willingly by their own free choice.

7. ***Respect for all subjects, potential and enrolled:*** The study subject should always be the first priority of the researcher. It is vital that their needs are put before the needs of the study and researcher. The subject has the opportunity to withdraw from the study at any time and the researcher must constantly monitor them during the study. It is also important that the subject is monitored after the study, to ensure no adverse effects have occurred.

What is the Importance of Confidentiality in Research Ethics?

As Columbia University states, **confidentiality** has always been a large cornerstone of the physician-patient relationship and it carries over to the researcher-research subject relationship as well. Confidentiality is defined as the protection of one's privacy[8] and is of the utmost importance when conducting research.

Often when conducting research, the researcher gathers very personal and important information about the subject. This information, if discovered by the public, could potentially lead to embarrassment or even worse, harm to the subject's status both socially and economically.[8] It is a privilege for the researcher to have the subject in their study, so it is key that they do everything possible to maintain the subject's confidentiality at all times.

What is Research Misconduct?

Research misconduct is defined as the 'fabrication, falsification or plagiarism in proposing, performing or reviewing research or in reporting research results.'[3] This means that the researcher cannot make up, manipulate or copy someone else's data in order to receive their desired results.

However, honest human error is not considered to be research misconduct. This is because there was no actual intention of deception by the researcher. As long as the inaccurate data was not created on purpose, it will not fall under the category of research misconduct.

What are the Ethics of Deceiving/Misleading Research Subjects?

As per the University of Washington, the vast majority of the time, it is not ethical to deceive research subjects. The independent party reviewing your study, likely the REB, must be provided with substantial evidence proving why deception is necessary for the study. If deception can be avoided, it should be. If it is decided that deception is the best method to carry out the study, so it is very important to the subject given a full explanation once the study is completed.[2] This is also known as a ***debriefing.***

A very commonly used example of deceiving patients is the use of a placebo. This is often a pill that is presented to the patient as a legitimate drug but is often no more than a sugar pill. The orthopedic version of a placebo is commonly referred to as a ***sham surgery***. This is when the surgeon makes an incision, but no actual surgery is performed. The patient is anesthetized during this process and is unaware that no legitimate surgical procedure took place. This is often used to test the legitimacy of a surgical procedure that has a debatable efficacy.[5]

A great example of the use of this technique is the study done by Sihvonen, et al.[5] In this study, the efficacy of arthroscopic partial meniscectomy was studied, as there is little proof showing how effective it actually is. To briefly summarize this study, some patients underwent the actual procedure, while others underwent a sham surgery. Twelve months after the procedure was performed, there was little difference in the result of either the arthroscopic partial meniscectomy or the sham surgery.

Definitions

Confidentiality: The protection of a research subject's privacy.

Debriefing: A thorough explanation of the objective and protocol of a research study provided to the research subject after the study has concluded.

Nuremberg code: Ten rules made after World War II that are known as the original guidelines for research ethics.

Research ethics: Rules for researchers to follow that separate acceptable and unacceptable behavior when conducting research.

Research ethics board (REB) or institutional review Board (IRB) or ethics committee (EC): The independent third party responsible for approving and monitoring all research studies under its jurisdiction.

Research misconduct: The fabrication, falsification or plagiarism in proposing, performing or reviewing research or in reporting research results.

Sham surgery: Similar to a placebo, this is when a subject believes that they had a surgical procedure performed but in reality it had not.

REFERENCES

1. Resnik D. What is Ethics in Research & Why is it Important? NIH. 2015.
2. Adams LA, Callahan T. Research Ethics. 2015.
3. Francis S. Developing a federal policy on research misconduct. Sci Eng Ethics. 1999;5(2):261-72. Available from http://www.aps.org/policy/statements/upload/federalpolicy.pdf.
4. National Institutes of Health. Pursuing potential research participants protections: guiding principles for ethical research. NIH; 2012. Available from http://www.nih.gov/health/clinicaltrials/highlights/2012-08-ethicalresearch. htm [Accessed November, 2012].
5. Sihvonen R, Paavola M, Malmivaara A, et al. Arthroscopic partial meniscectomy versus sham surgery for a degenerative meniscal tear. N Engl J Med. 2013;369(26):2515-24.
6. US Department of Health & Human Services (2005). Washington: The Nuremberg Code. Available from http://www.hhs.gov/ohrp/archive/nurcode.html.
7. Government of Canada Panel on Research Ethics. TCPS 2 Chapter 6. 2015. Available from http://www.pre.ethics.gc.ca/eng/policy-politique/initiatives/tcps2-eptc2/chapter6-chapitre6/.
8. Privacy and Confidentiality. Columbia University. N.p. Web. 2015. Columbia University. Privacy and Confidentiality. Available from http://ccnmtl.columbia.edu/projects/cire/pac/foundation/#1.

Why do we Need Patient Consent? Designing a Good Consent Form

Chuan Silvia Li, M Borate

Key Objectives

- Understand what patient informed consent is
- Understand why patient informed consent is important
- Understand the key steps in the informed consent process
- Understand the key components of the informed consent form
- Understand when revisions to an informed consent form is necessary
- Understand when waiver and alteration of informed consent forms is necessary.

What is Patient Informed Consent?

Informed consent serves as a voluntary agreement to participate in clinical research. It is not merely a form that is signed but is a process in which the subject has an understanding of the research and its risks. Informed consent is essential before enrolling a participant and ongoing once enrolled. Informed consent originates from the legal and ethical right the patient has to direct what happens to his or her body, and from the ethical duty of the physician to involve the patient in his or her healthcare. Informed consent must be obtained for all types of research involving human subjects, including diagnostic, therapeutic, interventional, social and behavioral studies and for research conducted domestically or abroad. Obtaining consent involves informing the subject about his or her rights, the purpose of the study, the procedures to be undergone and the potential risks and benefits of participation. Subjects in the study must participate willingly. Vulnerable populations (e.g. prisoners, children, pregnant women, etc.) must receive extra protections. The legal rights of subjects may not be waived and subjects may not be asked to release or appear to release the investigator, the sponsor, the institution or its agents from liability for negligence.[1]

Informed consent is described in ethical codes and regulations for human subjects research. The goal of the informed consent process is to provide sufficient information so that a participant can make an informed decision about whether or not to enroll in a study or to continue participation. The informed consent document must be written in language easily understood by the participant, it must minimize the possibility of coercion or undue influence, and the subject must be given sufficient time to consider participation.[1]

Why is Patient Consent Important?

Informed consent is important because it allows subjects to make an informed and voluntary choice to participate or refuse to participate in a project where they will be asked to take risks for the benefit of others.[2-8] In both research and clinical care, informed consent represents permission to intervene in a person's private sphere.[8] Moreover, trust is a motivating factor for research participation and thus we put this at risk if we allow false expectations and prove ourselves unworthy of this trust.[8] Finally, better information may decrease anxiety and seems to have at most a small negative effect on research recruitment.[8]

Voluntary informed consent is a requirement for the ethical conduct of human subjects research. Informed consent is the process through which researchers respect the fundamental ethical principle of individual autonomy. An autonomous individual is one who is capable of deliberation and personal choice. The principle of autonomy implies that responsibility must be given to the individual to make the decision to participate.[1]

Informed consent means that subjects are well-informed about the study, the potential risks and benefits of their participation and that it is research, not therapy, in which they will participate. Voluntary informed consent is absolutely essential not only for the safety, protection and respect of the subject, but also to protect the integrity of the research itself.[1]

What are the Key Steps in the Informed Consent Process?

Informed consent is more than a form; it is also a process. Information must be presented to enable persons to voluntarily decide whether or not to participate as a research subject. The informed consent process must be a dialogue of the study's purpose, duration, experimental procedures, alternatives, risks and benefits. The process of consenting is ongoing and must be made clear to the subject that it is his or her right to ***withdraw*** or ***opt-out*** of the study or procedure at any time, not only just at the initial signing of paperwork. The location where the consent is being discussed with the subjects, as well as the subject's physical, emotional and psychological capability must be taken into consideration. The informed consent process should ultimately ensure that the subject understands and really 'gets' what they are signing up for.[1] The elements of adequate informed consent include disclosure, understanding, decision-making capacity and voluntariness.[8]

Informed consent is an ongoing process that must occur ***before*** any clinical trial-related procedures are conducted. The process consists of a document and a series of conversations between the clinical trial participant and the principal investigator (PI) and delegated healthcare professionals, as appropriate. While the PI may delegate the task of administering and obtaining informed consent to a qualified individual, he or she is ultimately responsible for ensuring the process is conducted properly.[9] The key steps in an informed consent process include:

- The PI discusses the trial's risks, benefits and other aspects with the potential participant and/or authorized representative and, if required, the participant's legal representative, before the trial begins. Note that the discussion about the study should be presented in language that the participant and/or authorized representative understand easily.
- The PI gives the potential participant and/or authorized representative adequate time and opportunity to read

the consent form and ask questions about the study and discuss it with study investigators and/or family members.
- If the potential participant and/or authorized representative decides to get involved in the study, he or she provides voluntary consent by signing and dating the written informed consent document approved by the local ethics committee. A copy of the consent form should be provided to the subject and/or authorized representative upon conclusion of the consent process. The participant and/or authorized representative has the right to withdraw consent at any time without penalty, repercussions or reason.

What are the General Guidelines on Designing Patient Informed Consent Forms (ICFs)?

Investigators must follow the International Council on Harmonization (ICH) good clinical practice (GCP) guidelines.[2] Section 1.28 describes the informed consent process, while the requirements and process for obtaining the informed consent form from a clinical trial participant are explained in section 4.8.

Besides following ICH guidelines, investigators need to adhere to national and local regulatory requirements, sponsor requirements and privacy and personal data security regulations applicable in the country in which the study is being conducted.[9]

The informed consent document must be fully approved by an institutional review board (IRB) or an independent ethics committee (IEC) prior to its use with trial participants.

The informed consent form, which is a legal document, must include 20 ICH-required elements (section 4.8.10 of the GCP guidance).[2] They include the purpose, duration, risks, benefits, costs and additional expenses of the trial; a description of the trial procedures; alternative care options; and volunteers' rights.

What are Some Tips on Writing a Well-designed Patient Consent Form?

The informed consent form should be easy for prospective participants to understand and not sound legalistic or patronizing. The consent form should be written in the second person (i.e. 'you', 'yours') except the signature section should be in the first person singular (i.e. 'I', 'Me', 'My'). The informed consent form should use lay, plain and concise language not higher than an 8th grade level of English. This is the average reading level in North America and about the level of a daily newspaper. Terms such as 'randomization', 'double-blind' and 'placebo', should be explained in simple language, assuming no familiarity with a technical vocabulary. There are guides on the internet to help you find substitutes for words that are overly scientific or are professional jargon.[10] Patients may be put off enrolling in studies by the language used in informed consent forms and insisted upon by ethics committees.[11] A balance should be maintained between the readability of the patient consent form and the ethics committee requirements. Make sure the wording of the informed consent form does not exert any undue influence on the participant. Avoid the terms 'subject' or 'patient'; use instead the terms 'volunteer' or 'participant.' The form can be made easier to read by using headings and point form, when appropriate. The date and version number of the informed consent form and the page number should appear on the page.

People who do not speak the dominant local language should be provided with a translation of the informed consent document. An impartial witness, who speaks the dominant local language as well as the individual's language, should ensure that the person understands the form in its entirety before the person makes a decision. A person who speaks and understands the dominant local language, but does not read and write it, should have the contents of the informed consent explained to him or her by an impartial witness. This individual may then indicate consent by signing or making his or her mark on the form.

What are the Elements of the Consent Forms?

Whenever human subjects participate in a research study, they need to be given enough information to provide a truly voluntary and informed consent. Subjects must be provided the following information:[1,11]

Institution Logo or Letterhead

The logo of the institution or institutional letterhead should be used for the informed consent form.

Introduction

Clearly state that the study involves experimental research and what part of the study is experimental. State what is being studied and who is doing the research by listing the following:
- Full study title
- Name and the telephone number the PI/local PI
- Name of the institution/organization
- Name of the sponsor
- Funding source of the research study
- Date and version number of the consent document
- 24-hour telephone number and contact person for study participants in the event of a research-related injury or emergency.

On first mention, ensure that you provide all the names of drugs, including generic and brand names. If applicable, identify whether the sponsor also manufactures the study drug.

Purpose and Design of the Research Study

State the study's objectives, rationale and design. List the inclusion and exclusion criteria. Mention the approximate number of participants to be enrolled in the study. State why this participant has been chosen for this research. People often wonder why they have been chosen to participate and may be fearful, confused or concerned. Explain how the participants will be assigned to the study treatment, procedure or intervention (for example, randomly or blindly). Explain whether random allotment to a particular treatment is being used in the study design, the probability of receiving one treatment versus another and, if applicable, procedures for initiating and breaking the double-blinded allotment. Provide background information on the study as well as information about both licensed and investigational drugs. Within this section state explicitly that the research is experimental and may not benefit the participant.

Note: Many people have trouble understanding probability, so it is advisable to use frequency instead, e.g. state that five participants will receive the drug and five will be in the control group that does not receive the drug, rather than saying that you have a 50/50 chance of getting the drug.

Procedures Involved in the Research

Include a statement about the time commitments expected of the subject, including the duration of the overall research study, the duration from the screening visit to the last visit, frequency of visits and expected length of visits, if relevant. Describe the study test procedures to be followed, including details of all invasive procedures, as well as treatment regimens and dosage at visits. Specify clearly any possible inconveniences. Include a paragraph in this section on how to take the investigational medications, noting particularly, any special instructions with respect to scheduling, food restrictions or requirements and the storage of drugs. Offer plain language definitions for any technical terms used and identify any aspects of the study that are experimental. Identify who will pay for additional costs resulting from participation: travel expenses, daycare and so on. Describe the participant's responsibilities. Emphasize, as well, the importance of following the procedures of the trial and state the consequences of not following the procedures and how you define non-compliance. Use a chart for a schedule of visits, if appropriate. If applicable, state whether and how adherence will be monitored. State whether lab test results will be given to participants in real time.

Participant Withdrawal

State that participation in the study is voluntary and that the participant is free to leave the study at any time without penalty or affecting the healthcare at their institution. Describe why the study might be discontinued or why a participant might be withdrawn from the process. Describe any foreseeable circumstances and/or reasons under which the subject's participation in the trial may be terminated. Also specify, if applicable, what steps are being taken to monitor safety in the study. Describe the health consequences, if any, and that it is solely the participant's decision to leave the trial, as well as the procedures that the participants will be asked to follow. Make it clear, however, that the participant is under no obligation to follow any specific procedure to leave a trial.

Risks, Side Effects and Harms

Explain and describe all known or expected risks and discomforts to the participants and, when applicable, to an embryo, fetus or nursing infant. Provide enough information about the risks so that the participant can make an informed decision. Describe the level of care that will be available in the case of an adverse event so that harm does not occur and also describe who will provide this care and who will pay for it. Note that these include not only physical injury but also possible psychological, emotional, social, legal or economic harm, discomfort or inconvenience. Also note if any previous studies (on animals, as well as humans) revealed side effects and whether or not they were reversible. In order to help the volunteer assess these risks, use relative frequency percentages wherever possible and the sample size from which these percentages were derived. State that there may be risks unknown at this time. If available, provide information from similar drugs or drugs of the same class. State also that participants are entitled to and should receive updates about risks, side effects and potential harms as information becomes available. The subject or the subject's legally acceptable representative will be informed in a timely manner if information becomes available that may be relevant to the subject's willingness to continue participation in the trial. Also state that taking part in the study could prevent participants from taking part in future studies due to exposure to the study drugs. Also state, if applicable, that exposure to these drugs may make participants resistant to other drugs in the same class (e.g. protease inhibitors, non-nucleoside reverse transcriptase inhibitors) and suggest the strength of evidence indicating this.

Potential Drug Interactions

List the drugs that the participant will not be permitted to take during the course of the study, including street drugs and alcohol, if applicable. The list of street drugs should include street names and generic names of the drugs. Be careful to mention any over-the-counter medications, including complementary therapy, herbal and vitamin supplements, as well as any foods (e.g. grapefruit) that may interact with the study drugs. If there is insufficient information about potential drug interactions, this section should warn readers about this. If oral contraceptives are taken by the participant, explain why they may not be effective and note if there are any known or potential drug interactions between the study medications and oral contraceptives. Instruct readers that during the duration of the study, participants are asked to inform the study coordinator or investigator of any changes in their medications, including vitamins and herbal medicines or remedies.

Alternative Sources of Treatment

Advise the participants about comparable treatments, more established treatments that may be available to them or if no other treatments are available. Describe important potential benefits and risks of these alternative treatments. Inform participants that if any other treatments become available during the course of the study, they will be informed about them.

Continued Access

Indicate which of the study drugs will continuously be made available to the participants once the trial is over and for how long. If they will not be made available at the end of the trial, state this. Indicate whether or not participants will continue to have access to the drug if they withdraw or are withdrawn.

In addition, the monitors, the auditors, the IRB/IEC and the regulatory authorities will be granted direct access to the subject's original medical records for verification of clinical trial procedures and/or data, without violating the confidentiality of the subject, to the extent permitted by the applicable laws and regulations and that, by signing a written informed consent form, the subject or the subject's legally acceptable representative is authorizing such access.

Pregnancy/Childbearing Potential

State the risks associated with pregnancy and the study drugs, including all available information about the potential risk of fetal toxicity, based on completed animal studies or fetal toxicity of similar drugs. If no relevant information is available, a statement should explicitly note the potential fetal risks. State risks of breastfeeding while taking study drugs. State the effects on sperm and whether the duration of these effects are known. Recommend that participants continue to use acceptable methods of birth control after the study.

Potential Benefits

Explicitly state that no clinical benefits for the volunteer are guaranteed because the research is experimental nor are the possible expected benefits guaranteed to the individual human subject, if applicable. Describe the potential benefits of the research. Benefits may be divided into benefits to the individual, benefits to the community in which the individual resides and benefits to society as a whole as a result of finding an answer to the research question.

Reimbursement and Compensation

This section should include information on financial costs to the individual participating, including the reimbursement of costs of treatment, travel, childcare, money for wages, money lost due to visits to health facilities and any other anticipated expenses. The amount should be determined within the host country context. Mention only those activities that will be actual benefits and not those to which they are entitled regardless of participation. This section should also indicate whether compensation and/or treatment for study-related injury is available and describe these.

Sharing the Study Results

State that study staff will discuss the results of the study, once the study is over. Describe how participants will be informed of the results and specify which results will and will not be given to participants. If there is a plan and a timeline for sharing of information, include the details. Inform the participant that the research findings will be shared more broadly, for example, through publications and conferences.

Confidentiality

Explain how the research team will maintain the confidentiality of data. State that records identifying the participants will be kept confidential and, to the extent permitted by the applicable laws and/or regulations, will not be made publicly available. If the results of the study are published, the subject's identity will remain confidential. Describe also how confidentiality of the participant will be protected (e.g. by the use of codes rather than names on documents and labels). Name agencies that may have access to the data [e.g. Health Canada, Food and Drug Administration (FDA), drug company, data safety monitoring board and so on]. State if and when any agency would have access to study data by participant's name (rather than by ID number or birth date).

Future Research

Inform participants that explicit consent is required before investigators may use the information or samples obtained for research extending beyond the scope of this study.

Contact Person

Provide participants with the name and contact information of a local study coordinator, a physician and a local or national ethics review committee contact person (if applicable) who is involved, informed and accessible and that they can be contacted in case of any questions regarding the study. Identify the person to contact in case of study-related injury. In addition, a third party should be identified to answer any questions participants may have about their rights in a clinical trial. State also that the study has been approved by the IRB/IEC.

Incentives and Conflicts of Interest

Describe any incentives that the investigator, the participant's physicians or the research institution might receive for recruitment of participants and any other possible conflicts of interest.

Signature and Copy of the Informed Consent

It should be clear in this section that participation is voluntary and the consent form is not a contract and that the participant does not give up any rights by signing it. Rather, he or she is signing the form to indicate that he or she has read and understood the contents of the informed consent form. There should also be a sentence that restates that the participant can leave the study at any time without penalty or loss of benefits to which he or she is otherwise entitled.

The signature page should include the title of the study as well as a checklist of important things participants should be aware of, including key protocol-specific issues. Make sure to format your informed consent document so that the checklist fits on the page with the signatures of participants. It is recommended not to have a signature page with just the signatures.

The informed consent form should be signed and dated by the participant or by his or her legally acceptable representative and by the investigator or the person designated by the investigator conducting the informed consent discussion with the participant.

In case the participant or his or her legally acceptable representative does not speak the dominant local language or does not read and write, an impartial witness, who was present during the entire informed consent discussion, should sign and date the consent form.

A copy of the signed consent form must be given to the participant.

When do I Need to Revise an Informed Consent Form?

Informed consent documents must be revised any time new safety information becomes available or there is a change in trial procedures, participant compensation or personnel noted on the consent form.[2] The FDA and other regulatory agencies may require re-consenting of all currently enrolled study participants when a change is made to the consent form that may affect the participants' willingness to continue participation in the study. It is not necessary to distribute revised consent forms to study participants who have completed the research study.

Revisions to the informed consent document must be approved by an IRB/IEC again prior to its use and the informed consent process with the new information and documentation needs to be repeated with every clinical trial participant.[2] The participant is then required to sign the revised form.

When are Waiver and Alteration of Informed Consent Requirements Needed?

A waiver of one or more elements of informed consent or the needs of having informed consent process may be obtained from the IRB for some research projects that could not practically be done without an alteration to the required elements or for studies where required elements are not applicable.[1] In this case, an informed consent waiver should be submitted to the local IRB for review and approval.

When an IRB waives the requirement to obtain informed consent, it waives the entire requirement for the informed consent process.

Note: When the IRB grants an alteration of some or all of the elements of the informed consent (e.g. removes a required element of consent from the document), the process of obtaining informed consent is still required. Researchers interested in obtaining an alteration of the consent process should indicate clearly when submitting an IRB application.

More to Read

- ICH Steering Committee. ICH Harmonized Tripartite Guideline. 1996 May 1.
- CIOMS. Guideline 4: Individual Informed Consent. International Ethical Guidelines for Biomedical Research Involving Human Subjects. Geneva: CIOMS; 2002.
- Faden R, Beauchamp T. A History and Theory of Informed Consent. Oxford and New York: Oxford University Press; 1986.
- Wassersug RJ. Consent forms for clinical trials are too aggressive. BMJ. 2013 Aug 13;347:f4879.

Definitions

Informed consent: The process of providing sufficient information so that a participant can make an informed decision about whether or not to enroll in a study or to continue participation. It serves as a voluntary agreement to participate in clinical research.

Withdrawal: When the participant discontinues his or her participation in an ongoing research study. Subjects have the right to withdraw from research study at any time.

REFERENCES

1. Shahnazarian D, Hagemann J, Aburto M, Rose S. Informed Consent in Human Subjects Research. Office for the Protection of Research Subjects (OPRS). Univerisity of Southern California. 2013. Available at http://oprs.usc.edu/files/2013/04/Informed-Consent-Booklet-4.4.13.pdf (accessed 7 June 2015).
2. ICH Steering Committee. ICH Harmonized Tripartite Guideline. 1996 May 1.
3. The National Commission for the Protection of Human Subjects of Biomedical and Behavioral Research. The Belmont Report: Ethical Principles and Guidelines for the Protection of Human Subjects of Research. Washington, DC: Department of Health, Education and Welfare; 1979.
4. World Medical Association. Declaration of Helsinki: Ethical Principles for Medical Research Involving Human Subjects. 2000. Available at
5. Department of Health and Human Services. Rules and Regulations. Title 45, part 46; revised as of March 1983.
6. CIOMS. Guideline 4: Individual Informed Consent. International Ethical Guidelines for Biomedical Research Involving Human Subjects. Geneva: CIOMS; 2002.
7. Emanuel EJ, Wendler D, Grady C. What makes clinical research ethical? JAMA. 2000;283(20):2701-11.
8. Cahana A, Hurst SA. Voluntary informed consent in research and clinical care: an update. Pain Pract. 2008;8(6):446-51.
9. PPD. Investigator & Informed Consent. Available at https://www.ppdi.com/Participate-In-Clinical-Trials/Become-an-Investigator/Informed-Consent (accessed 7 June 2015).
10. World Health Organization. Informed Consent Form Templates. Available at http://www.who.int/rpc/research_ethics/informed_consent/en/ (accessed 7 June 2015).
11. Wassersug RJ. Consent forms for clinical trials are too aggressive. BMJ. 2013;347:f4879.

27

Collecting Data— it all Begins with a Good Data Form

Nikhita Singhal, Steve Rocha

Key Objectives

- Understand the purpose of data forms and their importance in conducting clinical research
- Learn the type of information and basic components to include in data forms
- Learn methods for preparing effective data forms that encourage accuracy and completion while minimizing errors and bias in data collection
- Understand the process for reviewing data forms and assessing their quality.

What is a Data Form and Why is it Needed?

A data form, generally referred to as a case report form (CRF), is a questionnaire or instrument utilized to structure and facilitate the collection of pertinent data regarding study participants in clinical research.[1] ***Source documents*** such as a patient's medical records, diagnostic test results or laboratory test reports may be used to complete CRFs.[1,2] The CRFs should accurately reflect the data from the source documents and should be reported legibly and in a timely manner. Once completed, the forms are sent to the coordinating center responsible for collecting the data.[1]

Data collection is a key aspect of clinical research. The data obtained is utilized to support or disprove hypotheses proposed within the study ***protocol*** and so it is vital to ensure that the correct data is measured and defined.[1] The quality of data collected depends upon the quality of the data collection instruments and so the development of CRFs represents a crucial step in the process of clinical research.[2,3] Regardless of the time and effort spent conducting the research, a meaningful analysis of results is not possible if the correct data is not collected; thus, data forms can have a significant impact on study success.[2,4]

What Kind of Information should be Gathered on a Data Form?

The data collected on a CRF is customized to each study protocol.[1] Before begin to develop any CRF, it is vital to have a firm grasp of the study's research objectives, research questions, the justification for the study and any existing literature on the topic.[5] It is also essential to be familiar with the research design, methods and analysis plan.

Each item on the data form should be thoroughly examined to ensure the information is necessary and required to address the previously determined research questions from the study protocol.[2] Finding a balance between collecting all necessary data and collecting extraneous information is integral. Avoid collecting redundant data, as this is a waste of valuable time and resources.[3,4] Instead, focus on collecting only the data which is necessary to address questions outlined in the study protocol and to provide accurate safety data. Each piece of data collected must have a specific purpose.[2]

What are the Components of a Good Data Form?

A good data form should be designed to gather the most complete and accurate information possible within the limits of available time and resources.[2] Study investigators should construct CRFs in a structured and standardized way to produce reliable, consistent and clean data for analysis. This is a rigorous procedure and requires careful planning and editing to ensure the data form is comprehensive and as useful as possible.

Data collected on CRFs often includes the following:
- Screening details or adherence to protocol inclusion criteria and exclusion criteria
- Patient demographic details (e.g. age, sex, height)

- Baseline medical history
- Diagnosis
- Concurrent medications
- Treatment details and modifications to experimental intervention (if applicable)
- Tracking of adverse events and other key outcomes
- Discharge details
- Subject follow-up.

Those preparing the data forms must take their questioning strategy into account when attempting to elicit information. In situations where subjective information is required, general and non-directive questions should be used.[6] In other cases, more specific and directive questions will be necessary.[6] For example, 'Have you experienced any light-headedness or dizziness since beginning of the treatment?' will result in a higher number of patients reporting this specific issue than simply asking, 'Have you experienced any problems since beginning of the treatment?'

The questions should be unambiguous and framed in a manner that limits the number of resulting ***data queries***.[1] At the same time, the prompts and instructions should be kept as concise as possible in order to ensure that they are read and followed by respondents. Long blocks of text may seem daunting or overwhelming and result in data being recorded incorrectly or not at all. Standard of care and site of workflow should also be taken into account when designing CRFs.[3,6] Respondents should be able to fill out the data form rapidly and easily. For this to occur, questions should be presented in a logical sequence.[2] It is vital to try to anticipate all possible clinical scenarios when creating checklists of answers, if any data cannot be collected due to the construction of the data form, it cannot be analyzed.[2]

Employing standardized templates reduces the time needed to develop, review and approve data forms.[1] It also facilitates collaboration and makes it possible to reuse validated instruments for similar studies in the future.[1] Additionally, the use of standards reduces training needed at each site and can expedite data entry.[3] However, there are some points to keep in mind when using standards. An item should not be included merely because it has been included in previous studies.[6]

The data collected must be necessary and relevant to each study's unique protocol. Additionally, it is important to obtain the written approval of the copyright holder in order to use an entire form or section of a form that has been copyrighted.[6] Even if the form you wish to reproduce is not copyrighted, obtain permission from the author of the original study.[6]

How do I Prepare a Well-designed CRF?

The design of data forms is just as important as their content. A well-designed data form improves the ease of use for clinicians or participants recording data and helps with comprehension and completion.[5]

Data forms should include a header and a footer to assist with organization. Typically, a header will contain the study name and number, site number, participant number and initials, form number and date.[5] The footer often includes the date, version number and page number.[5]

The following is a list of guidelines to follow when designing a CRF:

- Group related items into sections and label these sections with appropriate headings to describe their general content.[2]
- Use consistent formats, font style and font sizes throughout the CRF.[4] Size 10–14 point font is recommended to optimize readability.[5]
- Stress important words and phrases by bolding, italicizing or underlining them.[4]
- Avoid combining portrait and landscape page orientations.[4,6]
- Avoid overcrowding each page with questions. A clean, uncluttered layout is optimal for encouraging accurate data entry.[4,6]
- Provide clear visual cues such as boxes to clearly indicate where data should be recorded and in what format.[4] For example, rather than simply leaving a single line on which to record a participant's date of birth, provide a series of boxes followed by an indication of format (e.g. DD/MM/YYYY). (Table 27.1)
- Always specify the units of measurement for requested data.[4] For example, if requesting blood pressure, provide

Table 27.1: Comparing well-designed and poorly-designed data fields

Poorly-designed	Well-designed
Date of birth: _____	Date of birth: ☐☐/☐☐/☐☐☐☐ (DD/MM/YYYY)
Blood pressure: ____/____	Blood pressure: ☐☐☐/☐☐☐ (mmHg)
Temperature: _____	Temperature: ☐☐.☐(°C)

a set number of boxes followed by 'mmHg' to indicate expected values for the data to the respondent. This also aids with data interpretation and reduces the amount of manipulation required during data analysis.

- Specify the number of decimal places that should be recorded for a given item.[4] For example, one box, followed by a decimal point, followed by three more boxes indicates to the respondent that three decimal places are requested.
- Allow respondents to select options using check boxes rather than by circling answers whenever possible.[4]
- Organize questions in a manner that keep skips to a minimum.[4] Where skips are required, provide explicit instructions about what to skip and what not to skip in the appropriate places (i.e. if a section does not need to be completed given a certain response to a question, it should be clear at which item the user should begin recording the data to avoid errors of omission).[6]
- Avoid splitting related groups of questions concerning a single clinical study visit.[4,6] For example, information on a single adverse event should not be split and laid across multiple pages. This can complicate the data analysis later.

It should be noted that data forms may be produced in different formats, including paper or electronic documents.[1,4] However, regardless of the delivery method, data forms should adhere to the aforementioned guidelines.

How do I Avoid Introducing Bias or Errors in the Data Collected on Data Forms?

Gathering accurate data is of the utmost importance in clinical research. Following the design guidelines mentioned above will aid in minimizing errors in the collected data.

Other steps that can be taken to reduce errors revolve around the content of the questions and instructions. Ensure all questions are clear and unambiguous to respondents by employing simple, uncomplicated language and using terms that have the same meaning for all respondents.[2,6] Additionally, include a complete set of response options for each question (e.g. if necessary, include options such as ***Other***, ***None*** or ***Not applicable***).[6,7] The distinction between ***open-form items*** and ***closed-form items*** is also important in avoiding bias. Open-form items may be used when it is difficult to predict the responses that may be given to a question to avoid leading respondents toward certain 'permissible' responses.[3,7] Conversely, closed-form items are preferable when the responses should be structured and respondents may need to be reminded of all possible responses. Closed-form responses are also simpler to process in data analysis later.[6]

Whenever possible, CRF questions should be self-explanatory so as to avoid including separate instructions.[3] If instructions are necessary, make them as clear and concise as possible and place them on the form itself adjacent to the relevant section.[6] Including brief instructions and prompts on the data form increases the likelihood they will be read and followed by the respondent. This decreases the possibility of queries and facilitates data transcription and analysis. In the event that lengthier, more detailed instructions are required, they can be included in a separate document referred to as ***CRF completion guidelines***. This serves to decrease the number of pages in the CRF, reducing costs and also ensures the format of the page remains uncluttered.[3]

Lastly, avoid collecting derived or calculated data.[1,4] Instead, record only the raw data that will be used to make any calculations on the form. For example, rather than recording a participant's age, record their date of birth also. This can later be used to calculate age and will minimize errors in data analysis.

How do I Ensure the Prepared Data Form Follows Best Practices?

After developing any CRFs, the entire study team should review and approve them.[1,3] This provides a variety of perspectives and results in comprehensive feedback. Specifically, each member of the team should verify that the language used on the CRFs is consistent and comprehensible for the intended respondents. Reviewers should ensure that it is possible to collect all of the requested data. The data form must also completely capture all of the data that will be required for analysis and collect the data in an appropriate form for planned analysis.[3] Another point to keep in mind when reviewing CRFs is that data collection must occur in a manner that facilitates site completion.[3] Data forms that are too lengthy or cumbersome, place a burden on respondents and may negatively impact the study by reducing participation.

It is also helpful to review pilot and test data to ensure accuracy and analyzability.[1,8] Administering the data forms to real patients helps to ensure that every item on the form is easily comprehensible to the respondent, contains appropriate terminology and elicits a single response.[7,8] Furthermore, pilot testing provides insight into whether the data form is too much of a burden for respondents, in which case it will require further editing and review.

Data form development is a lengthy process and is the utmost importance to the success of any clinical study. It is best to develop data forms alongside the study protocol rather than hastily constructing them at the end of the process.[1,7] This collaborative effort can take months of planning and preparation, but it is paramount to collecting the highest quality data.[8]

Important Learning Points

- Case report forms (CRFs) guide data collection by providing a structured, standardized method for recording relevant information about study participants.
- Well-designed data forms are conducive to successful studies, as meaningful analysis cannot be conducted without high quality data.
- Carefully constructing unambiguous questions reduces confusion on the part of respondents and encourages accurate and specific data recording.

- Providing clear visual cues indicating preferred response format, facilitates the data collection and transcription process. Designing a clean, uncluttered data form is also a key point.
- It is essential to review prepared CRFs thoroughly to ensure that all data collection instruments are of high enough quality to produce appropriate data.

More to Read

- Bhandari M, Joensson A. Clinical research for surgeons. Stuttgart; New York: Thieme Publishing Group; 2008.
- Meinert CL. Clinical Trials: Design, Conduct and Analysis. 2nd edition. New York: Oxford University Press; 2012.

Definitions

Adverse event: Any unfavorable or unintended sign, symptom or disease associated with the use of a medical intervention under investigation.

Closed-form items: Questions that are completed using a defined list of permissible responses.[6]

Open-form items: Questions that do not have a defined list of permissible responses.[6]

CRF completion guidelines: A document providing unambiguous instructions on CRF completion in all practical scenarios.[3,4]

Data queries: Non-sensible or questionable data that must be explained.

Exclusion criteria: A set of characteristics that preclude potential subjects from participating in a clinical study.

Inclusion criteria: A set of characteristics that potential subjects must fulfill in order to participate in a clinical study.

Protocol: A document explaining the purpose, background, design, methods and organization of a clinical trial in detail.

Source documents: The original documents, data and records concerning study participants.

REFERENCES

1. Trocky N, Brandt C. Process of data management. In: Gad SC (ed). Clinical trials handbook. Hoboken: John Wiley & Sons; 2009.

2. Voorhees J, Scheipeter ME. Case report form development. In: Schuster DP, Powers WJ (eds). Translational and experimental clinical research. Philadelphia: Lippincott Williams & Wilkins; 2005.p.122-135.
3. Clinical Data Interchange Standards Consortium (CDISC). Clinical Data Acquisition Standards Harmonization (CDASH). Austin:CDISC;2008. Available from:http://www.cdisc.org/system/files/all/standard/application/pdf/cdash_std_1_0_2008_10_01.pdf.
4. Bellary S, Krishnankutty B, Latha MS. Basics of case report form designing in clinical research. Perspect Clin Res. 2014;5(4):159-66.
5. Bhandari M, Joensson A. Clinical research for surgeons. Stuttgart; New York: Thieme; 2008.
6. Meinert CL. Clinical Trials: Design, Conduct and Analysis. 2nd edition. New York: Oxford University Press; 2012.
7. Spilker B, Schoenfelder J. Data collection forms in clinical trials. New York: Raven Press;1991.
8. Weinstein JN, Deyo RA. Clinical research: issues in data collection. Spine (Phila Pa 1976). 2000;25(24):3104-9.

6. Getting the Word Out—Presentation and Publication

Section Outline

28. Creating an Impactful Slide Presentation
29. Writing a Good Clinical Research Paper
30. Making Sense of Reporting Guidelines
31. Submitting a Paper for Publication—A Guide to Success
32. Knowledge Translation 101—Maximizing Impact

28

Creating an Impactful Slide Presentation

Colm McCarthy, Mandeep Dhillon

Key Objectives
- Be able to identify the key elements of any presentation
- Understand the fundamentals of formatting a presentation
- Understand the important elements of giving a presentation
- Understand the usefulness and importance of presentations.

What is a Slide Presentation?

Regardless of their level of training or background, nearly everyone has observed a slide presentation. Slide presentations range from formal ***podium presentations*** at major conferences to the basis of most university level lectures, and are incredibly commonplace.[1,2] They are now so pervasive that it would be unusual for a major speaker at an event not to use a slide presentation. Nonetheless, it is important to understand the characteristics that differentiate a great slide presentation from a mediocre slide presentation.

Slide presentations contain slides that are projected and displayed on a large screen so that an audience can see them while they are explained by the presenter. In other words, slide presentations are a visual and oral presentation happening simultaneously. As such, the success of the slide presentation is dependent on both aspects and great slides can be ruined by a bad oral presentation or vice versa.[1,3]

Slide presentations are an opportunity for one to tell people about their work and create an association between it and themself. That is to say, the slide presentation heavily affects how people view both the speaker and their work.[4]

What is a Great Slide Presentation?

A great slide presentation engages the audience and conveys information to the audience in a clear, comprehensive and understandable manner. Knowing one's audience, however, is fundamental for a great presentation and a presenter should understand their audience and adjust their slide presentation accordingly.[3,4] A great presentation for one audience could be awful for another. In order to understand your audience, one can ask the following questions:

- ***Who:*** Is this a panel of experts, laypeople or individuals with moderate experience?
- ***What:*** What are the goals of my presentation? What do I want to give to the audience? Am I using appropriate vocabulary? How much background context is necessary?
- ***Where:*** What is the size of the audience and the venue? How large is the screen? How many screens are there? Will there be a microphone? Will there be a podium?
- ***When:*** How long should my presentation be? Will there be time for questions and discussion?
- ***How:*** Do I need to bring my own computer? Is my slide presentation compatible with the audiovisual equipment? How will my slide presentation be distributed afterwards?

What are Great Slides?

There are many software programs that can be used to prepare the slides for a slide presentation and Powerpoint, Keynote and Prezi are among the most common. The most important factors to consider when choosing a software program are the extent to which it is compatible with the audio-visual equipment in the venue in which one is presenting and the extent to which one can actually use it to make great slides.

Slides are a visual representation of the information being presented by the speaker. They can display charts, images, tables, plain text and videos. Great slides function as tools that augment the speaker's message while they are delivering it. Great slides are clear, concise, legible and not distracting.[1,2,4,5] When making slides, one should remember the acronym KISS (keep it simple stupid). To better understand each component of a slide one can consider the following aspects:

Background and Theme

Most software programs for slide presentations contain a default theme of black text on white background. While simple and clear, this theme might also be perceived as boring or uninteresting. Fortunately, most programs also come with a series of pre-prepared themes with varying fonts, text colors and slide background colors. One must be cautious, however, when selecting a theme (or making your own), as this is one of the easiest and most common ways of ruining a great slide presentation.[1,2]

One should be sure that their text is visible throughout the entire presentation, noting that sometimes the font colors change with bullet indentation.[2,5] Some themes have a variable hue of the background color and one must ensure that the text and images will be legible regardless of the color scheme.[2] One should also be sure to account for clashing colors (blue/red, red/green, blue/green, etc.) and consider that red and green, specifically often do not project well or cannot be perceived well even in non-color blind individuals.[1]

Finally, one should consider whether their audience will be in a dark room or a well-lit room. Dark backgrounds with light text are easier to view in dark rooms, while light backgrounds with dark text are easier to view in well-lit rooms.

Font

One should be sure to choose a font that is easily read. Times New Roman and Arial are classic legible fonts, while fonts such as Comic Sans or other are difficult to read and may be associated with childishness.[1,4,5] White font with a black outline is visible clearly on any background, but white font on a fading background from dark to light is easy to read only where the background is darkest.[1]

Text

A slide should have just enough text required to make the point.[2] Filling the slide with excessive text makes it difficult to read and confusing for one's audience.[5] As the number of lines of text increases, most programs automatically begin to decrease the font size. A good rule of thumb is to stop adding text before the font starts to change size to fit into the allotted space.

Graphics

Images, charts and tables are some of the most important and powerful tools in a great slide presentation. However, they can also ruin a slide when used poorly. Graphics should be easily understood at a glance.[1,2,5] When inserting an image, one should make sure that it is formatted to fit in the slide, that it maintains clarity and that it is not too small or pixelated.[1] For larger tables or charts, one might choose to highlight the important parts with either an abbreviated version or a pointer.[3] If one chooses to include videos, they should ensure that the videos are short, work properly and are capable of playing sound if appropriate.

Effects

Effects are a common pitfall for novice presenters. Many slide presentation programs offer the addition of sound effects, visual effects and other animations for each slide or for each bullet or graphics. These effects can be useful, for example, when posing questions to the audience because they provide a means of temporarily concealing the answers.[1,2] In general, however, excessive use of effects is at risk for being distracting.

Handouts

If one's slide presentation will be distributed after their presentation, it is necessary for the presenter to finalize their slides for both on-screen and printed handout use. Many themes, colored fonts, animations or other formatting changes do not convert well while printing in black and white.[6]

What is the Structure of a Great Slide Presentation?

The order and flow of the content plays a critical role in how a slide presentation will be perceived. Typical scientific slide presentations will contain a structure similar to this:
- Title slide with authorship and institution details
- Disclosures
- Learning objectives or goals

- Introduction and background context
- Methods and study design
- Results
- Limitations
- Implications
- Conclusions
- References.

How should a Great Slide Presentation be Delivered?

The most important part of delivering a great slide presentation is that "practice makes perfect". One should plan what they are going to say and how they will say it, then rehearse it thoroughly.[6] If one is fortunate enough to have peers to listen to their rehearsal several times, they should seek honest feedback and listen carefully. If one does not have peers to provide feedback, they might try rehearsing in front of a mirror.

Most slide presentation software applications have a presenter viewer that gives the presenter a different version of the slides than that which is being displayed to the audience. Often, the presenter viewer includes the previous, current and next slides, the author's notes and a timer. The previous, current and next slide allows one to know where they are in the presentation and where they going next, which may help to create smooth transitions between each section of the content. The author's notes section allows one to add additional cues and avoid the use of additional papers at the podium, which provides a clean and sleek appearance while presenting. The timer helps to keep one on track, which is essential for any good presentation.[4]

One can engage their audience by making eye contact and speaking clearly. Great slide presentations are an opportunity to really set oneself and one's work apart from others.[2] Whether a microphone is present or not, one should make sure that their volume is appropriate and they should take care to speak slowly and clearly.[4] If in doubt, it is usually best to slow down.

There is no faster way to lose an audience than by simply reading from the screen content that they have either already read or are currently reading themselves. One should discuss the content on their slides, but they should never read them directly.[2] Bullet points should be concise, while the speaker adds information and provides emphasis.[2,4]

It is also important to consider how one will address potential questions. Will they answer questions during the presentation, or will they wait until the end? During the presentation is often acceptable for lectures or other long presentations, while waiting until the end is typical for short scientific presentations.[4,5] If one chooses to answer questions during their presentation, they should consider how it might impact their ability to finish within their allotted time.

Humor can assist one in engaging their audience, but successful humor requires that one consider both their audience and themself. Inappropriate jokes can offend an audience and overly frequent jokes can be distracting.[7] If a presenter is not comfortable with incorporating humor directly, they might consider a funny graphic, such as a single frame cartoon.

Finally, it is useful to always have an extra copy of one's presentation saved on a portable device or available on an online server (including email). Technical problems can occur, but back up strategies can prevent disaster.

Important Learning Points

- Presenters should know their audience and venue before preparing their slides.
- Slides presentations should be compatible with a venue's audiovisual equipments.
- KISS: Keep it simple stupid.
- Distracting sound effects or animations should be avoided.
- Practice! Practice! Practice… and stay on time.
- Presenters should avoid reading directly from their slides.
- Handouts should be formatted appropriately for printing.

More to Read

Schmaltz RM, Enstrom R. Death to weak. PowerPoint: strategies to create effective visual presentations. Front Psychol. 2014;5:1138.

Definition

Podium presentation: A formal scientific presentation, either by invitation or by peer review at a conference or meeting.

REFERENCES

1. Schmaltz RM, Enstrom R. Death to weak PowerPoint: strategies to create effective visual presentations. Front Psychol. 2014;5:1138.
2. Harolds JA. Tips for giving a memorable presentation, Part IV: Using and composing powerpoint slides. Clin Nucl Med. 2012;37(10):977-80.
3. Wax JR, Cartin A, Pinette MG. Preparing a research presentation: a guide for investigators. Am J Obstet Gynecol. 2011;205(1):28.
4. Mayer K. Fundamentals of surgical research course: research presentations. J Surg Res. 2005;128(2):174-7.
5. Collins J. Education techniques for lifelong learning making a powerpoint presentation. Radiographic. 2004;24(4):1177-83.
6. Hardicre J, Coad J, Devitt P. Ten steps to successful conference presentations. Br J Nurs. 2007;16(7):402.
7. Kosslyn SM, Kievit RA, Russell AG, et al. PowerPoint presentation flaws and failures: A phsycological analysis. Front Psychol. 2012;3:230.

29. Writing a Good Clinical Research Paper

Sarah Resendes, Ashok Shyam

Key Objectives

- Understand the importance of writing clinical papers
- Learn how to organize a clinical paper by means of subject headings that reflect the scientific methods
- Learn what information is to be included in each subheadings
- Be provided with tips on effective clinical writing.

Why is Scientific Writing Important?

The evolution of medical practice depends greatly on the dissemination of knowledge. If beneficial treatments were discovered and never documented or shared with the rest of the medical community, the advancement of healthcare would be at a crawling pace, redundant experiments would be conducted needlessly and most importantly, patients would often receive less effective interventions than they would otherwise.

Writing and publishing clinical papers provides many benefits: lessons learned about improving practice can be shared with others, readers can provide helpful suggestions to the authors, it may provide a forum for debate or an impetus for change in medical practice and it may facilitate the formation of networks of individuals with similar interests.[1] Therefore, it is important that the results of clinical trials be documented and available for evaluation.

A well written clinical paper must provide its readers a comprehensive overview of how the study was conducted, the exact results attained and an accurate analysis of those results. It is important to realize that even exciting findings may not be accepted for publication if they are presented poorly, highlighting the importance of good clinical writing.[2] This chapter provides a basic guidelines for the writing of clinical papers.

What is the Basic Outline of the Clinical Paper?

A clinical paper serves as a description of the ***scientific method*** applied to a particular study question.[3] The scientific method has four stages: (1) recognition of a study question, (2) formulation of a hypothesis, (3) development of experiment(s) to reject or to accept the hypothesis and (4) interpretation and discussion of the results of the experiment.[3]

One can begin to write the clinical paper before the study is even carried out. In fact, this is the proper way to write scientific papers.[3] The conventional organization of a clinical paper is as follows: introduction, methods, results and discussion (IMRAD).[4] However, it would be difficult to write the paper in this order since, for example, the results of the trial and the discussion can be used to write the introduction, but results can only be attained after the study is carried out. Pollock et al.[5] provide the following writing sequence suggestion: methods, results, discussion and introduction (MRDAI). Including these subheadings in your clinical paper makes it easier to follow for the reader.

In short, the paper will state the question to be answered, how the answers will be attained, what the findings are, whether or not the question was answered and whether or not the findings of the study provoke further debate.[4]

Where Do I Start?

Once a study problem is established, a thorough literature search, as discussed in Chapter 11, must be undertaken so that the investigator is made aware of what other researchers have found on the topic (if anything).[3] Perhaps the problem has already been examined, eliminating the need to conduct the study altogether. If a literature search was not carried out, the investigator would be unaware of the background information that is already available on the topic and may be conducting the experiment needlessly, wasting resources and time. Likewise, a hypothesis can only be derived once the literature search has been conducted and the investigator has focused on exactly what the study question is.[3]

How do I Write an Introduction?

To begin the introduction section, it is important to include some background information on the study topic and a brief justification for completing the study. This section should outline what has been found in earlier studies and if no work has been done on the topic previously, information about the currently recommended treatments should be included. The crucial element of the introduction is outlining the objectives of the study and rationale for the research, including a specific research question.[4]

How do I Write a Method Section?

The methods section can be written prior to beginning a study, but may require modifications once the study has been completed.[3] This section is where the description of how the research was conducted is presented, including a thorough explanation of the study design, a description of the characteristics of the study participants, what experiments will be carried out (e.g. which interventions are being used), the measurements to be taken and a statistical analysis. If appropriate, it is also important to include a statement showing that ethics approval was obtained from the local Research Ethics Board/Institutional Review Board of each clinical site and informed consent was given by each subject in the trial.[4]

The description of the study design should indicate whether or not patients were randomized, if blinding was used, if control(s) were used (e.g. placebo), the parallel group or crossover design and a listing of all clinical sites were involved. The description of the study population should indicate the characteristics of the subjects (e.g. whether they were healthy, had a certain disease, etc.). It is important that you describe the characteristics of the patients in your study so that readers can compare them to the patients they treat in their own practice and with this information they can decide whether or not the results of your study are clinically relevant. This can be achieved by describing the patient eligibility criteria in the paper.

In this section explaining the interventions being tested, it is necessary to specify all aspects of the intervention in question (e.g. type and composition of drug, dosage, route of administration, etc.). Describing the measurements used entails indicating the endpoint(s) that deem an intervention as clinically effective or more beneficial than the alternative treatment. It is also necessary to outline which clinical procedures and tests are to be used in the study.[4]

The final subsection of the methods section should contain information on the statistical methods to be used for the analysis of the data.[3] It is important to indicate whether or not the intention to treat analysis was used and how losses to follow-up were analyzed. This practice helps to eliminate bias because it ensures that all data is accounted for each patient who was originally enrolled in the trial regardless of what happened to them thereafter.[6] Also, a justification of the sample size used for the study should be demonstrated using a sample size calculation. Overall, the methods section should be written in such a way that an independent investigator reading the paper could carry out the same study.[4]

How Do I Write a Result Section?

As one might assume, the results section can only be written after the study has been conducted and data were obtained. Data is the only thing displayed in the results section. Interpretation of the data and references to other studies should not to be included in the results and it should be included in the discussion.[3] In this results section, it is necessary to include the number of patients assigned for each intervention, how many were lost to follow-up or excluded (and the reasoning), any adverse events, demographics of the study population, the duration of the trial and whether or not the study deviated from the proposed protocol and why.[4] Using a flow diagram serves as an effective means of tracking the progression of patients throughout the study.

It is important to protect the identity of the patients who were involved in the study, therefore, no patient identifiers are to be included in the paper.[1] The use of figures, tables and graphs can be effective in organizing the data and making it easier to understand.[3] To avoid redundancy, it is important to avoid repeating the data that is presented in the tables.[4]

Statistics should be presented along with the data in order to attribute significance to the results[3]—statistics such as confidence intervals, standard deviations and standard error of the mean are useful here. When comparing two outcomes, statistical tests that assess whether or not differences are statistically significant should be carried out and reported.[3]

How do I Write a Discussion?

The discussion is meant to provide an interpretation of the results in order to highlight the clinical importance and significance of the findings. Repetition of the results should be avoided here.[4] The discussion section can also be started before the study is carried out, providing a concise overview of what other researchers have found on the topic previously. This information can be obtained from the literature review that was conducted as the first step of the writing process. The overview of the relevant literature should provide the reader with an understanding of how previous research relates to the present study.[3]

The central component of the discussion consists of an interpretation of the results. The writer should define the strengths and weaknesses of the study and also the clinical research implications of the study's findings.[4] Finally, conclusions are derived whereby the hypothesis is either accepted or rejected and the investigator may indicate if more research on the topic is necessary. One may choose to place the conclusion as a separate heading in the paper.[3]

How do I Write an Abstract?

Although the abstract is the first item presented in a paper, it is typically the last item written.[4] An abstract is a condensed version of the clinical paper, typically outlining the background, methods, results and conclusions of the study.[3] Most journals use structured abstracts and have a word limit (e.g. 250 words), so it must be concise and void of unnecessary elaboration.[3]

Are there other tips I should keep in mind while writing a clinical research paper?

When choosing a title for a clinical paper, it is good to keep it accurate, short and concise. The title is not the place to use informal terms, embellishments, question marks or exclamation points.[4] It is helpful to use ***medical subject headings (MeSH)*** which serve as keywords in your title so that it can be indexed and easily searched in an online database.[4]

The writing style should be as clear and concise as possible, making it easier to read and understand. A paper may considered to be well written when a reader who is entirely uninvolved in the study can understand everything in the paper.[1]

Having others to review your clinical paper is an excellent idea and can lead to the correction of inconsistencies, grammar and spelling errors. Use simple words and phrases, replace jargon words and only include necessary punctuation.[1]

It is important to be aware of who will be the target audience of the paper.[1] For example, a paper written for an audience of medical professionals will read differently than that intended for readers with no medical background. In this case greater emphasis must be placed on definitions and clarity of concepts that a medical professional may find basic.

For clinical papers reporting the results of randomized controlled trials (RCTs), the consolidated standards of reporting trials (CONSORT) statement is a useful tool to allow readers to evaluate the validity of the clinical trial on which the paper is based.[7] This consists of a checklist which identifies the key information to be included in the title, abstract, introduction, methods section, results section and discussion section and also includes a flow diagram tracking patient flow throughout the study.

Important Learning Points

- Begin the paper before you begin your study.
- Include subheadings throughout the paper.
- Write the paper in the following order: methods, results, discussion and introduction (MRDAI).

- Present the paper in the following order: introduction, methods, results and discussion (IMRAD).
- Conduct a thorough literature search in order to gain insight into what other researchers have found on the topic.
- The introduction outlines the objectives of the study and rationale for the research.
- The methods section should be written so that an independent investigator reading the paper could carry out the same study.
- Data is the only thing displayed in the results section.
- The discussion provides an interpretation of the results, not a repetition of the results.

More to Read

An example of a good clinical research paper:
- Randomized trial of reamed and unreamed intramedullary nailing of tibial shaft fractures. The Study to Prospectively Evaluate Reamed Intramedullary Nails in Patients with Tibial Fractures (SPRINT) Investigators. J Bone Joint Surg Am. 2008;90(12):2567-78.
- Pakes GE. Writing manuscripts describing clinical trials: A guide for pharmacotherapeutic researchers. Ann Pharmacother. 2001;35(6):770-9.

Definitions

Scientific method: A process of investigation that is the foundation of scientific inquest.[8]

Medical subject headings (MeSH): 'A controlled vocabulary thesaurus' developed by the National Library of Medicine that organizes sets of terms using keywords, facilitating the formation of literature searches with varying levels of specificity.[14]

REFERENCES

1. Dixon N. Writing for publication—a guide for new authors. Int J Qual Health Care. 2001;13(5):417-21.
2. Tomaska L. Teaching how to prepare a manuscript by means of rewriting published scientific papers. Genetics. 2007;175(1):17-20.

3. Van Way CW. Writing a scientific paper. Nutr Clin Pract. 2007;22(6):636-40.
4. Pakes GE. Writing manuscripts describing clinical trials: A guide for pharmacotherapeutic researchers. Ann Pharmacother. 2001;35(6):770-9.
5. Pollock AV, Evans ME, Wiggin NJB, et al. Writing your first scientific paper. In: Troidl H, Spitzer WO, McPeek B (Eds). Principles and practice of research. Strategies for surgical investigators, 2nd edition. New York: Springer-Verlag; 1991. pp. 391-403.
6. Minervation. (2009). The CONSORT Statement. [online] CONSORT website. Available from www.consort-statement.org/consort-statement/ [Accessed August 2009].
7. NC State University. (2004). LabWrite Glossary. [online] LabWrite resources. Available from www.ncsu.edu/labwrite/res/res-glossary.html [Accessed August 2009].
8. U.S. National Library of Medicine. (2009). Fact Sheet: Medical Subject Headings (MeSH®). [online] NIH website. Available from http://www.nlm.nih.gov/pubs/factsheets/mesh.html [Accessed August 2009]

30 Making Sense of Reporting Guidelines

Akhila Rachakonda, Kim Madden

Key Objectives

- Comprehend the importance of reporting guidelines and checklists in meeting appropriate standards for accurate reporting of health research
- Become familiar with the most common guidelines for reporting various types of research
- Understand that reporting guidelines will help researchers, healthcare professionals, journal editors, peer reviewers and all of those involved in the dissemination and uptake of health research.

Why do we Need Reporting Guidelines and Checklists?

The end goal of clinical research should be to effectively disseminate results to healthcare professionals and other stakeholders. This knowledge dissemination is effective only if the reporting of research methods, results and inferences are accurate. Accurate reporting is essential as published research could be integrated into a systematic review, meta-analysis, or the development of clinical guidelines after it is published. By using globally standardized research *reporting guidelines* and tools, information can be effectively communicated to *knowledge users* to enhance the pool of health evidence.[1]

Until the 1990s, there was no standardization of what should be reported in health research manuscripts. This lack of standardization led to problems with inadequate presentation of data, lack of complete information regarding research methods, selective reporting of results and omission or misinterpretation of various steps involved during conducting, collecting and synthesizing results.[1,2] For example, a systematic review of randomized trials in top orthodontics journals showed that some critical reporting elements are often missing from published randomized trials.[3] Only 5% of trials reported whether data analysts were blinded, 12% reported whether they used the *intention-to-treat* principle, 19% reported on the *external validity* of the trial and none reported on the degree of success of blinding.[3]

To improve the quality of reporting, now top medical journals like the British Medical Journal (BMJ), Journal of the American Medical Association (JAMA) and New England Journal of Medicine (NEJM) will not accept a clinical trial manuscript that does not follow standardized reporting guidelines.[4,5] Many journals also require the use of such guidelines for studies other than clinical trials as well. Even if the journal that you are targeting for your publication does not require the use of standardized reporting guidelines, it is a good practice to follow the guidelines anyway.

Which Guideline should I Use?

There are a number of reporting guidelines that are widely used among the top journals. Some common examples are given in Table 30.1.

All of the common reporting guidelines in Table 30.1 have some common elements. They all have standardized checklists to make it simple for those conducting and reporting the research to know what to report and how. Each reporting guideline suggests the use of a *flow diagram* to facilitate

Table 30.1: Commonly used reporting guidelines

Type of study	Reporting guideline
Randomized controlled trials	CONSORT
Systematic reviews and meta-analysis	PRISMA
Observational studies	STROBE
Protocol papers	SPIRIT
Diagnostic accuracy studies	STARD
Economic reviews	CHEERS

easy understanding of how the various groups involved in the study move from one point of the study to another. Flowchart 30.1 shows an example of a flow diagram for a hypothetical randomized controlled trial to illustrate what information should be included in such a flow diagram. The format of most of the reporting guidelines is similar in many ways in terms of the subheadings such as title of the project, introduction, methods, results, discussion and conclusion. Thoroughly understanding of any one guideline will help you to work easily through another.

CONSORT (Consolidated Standards of Reporting Trials) Statement

The CONSORT statement provides recommendations for reporting randomized trials. This evidence-based reporting guideline comprises a 25-item checklist and a flow diagram to help researchers accurately report all pertinent details of the design, data collection, analysis and interpretation of their study.[1,6] The checklist includes information on the title, abstract, introduction, methods (trial design, participants, interventions, outcomes, sample size, randomization, blinding, etc.), results (participant flow, recruitment, baseline data, outcomes, estimation, ancillary analyses, harms), discussion (limitations, generalizability, interpretation), registration, protocol and funding. This statement is almost universally accepted by peer reviewed medical journals, editors and reviewers.

PRISMA (Preferred Reporting Items for Systematic Reviews and Meta-analysis) Statement

The PRISMA statement is an evidence-based reporting guideline comprising a 27-item checklist and a flow diagram that helps authors in reporting systematic reviews and meta-analysis.[7] It helps to critically appraise systematic reviews and to measure the reporting quality of a review. This statement provides information on the title, abstract, introduction, methods (protocol, registration, data collection, risk of bias, summary measures), results (study characteristics, synthesis of results), discussion (summary of evidence, limitations, conclusions) and findings.

Flowchart 30.1: CONSORT flowchart for a hypothetical study of diabetics with frozen shoulder

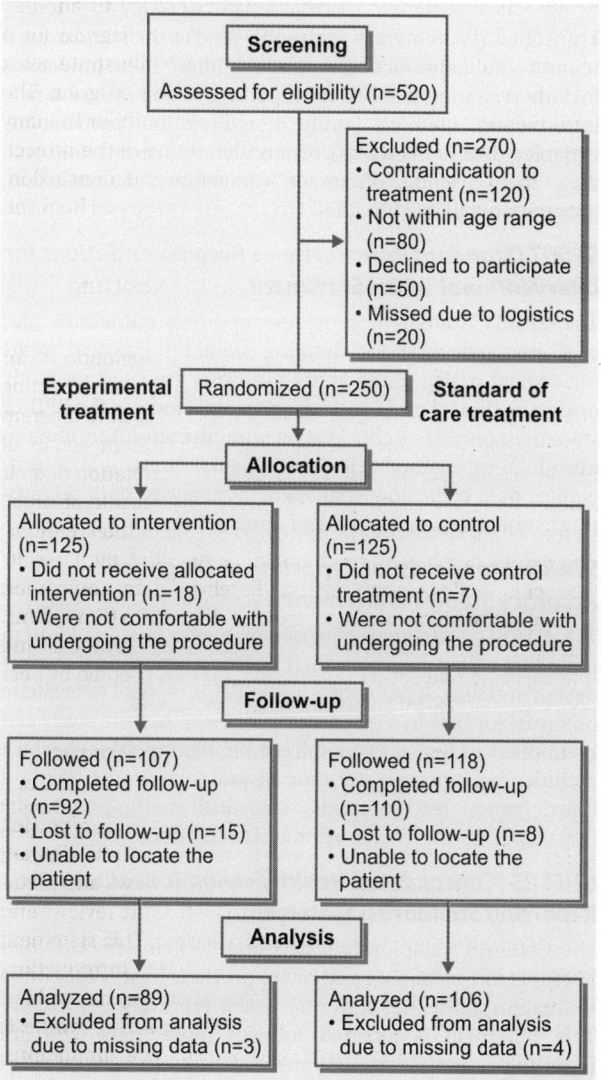

STROBE (Strengthening the Reporting of Observational Studies in Epidemiology) Statement

The STROBE statement is commonly used as the standardized reporting guideline for observational studies.[8] These guidelines include recommendations for reporting on the title, abstract, introduction, methods (study design, setting, participants, variables, data sources, bias), results (descriptive data, outcome data, main results), discussion (limitations, interpretation, generalizability) and funding.

SPIRIT (Standard Protocol Items Recommendations for Interventional Trials) Statement

The SPIRIT statement provides reporting guidelines and a 33-item checklist for defining standard protocol items for clinical trials.[9] These study protocols are used for study design in clinical trials and experimental studies. The SPIRIT statement provides a checklist on administrative information, introduction, methods (for participants, interventions, outcomes, data collection, management analysis, data monitoring), ethics, dissemination and appendices.

STARD (Standards for Reporting of Diagnostic Accuracy Studies) Statement

The STARD statement consists of a checklist of 25-item including a flow diagram which assists in reporting the study design and flow of patients.[10] It also helps readers to evaluate potential for bias in a given study and whether the study can be applied to a given generalized population. The checklist includes guidance on the title, abstract, keywords, method (participants, test methods, statistical methods), results (participants, test results, estimates) and discussion.

CHEERS (Consolidated Health Economic Evaluation Reporting Standards) Statement

The CHEERS statement consists of a 24-item checklist that attempts to consolidate and revise previous health economic evaluation guidelines into one useful reporting guideline.[11] This statement is targeted towards researchers who are reporting economic evaluations and editors/peer reviewers who are assessing reports for publication. The checklist consists of information on the title, abstract, introduction, methods (target population, setting, study perspective, comparators, time horizon, discount rate, estimating resources and costs, etc.), results (study parameters, incremental costs/outcomes, etc.), discussion (findings, limitations, generalizability, current knowledge), funding and conflict of interest.

Where can I Find More Information about Reporting Guidelines?

The Enhancing the Quaity and Transparency of Health Research (EQUATOR) network is an international organization that primarily focuses on raising awareness of the importance of accurate reporting of health research. The network maintains an online collection of various reporting guidelines including all the statements listed above. The reader can refer to this network for complete information. Website: www.equator-network.org

Being Aware of Reporting Guidelines

It is of utmost importance that authors, peer reviewers, journal editors and other knowledge users are aware of the common reporting guidelines for various study designs. Standardized reporting as per the guidelines facilitates the acceptance of manuscripts for publication in peer reviewed journals and helps future researchers to be able to produce better systematic reviews, meta-analysis and clinical guidelines.

Definitions

External validity: The extent to which a study can be generalized to other populations or situations.

Intention-to-treat analysis: Includes all randomized patients in the groups in which they were randomly assigned, regardless of their adherence with the entry criteria, treatment they actually received and subsequent withdrawal from treatment or deviation from the protocol.

Knowledge users: Groups of people for which the results of a study are likely to be useful for making clinical decisions, such as patients, healthcare professionals and policy makers.

Reporting guidelines: Tools developed to guide researchers on reporting research accurately and in a standardized manner.

Study flow diagram: A visual representation of the numbers of patients at each stage of a study, including screening, allocation, follow-up and analysis.

Trial registration: The act of recording information about a planned trial in an official trial registry [such as clinical trials government or European Clinical Trials database (EudraCT)] to improve transparency regarding reporting of clinical trials.

REFERENCES

1. Begg C, Cho M, Eastwood S, et al. Improving the quality of reporting of randomized controlled trials. The CONSORT statement. JAMA. 1996;276(8):637-9.
2. Moher D, Dulberg CS, Wells GA. Statistical power, sample size and their reporting in randomized controlled trials. JAMA. 1994;272(2):122-4.
3. Lempesi E, Koletsi D, Fleming PS, et al. The reporting quality of randomized controlled trials in orthodontics. J Evid Based Dent Pract. 2014;14(2):46-52.
4. Altman DG. Better reporting of randomised controlled trials: the CONSORT statement. BMJ. 1996;313(7057):570-1.
5. Rennie D. How to report randomized controlled trials. The CONSORT statement. JAMA. 1996;276(8):649.
6. Schulz KF, Altman DG, Moher D, et al. CONSORT 2010 statement: updated guidelines for reporting parallel group randomised trials. BMJ. 2010;340:c332.
7. Moher D, Liberati A, Tetzlaff J, et al. Preferred reporting items for systematic reviews and meta-analyses: the PRISMA statement. BMJ. 2009;339:b2535.
8. Von Elm E, Altman DG, Egger M, et al. The strengthening the reporting of observational studies in epidemiology (STROBE) statement: Guidelines for reporting observational studies. BMJ. 2007;335(7624):806-8.
9. Chan AW, Tetzlaff JM, Altman DG, et al. SPIRIT 2013 Statement: Defining standard protocol items for clinical trials. Ann Intern Med. 2013;158(3):200-7.
10. Bossuyt PM, Reitsma JB, Bruns DE, et al. Towards complete and accurate reporting of studies of diagnostic accuracy: the STARD initiative. Standards for reporting of diagnostic accuracy. BMJ. 2003;326(7379):41-4.
11. Husereau D, Drummond M, Petrou S, et al. Consolidated health economic evaluation reporting standards (CHEERS) statement. BMJ. 2013;346:f1049.

31

Submitting a Paper for Publication—A Guide to Success

Patrick Thornley

Key Objectives

- Learn how to select which journal to submit your research paper to
- Learn how to prepare a manuscript for submission
- Learn how to navigate the online submission process
- Learn how to effectively respond to reviewers' comments.

Summary

Scientific research is only useful to the scientific community if novel and methodologically rigorous research results are reported and published. Publication of research in a scientific journal is thus a critical aspect of participating in the research process.[1] However, with an ever-increasing number of research study submissions to academic journals, there is a rising rate of rejected research studies.[2] Acceptance rates are as low as 10% for some journals.[1] In Chapter 29, we discussed the core components of a good research paper and the importance of these components for achieving publication. In this chapter we will discuss how to select which journal to submit your research paper to and how to navigate the online submission process successfully.

How do I Select Which Journal to Submit my Research Paper to?

Deciding where to submit your research paper for ***peer review*** and publication is not an easy process. There are two general approaches—some researchers advocate selecting a target journal at the outset of writing and following their style requirements,[3] while others advocate a simplified, free-flowing technique that involves reformatting to follow the style requirements of a particular journal later on.[4] The second approach is far easier for inexperienced researchers, but both methods still require that you select a target journal.

You should consider whether your research study has a major finding and whether it is of widespread medical interest.[5] If so, a journal with broad areas of interest and diverse readership may be appropriate. If not, consider submitting to a subspecialty journal that has previously published papers with topics and designs similar to your own. Senior colleagues and well-published mentors can often assist in identifying potential journals for your work.

Journal impact factors are a measure of the average number of citations of articles published in a given journal over the past 2 years and they represent a good starting point for new researchers. Journals with higher impact factors generally have higher editorial standards and are more competitive, but they are also more likely to lead to effective translation of important science.

If you are unsure about whether your research study would fit in the scope of a journal, consider contacting the editor directly, outline the nature of your research and assess their interest in publishing your manuscript.[3] Most editors will not make a formal decision before seeing a copy of your manuscript, but appraising their interest early can sometimes avoid a prolonged review that would ultimately end in rejection.[2,3]

Lastly, beware of predatory journals that do not have adequate peer review processes, are not indexed in major databases and charge excessive publication fees.[6] Scholars who are newer to academic research are at particular risk, especially those scholars conducting research within developing nations. If considering submitting your research to an open access journal, consult the Directory of Open Access Journals for a list of credible open access journals. Be sure to cross-reference those journals which you are considering to submit against blacklisted journals on "Beall's List."[6]

How do I Prepare my Manuscript for Submission?

To prepare your manuscript for submission, review the 'Instructions for Authors' for that particular journal. The importance of strict adherence to these author instructions and emphasis on attention to detail during this process cannot be emphasized enough. Many journals receive very high volumes of submissions for each publication edition and failure to follow the author instructions for a given journal can lead to a quick rejection.

Preparing for submission involves formatting your manuscript and formatting or completing the supporting tables, figures, appendices and any conflict of interest or disclosure statements.[4]

Abstract

Most journals require the abstract to be submitted separately from the manuscript. The two most important details to consider are the maximum word or character count and whether there are any required headings or subheadings. Some journals will also ask that you assign a level of evidence based on their guidelines.[4]

Keywords

Keywords are individual words or short terms (three words or less), which describe the topic of your research. Keywords should not simply repeat your study title. Each journal will have a different maximum number of keywords you may use, which researchers in the same field may employ to access your study when conducting literature searches.[4] Think of the keywords which helps to increase the exposure of your article and choose terms wisely to maximize the chance that readers will find your paper and ultimately read your publication.

Title Page

Each journal will differ slightly in their instructions, but you will be expected to have on a single page—the full title of the manuscript, a list of all authors (arranged in order) along with a list of their institution affiliations. Lastly, you will also be asked to indicate the corresponding author, which is usually the first or supervising author. Some journals will request that you also submit a blinded title page in order to facilitate blinded peer review.

Cover Letter

Cover letters are not mandatory for most journals, but they are highly advisable because they provide an opportunity to introduce your work and address any important unusual aspects of it.[4] Address this letter to the Editor-in-Chief and use institutional letterhead with the date and the contact information of the corresponding author.

> *"Dear Dr. [name] and the editorial team at [journal name],*
>
> *Please find attached for your review, our manuscript entitled [title] for consideration of publication in a future issue of [journal you are submitting to].*
>
> *[Include two succinct paragraphs outlining your research, your key findings and why it would be of interest for the readership of the journal].*
>
> *On behalf of the authors, I, [corresponding author], had full access to all the data in the study and take responsibility for the integrity of the data, the accuracy of the data analysis and the decision to submit for publication. I was involved in all aspects of study conception and design, data acquisition, data analysis and interpretation, drafting the manuscript and critically revising the manuscript for intellectually important content. [Include the efforts in the manuscript for all other authors].*
>
> *This manuscript has not been previously submitted elsewhere. [Outline if any funding was received for this project and that all authors have completed their conflict of interest statements].*
>
> *We wish to thank you and the rest of your editorial team for your review and consideration of our manuscript for publication in your journal in advance.*
>
> *Sincerely,*
> *[Corresponding author]"*

Manuscript

Ensure that all short forms and abbreviations have been explained, all numbers are consistent between the abstract, main text, figures and tables,[7] and that the word counts and formatting follow the ***Instruction to Authors***. Re-read your manuscript several times to ensure clarity and a logical flow. Remove the abstract, figures and tables and save them as individual files to upload separately.

Tables and Figures

Each journal will indicate the file type in which they wish to have each table and figure submitted. Authors should recognize that images sometimes look clear on a personal computer screen but suffer from poor quality and pixelation if their file type or resolution is changed. Review the quality of your images on at least one other computer screen separate from your own after formatting.[1]

Supporting Documents

Most journals require all authors listed on the manuscript to complete confirmation of authorship as well as a conflict of interest (COI) statement. Consult the International Committee of Medical Journal Editors (ICMJE) if you are uncertain whether an individual should be listed as an author or a contributor on your paper.[8] Most scientific fields consider the first author as the most important contributor and the last author as the most important supervisor.[9] Many journals require a transfer of copyright agreement with your initial submission or upon acceptance for publication.[4]

How do I Navigate the Online Submission Process?

The vast majority of academic journals now operate solely via electronic manuscript submission systems. Each journal will have their own preferred electronic submission system, outlined in the author instructions section of their web page. If you are a first time user of this submission system, you will first need to create a username and a password and then follow the prompts for completing your account. Once logged in, the system should guide you through the phases of a general submission process:
- ***Type of study:*** Select the type of study that you are submitting.
- ***Title:*** Enter the full title of your study.

- ***Running title:*** Enter an abbreviated title, which will appear at the top of each page of the article.
- ***Abstract:*** Copy and paste your abstract into a textbox. This ensures your abstract conforms to the outlined word count for abstract submissions to the journal. Review your abstract within the textbox as formatting often changes during the transfer process from your word processor.
- ***Authors and institutions:*** It is also important to pay attention to the order in which the authors appear in this section as this will be the order in which the authorship appears on your manuscript. If you are the first author on this paper, then your name should appear beside authorship order "1".
- ***Reviewers:*** Many journals will afford you the opportunity to recommend two to three reviewers to review your study. You may also have the opportunity to indicate any reviewers you wish not to review your paper for risk of potential conflict of interest. Note that recommending reviewers is not a mandatory process for most journal submissions.
- ***Study details/comments section:*** Attach or copy and paste your cover letter. You may also be asked to indicate your total word count, number of tables and number of figures in this section and you may be asked whether you have previously submitted elsewhere, received ethics approval and are willing to attach transfer of copyright agreements and a conflict of interest statements for all authors.
- ***File upload section:*** Upload each file of your submission, including the separate files for your tables and figures. Most submission portals will allow you to add figure or table legends after uploading each document. Ensure that all uploaded files contain appropriate titles (e.g. "[Manuscript Title]_Figure 1").[1]
- ***Review and submit:*** The submission portal often allows you to view a final proof of your submission before confirming it. Review this proof in exquisite detail because it is your last chance to detect errors, which can be revised and re-uploaded with corrected files prior to submission.
- Monitor the status of your submission through peer review using the submission portal.

How do I Effectively Respond to Reviewers' Comments?

If you are asked to submit revisions, consider the reviewer's comments thoughtfully and try to apply them objectively to your work in order to improve the quality of your manuscript. If you disagree with a reviewer's comments, address it clearly and politely.

Solicit feedback from your co-authors. Create a document that outlines your responses to each comment sequentially and any changes made to your manuscript. The 'Instructions to Authors' will include direction about whether to highlight the changes in your manuscript and if yes then how to do so.[3]

Important Learning Points

- Identify a journal whose areas of interest and readership match your research.
- Pay close attention to the 'Instructions for Authors' when preparing your manuscript for submission.
- Double-check all aspects of your work, including the spelling of author names, the quality of your images, word counts and formatting.
- When responding to reviewer's comments, address each comment sequentially in an objective and polite manner.

More to Read

- Bhandari M, Joensson A, Borris LC. Getting your research paper published: A surgical perspective. New York: Thieme Medical Publishers Pvt Ltd; 2011.
- Cals JW, Kotz D. Writing tips series–effective writing and publishing scientific papers. J Clin Epidemiol. 2013;66:585. Part I-XII.

Definition

Peer review: A process that many, if not most, scientific journals use to ensure that journal articles are of adequate quality for publication. Usually two or more experts in the discipline evaluate and comment on the submitted manuscript and the authors have a chance to revise the manuscript based on the peer reviewer's comments.

REFERENCES

1. Hall PA. Getting your paper published: an editor's perspective. Ann Saudi Med. 2011;31(1):72-6.
2. Fonseca VA. How to get your paper published paper: An editor's perspective. J Diabetes Complications. 2014;28(1):1-3.
3. Guyatt GH, Haynes RB. Preparing reports for publication and responding to reviewers' comments. J Clin Epidemiol. 2006;59(9):900-6.
4. Bhandari M, Joensson A. Getting your research paper published–a surgical perspective. New York: Thieme Medical Publishers Pvt Ltd; 2011.
5. Dimitroulis G. Getting published in peer-reviewed journals. Int J Oral Maxillofac Surg. 2011;40(12):1342-5.
6. Bohannon J. Who's afraid of peer review? Science. 2013 4;342(6154):60-5.
7. Kloner RA. A brief review of useful tips for publishing your scientific manuscript. J Cardiovasc Pharmacol Ther. 2013;18(3):197-8.
8. International Committee of Medial Journal Editors (ICMJE). Defining the role of authors and contributors. April 15 2014. Available: http://www.icmje.org/recommendations/browse/roles-and-responsibilities/defining-the-role-of-authors-and-contributors.html.
9. Cals JW, Kotz D. Writing tips series–effective writing and publishing scientific papers. J Clin Epidemiol. 2013;66:585. Part I-XII.

32. Knowledge Translation 101—Maximizing Impact

Austin MacDonald, Vijay Shetty

> **Key Objectives**
> - Be able to define what knowledge translation is
> - Understand the steps involved in the 'knowledge-to-action' framework
> - Understand the importance of knowledge translation
> - Learn about the barriers to knowledge translation.

What is Knowledge Translation?

There exist many terms to describe the process of putting research knowledge into action.[1] The Canadian Institutes of Health Research (CIHR) defines knowledge translation as 'a dynamic and iterative process that includes synthesis, dissemination, exchange and ethically-sound application of knowledge to improve the health of Canadians, provide more effective health services and products and strengthen the healthcare system.'[2] In simple terms, knowledge translation is the process of taking disseminated knowledge and actually applying it to clinical practice.[1] Terms synonymous with knowledge translation include implementation science, research utilization and knowledge exchange.[1]

What is the Knowledge-to-Action Framework?

Knowledge translation is essentially the process of moving from knowledge to action.[3] Graham, et al.[4] conceptualized this process by developing the ***'knowledge-to-action'*** cycle, which is a conceptual framework that amalgamates traits found among a review of guidelines for applying research to clinical settings.

The 'knowledge-to-action' cycle consists of two key steps of knowledge translation. The *first step* is knowledge creation, which can be further considered as knowledge inquiry, knowledge synthesis and knowledge tools. The *second step* is the action cycle, which is the application of the knowledge to clinical settings. As knowledge moves from the inquiry phase to the action cycle phase, it becomes refined and increasingly clinically relevant.[3]

Knowledge Creation

Graham, et al.[4] describe knowledge creation as a funnel, whereby the endless amount of studies are filtered into the clinically relevant and useful information. Knowledge inquiry is the process of producing primary research studies and primary research can range from level I *randomized controlled trials (RCTs)* to level IV *case studies*. There exist an almost endless amount of clinical research produced in the world with varying accessibility and validity and the need for appraisal and further refinement is paramount.

Knowledge synthesis is the assessment and amalgamation of primary research into *systematic reviews*, with or without *meta-analysis*. Systematic reviews aim to combine and summarize the evidence on a specific topic in order to demonstrate overall outcomes and they are discussed further in chapter 11. High quality systematic reviews also include an element of critical appraisal, whereby they address the quality of the evidence in the studies that they review.[4]

Knowledge tools use systematic reviews to create practical clinical decision-making tools.[4] These tools include guidelines, decision aids and rules of care pathways.[4] The main purpose of knowledge tools is to present the information in a fashion that allows end-user application. Knowledge tools should provide explicit recommendations to clinicians, policy-makers and other stakeholders in order to effectively influence healthcare and they should be clear, concise and relevant.[4]

The Action Cycle

The action cycle consists of several phases, each of which are dynamic and may be influenced by the knowledge creation process.[1,4] These steps in the action cycle include: identifying the problem; identifying, reviewing and selecting the knowledge to implement; adapting or customizing the knowledge to local context; assessing the determinants of knowledge use; selecting, tailoring, implementing and monitoring interventions related to knowledge translation; evaluating outcomes or impacts of using the knowledge; and determining strategies for ensuring sustained use of knowledge.[1]

Identifying a problem and choosing relevant clinical research evidence is the first main step.[4] After this has been done, the evidence must be made relevant in a local context by considering how to apply it in the specific setting that is being discussed.[4] Generic recommendations, without context to local settings and population, will rarely be widely accepted.[4] Next is the assessment of barriers to the implementation of the knowledge, discussing strategies to overcome these barriers and identifying methods/strategies which is already in place to help.[4]

The planning and execution of the interventions should allow maximal awareness and promotion of the changes to the players that are involved.[4] Change is more likely to occur across a group if the knowledge tools being implemented are well-planned, promoted and focussed.[4] The ***action cycle*** does not stop after the interventions have been implemented. To be effective, the interventions must be continuously monitored and assessed, in order to determine how successful the intervention was.[4] Measurements of success should usually include an assessment of extent of the knowledge use and of the target outcomes.[4] If the intervention was not effective, potential barriers should be considered and the intervention should be modified.[4] The action cycle illustrates that assessment, evaluation and modification can occur constantly in order to optimize outcomes.[4]

The final step of the action cycle is to determine the sustainability of the knowledge. Similar to the evaluation of the implementation of the knowledge, barriers should be evaluated and the interventions should be modified to ensure long-term sustainability.[4] The evaluation of sustainability can provide feedback to the other steps in the action cycle.[4]

Why is Knowledge Translation Important?

Healthcare systems are constantly being challenged to apply evidence-based recommendations and improve patient outcomes, but evidence-based recommendations are often not applied effectively.[1,5] Straus, et al.[1] reported that evidence-based recommendations are not followed at many levels across the healthcare system, including healthcare providers, policymakers and even patients. Failure to follow evidence-based recommendation may lead to inefficient use of resources in resource-limited healthcare systems.[4] Schuster, et al.[6] demonstrated that only 60–70% of patients in the United States were managed according to the evidence-based recommendations.

It is becoming well-known that medical research is not being implemented in a timely fashion in clinical settings.[4,7] Healthcare systems across the world are beginning to emphasize evidence-based and cost-effective approaches to clinical practice.[4] By increasing the use of high-quality evidence, clinicians can improve the quality of healthcare and patient outcomes while reducing cost, unnecessary interventions and adverse effects.[3] Knowledge translation is an emerging and rapidly-growing field.

What are the Barriers to Effective Knowledge Translation?

There exist several barriers to effective knowledge translation and occur at all steps in the knowledge-to-action cycle.[1] In addition to lack of research training and funding for clinicians, the most important barrier to effective knowledge translation is the sheer volume of research produced each year. It is impossible for clinicians to synthesize and appraise all of the evidence that is relevant to their practice.[1,8] Systematic reviews often do not give clear recommendations to inform guidelines or influence practice.[1]

Barriers can occur at every level of the healthcare system.[1] They can include financial barriers at the system level, available equipment and human resources at an organizational level, adherence to practice guidelines by individual physicians and even adherence to physicians' recommendations by the patients.[1]

Important Learning Points

- Knowledge translation is the process of taking research findings, refining them and applying them to clinical practice.
- The knowledge-to-action cycle involves knowledge creation (which includes knowledge inquiry, knowledge synthesis and knowledge tools) and the action cycle.
- Knowledge translation is critical to ensure the implementation of high-quality evidence-based recommendations and optimize outcomes for patients in resource-limited health-care systems.
- There are many barriers to knowledge translation and they must be addressed in order for proper knowledge to action implementation.

More To Read

- Graham ID, Logan J, Harrison MB, et al. Lost in knowledge translation: time for a map? J Contin Educ Health Prof. 2006;26(1):13-24.
- Straus SE, Tetroe J, Graham I. Defining knowledge translation. CMAJ. 2009;181(3-4):165-8.

Definitions

Case study: In medicine, a case study is a detailed report about a single patient that clearly describes what the patient presented with, any interventions, treatments done and outcomes and follow-up.

Knowledge-to-action cycle: The process of applying primary research knowledge to clinical settings. Consists of two main steps: knowledge creation, further broken down into knowledge inquiry, knowledge synthesis and knowledge tools; and the action cycle.

Meta-analysis: Statistically combining quantitative data from several studies to yield a single pooled summary estimate.

Randomized controlled trials (RCTs): A study design to determine a cause-effect relationship between treatment groups and/or control group. RCTs involve randomization process to assign patients to each group.

Systematic review: The identification, selection, appraisal and summary of primary studies that address a focused clinical question using methods to reduce the likelihood of bias.

REFERENCES

1. Straus SE, Tetroe J, Graham I. Defining knowledge translation. CMAJ. 2009;181(3-4):165-8.
2. Canadian Institutes of Health Research. (2010) More about knowledge translation at CIHR. Website. Available from: www.cihr-irsc.gc.ca/e/39033.html. Accessed 2015 Apr 27.
3. Menear M, Grindrod K, Clouston K, et al. Advancing knowledge translation in primary care. Can Fam Physician. 2012;58(6):623-7.
4. Graham ID, Logan J, Harrison MB, et al. Lost in knowledge translation: time for a map? J Contin Educ Health Prof. 2006;26(1):13-24.
5. Kohn LT, Corrigan JM, Donaldson MS. To Err is human: building a safer health system. Washington (DC): National Academies Press (US); 2000.
6. Schuster MA, McGlynn EA, Brook RH. How good is the quality of healthcare in the United States? Milbank Q. 2005;83(4):843-95.
7. Waddell C. So much research evidence, so little dissemination and uptake: mixing the useful with the pleasing. Evid Based Ment Health. 2001;4(1):3-5.
8. Russell G, Geneau R, Johnston S, Liddy C, Hogg W, Hogan K: Mapping the future of primary healthcare research in Canada–A report to the Canadian Health Services Research Foundation. Ottawa: Canadian Health Services Research Foundation; 2007.

Glossary

A priori: A method of defining the aspects of the treatment and outcomes that will be analyzed, prior to beginning a clinical trial.

A priori hypothesis: A hypothesis generated which is takes place before the research study.

Absolute risk: The overall risk difference between receiving an intervention versus not.

Adjudication: When an outcome is determined by an independent person or group of individuals who are not involved in the study.

Adverse event: Any unfavorable or unintended sign, symptom or disease associated with the use of a medical interventions under investigation.

Allocation concealment: Methodological strategy to make sure that the person who is enrolling the participants in a randomized trial is unaware of to what study arm for the next participant will be assigned to.

Analysis of variance (ANOVA): A statistical test to determine, if there are any differences between the means of three or more groups.

Analytical studies: Studies that test a specific hypothesis about the relationship of a disease to a putative cause, by relating a particular exposure of interest to the disease or outcome of interest.

Anchor-based method: This method uses a reference as an anchor to determine if the changes in outcome are clinically important or not.

Anecdotal clinical evidence: Case-based information on a small number of patients.

Area under the ROC curve: The area used for determining the accuracy of a diagnostic test.

Ascertainment bias: It occurs when the results or conclusions of a trial are systematically distorted by knowledge of which intervention each participant is receiving.

Attrition bias: Systematic differences between the groups under study due to participants' withdrawals.

Benefit: Anything that results that is of value.

Bias: Systematic deviation from the underlying truth because of a feature of the design or conduct of a research study.

Binary data: It can only be classified as two categories like yes or no.

Biological plausibility: The proposal of a cause-and-effect relationship that is consistent with existing biological and medical knowledge.

Blinding (diagnostic studies): The index test and reference standard are assessed by interpreters who are unaware of the results of the other investigations.

Blinding (treatment studies): Condition of patients, clinicians and researchers participating in a study of being unaware of which participant were allocated to the intervention and control arm.

Bonferroni correction: A statistical method used to correct the consequences of multiple testing or multiplicity.

Case report form (CRF): A questionnaire used to collect data from each participant in a clinical trial.

Case report: A detailed description of the clinical experience of individual study subjects.

Case series: A collection of related case reports, consisting of patients with similar diagnosis and undergoing in the same treatment.

Case study: In medicine, a case study is a detailed report about a single patient that clearly describes what the patient presented with, any interventions and treatments done, outcomes and follow-up.

Case-control study: A study design in which a group of people with a certain disease, state or condition are identified first and then compared to a group without the disease, state or condition.

Categorical data: Data values fall into unordered categories or classes.

Certainty in the evidence: To what extent the estimates of effect or association for a particular outcome are close to the truth.

Clinical effectiveness: The application of interventions which have been shown to be efficaciously to appropriate patients 'in a timely fashion to improve patients' outcomes and value for the use of resources.

Clinical recommendations: Recommendations created by a development group that provide insight into the appropriateness and validity of any given intervention or treatment modality.

Clinical research nurse: Research professionals that focus on the care of patient participants, typically work in a hospital or medical facility setting.

Clinical trial monitor: Research professionals responsible for numerous activities in all phases of a clinical trial.

Clinical trial: A method of research designed to test an investigational product/device on human participants.

Closed response format: A survey response format that provides pre-coded responses for the respondent to choose from.

Closed-form items: Questions that are completed using a defined list of permissible responses.

Cochrane Collaboration: A non-profit organization that aims to provide current and readily available healthcare information worldwide.

Cohen's d: A common measure of effect size, i.e. the difference between two means divided by the standard deviation.

Co-interventions: Interventions other than the one under study that may affect the outcome of interest and when differentially applied, may introduce bias.

Comparison group: A group in a randomized controlled trial that receives no treatment.

Confidence interval (CI): The range of values within which there is a given probability that the true values lies. Usually, a 95% confidence interval is provided.

Confidentiality: The protection of a research subject's privacy.

Confounding bias: This type of bias is due to spurious associations resulting from imbalance in prognostic factors between groups.

Confounding variable: A variable or factor that is correlated with both the outcome and exposure. It therefore may appear to be directly causing the outcome because its value fluctuates in synchrony with the causative exposure.

Construct validity: The range of scores from the tool that are consistent with the hypothesis which is proposed before the test.

Content validity: The extent to which the items of the measurement instrument adequately reflect the construct being measured.

Continuous data: Data that represent measurable quantities but are not restricted to taking on certain specified values.

Contract research organization (CRO): A person or organization (commercial, academic, etc.) contracted by the sponsor to perform one or more of a sponsor's trial related duties and functions.

Correlation: The degree of which two continuous variables vary together.

Cost benefit analysis (CBA): A form of health economic evaluation in which the benefits are expressed in monetary terms.

Cost minimization analysis (CMA): A form of health economic evaluation where two comparative procedures with equivalent health outcomes are compared.

Cost utility analysis (CUA): A form of cost-effectiveness analysis where benefits are measured in terms of a utility measure such as the quality-adjusted life year (QALY).

Cost: The economic definition of cost (also known as opportunity cost) is the value of opportunity forgone (strictly the best opportunity forgone) as a result of engaging resources in an activity. Note, that there can be a cost without the exchange of money.

Cost-effectiveness analysis (CEA): A form of health economic evaluation where benefits are measured in terms of natural, disease-specific units such as cases which are successfully treated or the number of stroke averted.

CRF completion guidelines: A document providing unambiguous instructions on CRF, completion in all practical scenarios.

Criterion validity: The extent to which the scores of a utility outcome tool are an adequate reflection of the ***gold standard.***

Critical appraisal: Systematically judging the validity, applicability and methodological quality of research.

Data and safety monitoring board (DSMB): An independent group of experts that monitor and assess the collected data for patient safety and determine if it is safe for the clinical trial to continue or not.

Data queries: Non-sensible or questionable data that must be explained.

Data-dredging: The use of data mining is to identify statistically significant results within a data set that only occur by chance.

Debriefing: A thorough explanation of the objective and protocol of a research study, provided to the research subject after the study has concluded.

Decision-analysis: Explicit quantitative mathematical approach for prescribing conditions under conditions of uncertainty.

Delphi method: This method relies on the opinion of a panel of experts to reach a consensus on the minimal clinically important difference based on the best available evidence.

Demand: The quantity of a good buyers who wish to purchase at each conceivable price.

Dependent variable: The event being studied and expected to change with changes in the independent variable.

Descriptive studies: Studies that focus on describing the distribution of a disease in relation to factors such as age, location and sex.

Detection bias: Intention to look more carefully for an outcome in one of the intervention groups.

Direct costs: All resources that are consumed in the provision of a health promotion program. These may be incurred by the health promotion service, community or clients.

Discount rate: The rate chosen to express the strength of preference over the timing of costs and benefits (see discounting and time preference).

Discounting: The most widely accepted method of incorporating the time preference into the evaluation of a program when the costs and benefits do not occur at the same point of time.

Distribution method: This method uses statistical measures of spread to estimate the minimal clinically important difference.

Dose-response gradient: The demonstration of an incremental increase in response to a given treatment modality, as a result of incrementally increasing the dose.

Double-blinded study: A clinical trial in which both the patient and physician/investigators are masked from knowing which treatment group the patient is receiving.

Economic evaluation (economic appraisal): The comparison of alternative courses of action in terms of their costs and consequences, with a view of making a choice.

Effect size: The magnitude of strength of an association.

Effectiveness: The extent to which program achieve their objectives, in real-life settings.

Efficiency: Maximizing the benefit to any resource expenditure or minimizing the cost of any achieved benefit.

Eligibility criteria: The characteristics that will include or exclude potential participants.

Ethics approval: Any study involving living participants requires the approval of an ethics committee.

Ethics committee (EC): A committee that formally monitors all the research projects to make sure that they meet to ethical and scientific standards.

Evidence-based medicine (EBM): The integration of clinical expertize, patient values and the best research evidence into the decision making process for patient-care.

Exclusion criteria: A set of characteristics that preclude potential subjects from participating in a clinical study.

Exposure: Something where patients are exposed that may affect their health. This could either be a putatively harmful intervention or a beneficial one.

External validity: The extent to which a study can be generalized to other populations or situations.

Fisher's exact test and Chi-Square (χ^2) test: Statistical tests that determine how expected proportions are compare to observed proportions.

Forest plot: Graphical presentation that illustrates the magnitude of treatment effect or association between an experimental and control group. It is the most common graphic representation of meta-analysis.

Funding agency: Organizations that provide funding for research studies. An application must be completed, which is then reviewed by a committee that decides whether or not to award a researcher a grant.

Gold standard: A method having established or widely accepted accuracy for determining a diagnosis and providing a standard to which a new diagnostic test can be compared.

Grey literature: Reports that are produced by all levels of government, academics, business and industry in print and electronic formats but that are not controlled by commercial publishers.

Hawthorne effect: Refers to the phenomenon, where subjects tend to improve specific behaviors when they know they are being studied.

Health economics: The study of how scarce resources are allocated among alternative uses for the care of sickness and the promotion, maintenance and improvement of health, including the study of how healthcare and health-related services, their costs and benefits and health itself are distributed among individuals and groups in society.

Health economists: Individuals who study health economics.

Health: A state of complete physical, mental and social wellbeing and not merely the absence of disease or infirmity.

Hierarchy of evidence: A ranking system for health research where a variety of factors are considered, including study design and methodology, validity and quality of research. The ranking system consists of 5 levels, 1 being the highest quality of evidence and 4 or 5 being the low quality evidence.

Imprecision: Imprecision refers to the statistical assessment (typically confidence intervals) surrounding the measure of effect. If confidence intervals or other provided measures of variance are very large, the results may suffer from imprecision.

Incidence: The number of new cases of disease or outcome as a percentage of the total number of subjects in the group.

Inclusion criteria: A set of characteristics that potential subjects must fulfill in order to participate in a clinical study.

Inconsistency: Inconsistency refers to the heterogeneity of the estimated outcome effects from multiple studies. If results from multiple studies are variable even though they had the same research question, this may represent inconsistency.

Incremental cost-effectiveness ratio (ICER): Obtained by dividing the difference between the costs of the two interventions by the difference in the outcomes, i.e. the extra cost per extra unit of effect.

Independent variable: The variable that is being manipulated, i.e. expected to cause changes in the dependent variable.

Index test: The test under the evaluation in a study of a diagnostic test. It includes information gathering from the history, physical examination, function tests, laboratory tests, imaging tests and histopathology.

Indirect costs: These relate to the losses to society incurred as a result of participating in the program, such as the impact on production, domestic responsibilities, social and leisure activities.

Indirectness: It refers to the consistency across, included study research questions/ PICO statements. Studies included in the same body of evidence should all address the same research questions through a similar PICO statement (e.g. studies should all include the same patient population, intervention, comparator/control and outcomes) and if there is variability between studies, indirectness should be considered.

Informed consent form: A form signed and dated by a subject who voluntarily confirms his/her willingness to participate in a clinical trial. This form is signed and dated after the patient is informed all aspects of the trial that are relevant to the subject's decision to participate.

Informed consent: The process of providing sufficient information so that a participant can make an informed decision about whether or not to enroll in a study or to continue participation. It serves as a voluntary agreement to participate in a clinical research.

Institutional Review Board (IRB): A committee that formally monitors all research projects to make sure that they meet ethical and scientific standards.

Intention-to-treat analysis: Includes all randomized patients in the groups to which they were randomly assigned, regardless of their adherence with the entry criteria, regardless of the treatment they actually received and regardless of subsequent withdrawal from treatment or deviation from the protocol.

Interaction: A statistical test used to determine whether treatment effects differ across the subgroups.

Internal consistency: The degree of interrelatedness to which each individual test item measures the same construct.

Internal validity: It is the ability of the study results to support a cause-and-effect relationship between the treatment and the observed outcome. In other words, the observed difference in outcome between groups is attributable only to the effect of the intervention under investigation.

International Conference on Harmonization of Good Clinical Practice (ICH-GCP): The ICH-GCP guideline was developed to provide a unified standard for the European Union, Japan and United States, as well as those of Australia, Canada, the Nordic countries and the World Health Organization (WHO). Good clinical practice (GCP) is standard for the design, conduct performance, monitoring, auditing recording analyses and reporting of clinical trials that provides assurance that the data and reported results are credible and accurate and that the rights, integrity and confidentiality of trial subjects are protected.

Inter-rater reliability: The degree of agreement between scores given to patients by two or more raters.

Interval data: Interval data is classified into categories where we know not only the order, also the exact differences are known between the values, but there is no true zero.

Intra-rater reliability: The degree of agreement across different times with respect to a single rater.

Item: A question in a survey. It is comprized of two components: stem and response format.

Knowledge-to-action cycle: The process of applying primary research knowledge to clinical settings. Consists of two main steps: **knowledge creation**, further broken down into knowledge inquiry, knowledge synthesis and knowledge tools; and **the action cycle**.

Knowledge users: Groups of people for which the results of a study are likely to be useful for making clinical decisions, such as patients, healthcare professionals and policymakers.

Language/country bias: Bias due to only including in a systematic review studies published in certain languages or countries.

Latency period: The period of time between a specific exposure and the development of symptoms of a diseases.

Likelihood ratio: The relative likelihood that a given test would be expected in a patient with a condition of interest, as opposed to one without the condition.

Linear regression: A statistical analysis to predict a continuous dependent variable based on one or more independent variables.

Logistic regression: A statistical analysis to predict a binary dependent variable based on one or more independent variables.

Magnitude of effect: The extent of impact that the intervention has on the population.

Markov model: A particular type of decision analysis that allows the transfer between the different health states over a period of time.

Mean difference: Statistic that measures the absolute difference between the mean in two groups that are compared. This difference in means can be used as summary statistic in meta-analysis for continuous outcomes that were measure using the same scale among included studies.

Mean: The sum of values divided by the number of values in the data set.

Measure of central tendency: Measure that describes the central position of the data set using a single value.

Measurement error: The difference between the true value and the value obtained from a certain measurement.

Measuring instrument: An instrument that shows the extent or degree of something; ensures accuracy in measurement.

Median: It is the number in a data set that falls in the middle so that half of the values lie above and below this number.

Medical Subject Headings (MeSH): A **controlled vocabulary thesaurus** developed by the National Library of Medicine that organizes sets of terms using keywords, facilitating the formation of literature searches with varying levels of specificity.

Meta-analysis: Statistically combining quantitative data from several studies to yield a single pooled summary estimate.

Micro-costing: An estimate is made for each element of resource which is using within the program and a unit cost is derived for each.

Minimal clinically important difference: A difference that would be considered meaningful and worthwhile by a patient and one that would make them consider for repeating the treatment if it their choice to make again.

Missing participant data: Outcome data for trial participants whose status on the outcome of interest is unknown.

Mode: The value that occurs most frequently in a data set.

Multiplicity: The act of testing multiple hypotheses simultaneously. It also referred to as multiple testing.

Narrative review: An article that reviews literature (such as a book chapter) that is not conducted by using methods to minimize bias and is not reproducible.

Negative predictive value: The proportion of patients with a negative test who truly do not have the condition (d/c+d).

Nominal data: Nominal data is classified into categories, but does not have an inherent order or scale.

Non-responder bias: When differences in the characteristics of responders and non-responders leads to inaccurate results and inferences. This is usually a concern when response rate is too low.

Nuremberg Code: 10 rules made after WWII that are known as the original guidelines for research ethics.

Odds ratio: The ratio of the odds of development of disease in exposed individuals to the odds of development of disease in non-exposed individuals.

Open response format: A survey response format that allows the respondent to respond in their own words.

Open-form items: Questions that do not have a defined list of permissible responses.

Opportunity cost: The cost of a unit of a resource is the benefit that would be derived from using it in its best alternative use.

Optimal information size: The number of patients required to develop an adequately powered randomized controlled trials.

Ordinal data: Ordinal data is classified into categories and has an inherent order.

Outcome: An indicator of health status that will be used to assess the difference between the treatment and/or control groups.

Paired t-Test: A statistical test to determine if there is a difference between two means using paired data.

Patient-important outcome: An outcome that is valued by the patient as well as the physician.

Peer review: A process that many, if not most, scientific journals use to ensure that journal articles are of adequate quality for publication. Usually, two or more experts in the discipline evaluate and comment on the submitted manuscript and the authors have a chance to revise the manuscript based on the peer reviewers' comments.

Performance bias: Systematic differences are introduced to the intervention or control group in the clinical care that they receive or other factors that these groups may be exposed to, aside from the interventions under study.

Perspective: The point of view from which an analysis is carried out. The social welfare perspective consider costs and benefits from the point of view of society.

PICO: Refers to patient/population, intervention, comparator and outcomes. It is a tool used to identify the research questions of a project.

Pilot study: A small scale preliminary study conducted before the main research in order to check the feasibility or to improve the design of the research.

Pilot-testing: Administering the survey to a sample of the target population to identify any changes that need to be made. This is done before the main administration takes place.

Placebo: Biologically inert substance that is as similar as possible to the active intervention. Placebo allows implementing blinding.

Podium presentation: A formal scientific presentation, either by invitation or by peer review, at a conference or meeting.

Population of interest: The specific group of people that the researcher is interested in making inferences about from the study.

Positive predictive value: The proportion of patients with a positive test who have the condition (a/a+b).

Post-hoc analysis: The act of creating and testing hypotheses after the research study has been conducted.

Glossary

Post-test probability: The probability of having the target condition after the application of a diagnostic test.

Power: The probability of rejecting a false null hypothesis. It is inversely proportional to Type II error (β).

Present values: The today's value of future costs or benefits (after adjusting by discounting).

Pre-test probability: The probability of having the target condition before the application of a diagnostic test.

Prevalence: The total number of cases of a disease that exist at a given point of time.

Primary outcome: The observation that is most clinically relevant in determining the effect of the intervention on key variables in the study; the outcome of greatest importance.

Principal investigator (PI): The person that assumes responsibility for the conduct of a clinical trial.

Prognostic balance: Balance achieved by randomizing participants to the study arms in relation to their biological, psychological and social characteristics, which confer increased or decreased risk of a favorable or unfavorable outcome. In addition, other unknown characteristics that may influence the outcome are also balanced by randomization.

Prognostic factors: Baseline factors or characteristics of a subject which may influence their risk of developing the outcome of interest. These can unfortunately act as confounders when they are not balanced between the groups in the study.

Prognostic imbalance: A lack of similarity of prognostic characteristics between the groups being studied. For example, if age is a prognostic factor then great differences in the age distribution of participants between the two groups would be considered prognostic imbalance.

Protocol: A document describing the purpose, background, design, methods and organization of a clinical trial.

Publication bias: Bias due to the selective publication of research depending on the direction of the study results and whether they are statistically significant.

Qualitative interaction: The treatment effect is beneficial to one subgroup and harmful to another.

Quality-adjusted life years (QALYs): Calculated by adjusting the estimated number of life-years, an individual is expected to gain from an intervention for the expected quality of life in those years. The quality of life score will range between 0 for death and 1 for perfect health, with negative scores being allowed for states which is considered worse than death.

Quantitative interaction: The treatment effect is beneficial or harmful to all subgroups but the magnitude of the effect is different across the subgroups.

Random allocation: Allocation of participants to groups under comparison by random chance.

Random error: Unavoidable influence of chance in any measure conducted. The larger the sample size, the smaller the random error and the more precise the results.

Random sampling: A sampling technique in which individuals for a study sample are selected by chance.

Randomization: Allocation of participants to groups under comparison by random chance.

Randomized controlled trials (RCTs): A study design to determine a cause-and-effect relationship between treatment groups and/or control group. RCTs involve randomization process to assign patients to each group.

Rate: The number of events in those at risk for the event divided by the total follow-up person time.

Ratio data: Ratio data is continuous data that has order, a meaningful scale and there is a true zero.

Receiver-operator curve: A graphical method for determining the best cut-off for a diagnostic test.

Recursive search: The process of reading the reference lists of studies included in a review to determine whether or not they should also be included in the review.

Reference standard: The best available method for establishing the presence or absence of the condition of interest and serves as the ***truth*** in a study of a diagnostic test. It can include laboratory tests, imaging tests, pathology and clinical follow-up.

Regression: A statistical method used to determine whether relationships exist between specified variables or not.

Relative risk: The ratio of the risk of disease in exposed individuals to the risk of disease in non-exposed individuals.

Reliability: The consistency of the data and its interpretation.

Reporting guidelines: Tools developed to guide researchers on reporting research accurately and in a standardized manner.

Research coordinator: The **hub** of the clinical trial; liaises between principal investigator, clinical research team, sponsor, sites and study-subjects.

Research Ethics Board (REB): A committee that formally monitors all research projects to make sure that they meet ethical and scientific standards.

Research ethics: Rules for researchers to follow the separate acceptable and unacceptable behavior when conducting research.

Research misconduct: The fabrication, falsification or plagiarism in proposing, performing or reviewing research or in reporting research results.

Research question: The question that the investigator(s) intend to answer using research methodology. Developing a clear research question is the first step in conducting a research project.

Residual confounding: Refers to the fact that some unaccounted prognostic characteristics remain unbalanced even after statistical adjustment and attempts at balancing between groups. It is due to the presence of prognostic factors that are unknown to the investigator; this is inevitable in cohort studies.

Resources: Things that contribute to the production of output. Money gives a command over resources but is not a resource per se.

Response format: The component of a survey item that provides the framework for the answer.

Risk of bias: The potential of a study to have been adversely impacted by unintended or non-ideal circumstances.

Sample size: The number of participants or experimental units included in a clinical research study.

Sampling error: The probability that the sample is not representative of the population from which it is drawn.

Sampling: The method employed by the researcher for selecting individuals for the study sample.

Scarcity: There will never be enough resources to satisfy human that wants completely.

Scientific method: A process of investigation that is the foundation of scientific inquest.

Secondary outcome: An outcome believed to be related to the primary outcome and is used in addition to the primary outcome.

Selection bias: Presence of any systematic difference between the baseline characteristics of participants allocated to the groups under the study in a randomized controlled trials.

Selective citation bias: Bias, due to only including articles that contain certain results in a systematic review.

Selective outcome reporting: Inclination of authors to differentially report research results depending on their relevance rather than what it was actually measured.

Self-administered survey: Surveys that are administered with no personal interaction between the surveyor and respondent while being conducted.

Sensitivity analysis: A process through which the robustness of an economic model is assessed by examining the changes in results of the analysis when key variables are varied over a specified range.

Sensitivity: The proportion of patients with a given condition who have a positive test (a/a+c).

Sham surgery: Similar to a placebo, this is when a subject believes that they have had a surgical procedure performed but in reality it had not.

Single-blinded study: A clinical trial in which only the patient is unaware of the treatment group, he/she is a part of.

Smallest effect size of interest: The difference between study groups that the investigator determines to be of scientific and clinical interest.

Source documents: The original documents, data and records concerning study participants.

Specificity: The proportion of patients truly free of a given condition who have a negative test (d/ b+d).

Spectrum bias: When the patients enrolled in the research study and do not represent the appropriate patient population.

Spurious result: A wrongful inference suggesting two events or variables have a causal relationship, when in fact they do not. It is also known as Type I error.

Standard deviation: The standard deviation is the average difference between each value in the set and the cumulative mean.

Standardized mean difference: Meta-analytic summary statistic used when the included studies assess the same outcome but measure them in a variety of ways. To solve this, it is necessary to standardize the results of the studies in a uniform scale to be combined. This statistic represents the effect size of the intervention expressed in standard deviation units.

Stem: The question or statement component of an item in a survey.

Stopping rule: It is a part of the interim analysis and is used as a guide to terminate the clinical trial as soon as there is an indication for one of the treatment groups being inferior to the other.

Stratified randomization: The act of subgrouping a patient population based on a certain variable prior to randomly allocating them to a treatment group.

Study design: The methodology behind a clinical study, which can be defined and based on the characteristics of the study (randomization, control groups included, etc.)

Study flow diagram: A visual representation of the numbers of patients at each stage of a study, including screening, allocation, follow-up and analysis.

Study rationale: A detailed explanation of the reasons that why research on given topic is necessary.

Subgroup analysis: Act of comparing treatment effects between subgroups to identify any differences.

Subgroup: A population within the study sample that can be categorized by some sort of differential quality; ideally a baseline characteristic.

Surrogate outcomes: An outcome that is closely related that is used to make inferences about the outcome in question.

Surveillance bias: It occurs when the assessors follow and examine one cohort more closely than the other. This can be avoided by blinding assessors to which group is receiving the exposure.

Survival analysis: A statistical analysis to predict the time to an event-based on one or more independent variables.

Systematic review: The identification, selection, appraisal and summary of primary studies that address a focused clinical question using methods to reduce the likelihood of bias.

Test-retest reliability: The reliability of a test administrated at different times.

Time lag bias: The rapid or delayed publication of research findings, depending on the nature and direction of the results.

Time preference: Individuals are not indifferent to the timing of costs and benefits, preferring benefits sooner and costs later.

Trial registration: The act of recording information about a planned trial in an official trial registry (such as clinicaltrials.gov or EudraCT database) to improve transparency regarding reporting of clinical trials.

t-Test: A statistical test to determine if there is a difference between two means.

Type I error: Incorrect rejection of the null hypothesis and concluding a relationship exists between two variables when in fact it does not. It is also known as a spurious result.

Type II error: Incorrect acceptance of the null hypothesis and concluding no relationship exists between two variables when in fact it does.

Utility: A measure of the ***satisfaction*** (benefit) obtained from the consuming goods and services.

Validity: How well the data collected by the survey instrument reflects what the researcher set out to measure.

Variability: The standard deviation of an outcome of interest within the study population.

Verification bias: Bias caused by the results of the diagnostic test, which can influence whether the patients are assessed with the reference standard or not.

Weighted analysis: Taking into account the sample size and number of events of the studies included in a meta-analysis; bigger studies have a greater effect on the overall result than smaller studies.

Willingness to pay (WTP): This technique asks people to state explicitly the maximum amount they would be willing to pay to receive a particular benefit. It is based on the premise that the maximum amount of money an individual is willing to pay for a commodity which is an indicator of the value to them of that commodity.

Withdrawal: When the participant discontinue his or her participation in an ongoing research study. Subjects have the right to withdraw their participation from research study at any time.

Index

Page numbers followed by f and t indicate figures and tables, respectively.

A

Academic institutions 24
Accumulation of trials 12
Allocation concealment 165, 173
American medical association 325
Analytical studies 38
Anchor-based method 224
Anecdotal clinical evidence 96, 106
Arm, disability of 211, 214
Arthroscopic partial meniscectomy 281
Ascertainment bias 43, 49
Attrition bias 168, 173
Authors, instruction to 334

B

Background context 313
Barriers, assessment of 341
Bias
　assessing risk of 170
　in body of evidence 104
　in randomized controlled trials 163
　type of 164t
　risk of 170, 174, 176, 178, 186
Bibliographic database 16
Binary
　data 242, 250
　outcomes 231, 237
Biological plausibility 257, 260
Bloodletting 4
Body of evidence, certainty in 103
Bonferroni correction 256, 260
Breastfeeding, risks of 292
Budget and timeline 195

C

Canadian agency for drugs and technologies in health 120
Canadian institutes of health research 339
Cancer stages 242
Case-control study 63
Causation, evidence of 58
Central tendency, measure of 243, 250

Childbearing potential 291
Chi-square test 250
Chronic myofascial pain syndrome 57t
Classical test theory 149
Clinical case
  series 72
    limitations of 74
    strengths of 73
Clinical expertise, integration of 10
Clinical heterogeneity 17
Clinical research
  associate 270
  nurse 270-272
    roles of 270
  process of 298
  proposal 191
Clinical superiority trial 234
Clinical trial
  aspects of 271
  efficiently 267
  monitor 269, 272
  site selection 270
Closed response format 82, 88
Closed-form items 304
Clustered samples 239
Cochrane
  collaboration 7
  library databases 16
  review 16
  risk of bias tool 170, 171t
Cohort study 36
  disadvantage of 56
  rank 55
Cohorts prior, selection of 56
Common statistical tests 247t
Commonly used reporting guidelines 325t
Comparison group 74, 78
Concurrent medications 299
Conducting literature search 16
Conducting systematic review, process of 96
Confounder, exposure and outcome, relationship between 58f
Confounding bias 56-58, 60, 61
Consensus-based standards 159
Consent document, version number of 288
Consent forms, elements of 287
Consolidated health economic evaluation reporting standards 125
  statement 328
Construct validity 209, 215
Content validity 208, 215
Contingent valuation 121
Contract research organization 269, 272
Control group 41, 42
Controlled trials 40
Correlation analysis 248
Cost benefit analysis 111, 113, 126
Cost-effectiveness analysis 112, 113, 126
  plane 114

Cost-minimization analysis 111, 112, 126
Costovertebral angle 136
Cost-transfer, accounts for 118
Cost-utility analysis 112, 115, 126
Cover letter 334
Credible systematic reviews 103
Criterion validity 209, 215
Critical appraisal 19
Critically appraise
  case-control studies 67
  literature 17
  published economic evaluation 124
Cruciate ligament, anterior 137
Curriculum vitae 192

D

Data
  analysis 195
  and safety monitoring board 47, 49, 196
  collection plan 195
  monitoring committee 196
  queries 299
Data-dredging 254, 260
Debriefing 281
Deceiving/misleading research subjects, ethics of 280
Decision-analysis 126
Delphi method 224
Demand 126
Dependent variable 195, 198
Descriptive statistics 243
Descriptive studies 38
Design requirements 160
Detection bias 167, 173
Determining survey composition 82
Deterministic sensitivity analysis 124
Diabetics with frozen shoulder, hypothetical study of 327
Diagnosis and diagnostic tests, probability of 135*f*
Diagnostic accuracy studies 325*t*
  statement, standards for reporting of 328
Diagnostic test 41, 136
  properties of 141*t*
  study 133
    basics of 133
Direct costs 126
Discharge details 299
Discrete choice experiment 122
Disprove hypotheses 297
Distribution method 224
Dose-response gradient 182, 185
Double-blind study 43, 50
Drug 265
  composition of 319
  development of new 24

E

Economic
  appraisal 126

evaluation 126
basics of 110
reviews 325*t*
Education and research 12
Efficient study design 74
Enroll, order to 279
Ensuring investigator product compliance 271
Ensuring running, capable of 267
Equivalence interval 229
Ethical concerns 48
Ethical considerations 196
Ethically sound 74
Ethics
approval 191, 198
committee 268, 273, 277, 281, 287
European organization for research and treatment of cancer core quality of life questionnaire 121
Evidence
different types of 35
limitations, conclusions, summary of 326
hierarchy of 23, 33, 38, 40, 64
Evidence-based
clinician 14
medicine 3, 9, 13, 14, 22, 24, 28, 33, 64
origins of 3
virtues of 9
Existing video-assisted thoracic surgery 114
Experiment, development of 317

F

Fair subject selection 278
FDA regulation, according to 266
Federal regulations, code of 266
Fetal
chromosomal abnormalities 135
toxicity of similar drugs 292
File upload section 336
Fisher's exact 246
test 250
Floor and ceiling effects 82
Food and drug administration 293
Forest plot 100, 107
Formula, calculation by 232
Function tests 146
Funding agency 191, 198

G

Generic and disease-specific outcome tools 211
Generic outcome tools 209, 210
Good clinical practice 272, 286
Good data form, components of 298
Great slide presentation 310
Grey literature 98, 107

H

Hand, disability of 211, 214
Hawthorne effect 60, 61
Health 110, 126

economic 18, 110, 126
  and health economic evaluation 110
  evaluation, types of 111
  measurement instruments, selection of 159
  outcomes, monetary value for 121
  research, transparency of 329
  state valuations 122f
  utilities index 121, 213
Healthcare
  advancement of 316
  quality of 342
Health-related quality of life 120
Heterogeneous sample of people 151
Hip fractures, risk of 64
Hypothesis
  formulation of 317
  generation 73
  testing 219t, 229, 246
Hypothetical data for meta-analysis 101t
Hypothetical meta-analysis 102f

I

Iatrogenic harm 18
Imaging tests 146
Incident cases 65
Incremental cost-effectiveness ratio 114, 127

Independent ethics committee 286
Indirect costs 122, 127
Indirect method 121
Individual autonomy, principle of 284
Individual studies, summary of 22
Individual without disease 140
Information provided 232
Informed consent 279, 295
  form 268, 272
    alteration of 283
  serves 283
Institutional review board 268, 273, 277, 281, 286, 318
Instrument development 81
Interest, conflict of 335
Interim analysis 45
Internal consistency 207, 215
International committee of medical journal editors 335
International conference on harmonization of good clinical practice 270, 272
International council on harmonization 286
Interpreting health economic evaluation results 115f
Inter-rater reliability 215
Intervertebral disc herniation 26
Interviewer bias 86

Intraclass correlation coefficient 157, 160, 239
Intra-rater reliability 207, 215
Involves symptomatic pain 15

J

Jewett hyperextension orthosis 17

K

Kappa statistic, categories for 157t
Knowledge
　creation 340, 343
　dissemination of 316
　implementation of 341
　purpose of 340
　translation 339
　　barriers to effective 342
　　important 342
　　plan 196
　users 329
Knowledge-to-action 339
　cycle 343
　framework 339

L

Language/country bias 99, 107
Life and health utility outcome tool 205
　common quality of 205
　types of 209
Literature on topic 298
Literature review 193
Logistic regression 247, 250
Low-density lipoprotein 65
Low-quality evidence 34
Lung cancer 118

M

Magnetic resonance imaging 137, 214
Manuscript 334
　for publication 270
Markov model 117, 127
Mean and standard deviations 244f
Meaningful analysis 303
Measurement error 150, 161, 206, 215
Measuring instrument 202, 204
Medical
　charts, previous 67
　evidence, hierarchy of 55
　history, baseline 299
　literature 21
　　plenty of 22
　　uses of 21
　　quality of 21, 23
　subject headings 321, 322
Medicine, conventional 10
Medicolegal issues 12
Merits and concerns 48
Meta-analysis, basics of 95
Minimally-invasive deformity surgery, effect of 73
Missing participant data 173
Mnemonic SnNOut 138

Monitoring patient safety and wellbeing 271
Musculoskeletal disorder 57t

N

Narrative and systematic reviews, comparison between 97t
Narrative review 96, 107
    for informing decision-making 106
National institutes of health 275
Navigate online submission process 335
Necessary regulatory documents 270
Negative predictive value 138
Negative test 140
Negligence, liability for 284
New England journal of medicine 325
Newer antibiotic drugs 10
Non-cardiac conditions 66
Nonpharmacological trial 48
Non-responder bias 85, 89
Novel procedure or treatment 73
Novel robotic-assisted thoracic surgery 114
Novel surgery 118
Null and alternative hypothesis of clinical superiority 230t
Number of clinical trials 270

Nuremberg code 281
    creation of 276

O

Observational studies 325t
Observer effect 60
Observer expectancy 59
Open fractures, treatment of 72
Open response format 89
Opportunity cost 118, 127
Optimal information size 180, 186
Orthopedic
    RCTS, evidence in 26
    research 25
    spine 15
        surgeon 14
    surgery 14, 17
        literature 24
Oxford hip score 120

P

Pain
    improvement in 18
    resolution of 18
Paired t-test 248, 250
Participant withdrawal 289
Patient
    demographic details 298
    health, information on 133
    important outcome 204
    informed consent 283
    population 15
Patient-important outcomes 202

Patient-rated wrist evaluation 215
Penicillin, discovery of 10
Performance bias 166
Pharmacy, doctor of 267
Philosophy, doctor of 267
Physical
　examination 146
　injury 290
Physicians, important for 3
Pilot-testing 83, 89
Placebo 78, 167, 173, 318
　ethics of 74
Plagiarism in proposing 280
Playing, capable of 312
Podium presentation 309, 315
Pooled standard deviation 249
Positive predictive value 138
Positive test 139
Post-hoc analysis 254, 260
Post-test probability 134, 146
Potential benefits 292
Potential drug interactions 290
Practice makes perfect 313
Pragmatic reflection of clinical practice 73
Pregnancy 291
Pregnant women, sample of 135
Prepare manuscript for submission 333
Pre-test probability 134, 141, 146
Priori hypothesis 253, 260
　small number of 253
Probabilistic sensitivity analysis 124
Prognostic
　balance 166, 173
　factors 55, 61
　　balance of 41
　　imbalance 56, 61
Prospective cohort study 53, 54
　limitations of 55
Protocol and case report form development 270
Protocol papers 325t
Psychological capability 285
Publication
　bias 99, 107
　standard criteria for 21

Q

Qualitative interaction 257, 260
Quality adjusted life years 120, 127
Quality improvement 12
Quantitative interaction 260
Quickdash 214

R

Radiographs/imaging, previous 67
Random allocation 165, 174
Random assignment 42
Random error 102, 107
Random sampling 85, 89

Randomized controlled trial 7, 8, 9, 25, 33, 35, 53, 63, 72, 98, 116, 178, 321, 325t, 340, 343
Rating publication bias 179
Rating study limitations 178
RCT in orthopedics 25
RCT study designs 45
Recall bias 68
Receiver operating characteristic curves 143
Region/disease-specific outcome tools 210
Reliability 150
 basics of 149
 coefficient 150
 study 159
  characteristics of 155
 versus validity 153f
Renaissance era 4
Reporting bias 169
Reporting guidelines 324, 329
 being aware of 329
Reporting trials
 consolidated standards of 25, 47, 321
 statement, consolidated standards of 326
Research coordinator 267, 273
 responsibilities of 268
 roles of 267
Research ethics 275, 281
 board 268, 273, 275, 277, 281, 318
 main pillars of 278
 origins of 276

Research involving human subjects, types of 283
Research method 84
Research misconduct 280, 281
Research protocol 189
Research question 19, 80, 84, 89, 177
Research study
 funding source of 288
 purpose and design of 288
Research, understanding of 283
Research-related injury 288
Residual confounding 57, 61
Respondent bias 86
Response format 81, 89
Retrospective cohort study 54
Retrospective design 75
Retrospective studies 63
Reviewing eligibility criteria 271
Rheumatoid arthritis 214
Right study design 31
Roland-Morris disability questionnaire 17
R-squared value 248
Running title 336

S

Safety of human participants, guidelines for 270
Sample selection 41
Sample size estimations 234f, 236f
Sampling bias 57, 59

Sampling error 85, 89
Sampling technique 85, 89
Scientific method 317, 322
Scientific validity 278
Screen studies 98
Scurvy 5
Section outline 189
Selecting alpha and power, effects of 221
Sensitivity
   analyses 124, 128
   and specificity 137
Serum 136
Sham procedure 167
Sham surgery 281
Shoulder, disability of 211, 214
Single-blinded 43
   study 50
Smoking 118
Sound rationale 253
Source documents 304
Spectrum bias 135, 147
Spinal stenosis 26
Spine patient outcomes research trial 26
Spurious result 254, 261
Standard deviation 225, 232, 243, 251
Statistical
   methods 160
   power 64
Stopping rule 45, 50
Stratified randomization 255, 261
Study
   comparability 119
   design 45, 176, 186, 194
      types of 34
   details/comments section 336
   flow diagram 330
   limitations of 85, 195
   population, demographics of 319
   question 116
   rationale 193, 198
   results, sharing 292
   themselves, types of 12
Subgroup analyses 252, 261
   from different studies, compare results of 259
   performed 257
   reported 258
Subjective data 67
Sudden occlusion syndromes 9
Supporting documents 335
Surgical interventions 112*f*
Surgical treatments, participants to 26
Surgical trials, randomization in 27
Surrogate outcome 181, 186
Survey 79
   administration 86
   design 86
   developed 80
   development of 80
      steps in 81*f*
   important in clinical research 80
   research, quality of 87
   results reported 84
Survival analysis 249, 251

Symptomatic atherosclerotic disease 9
Systematic methodology 13
Systematic review 22, 95, 96, 108, 340, 344
 advantages of 98
 and meta-analysis 325*t*
 basics of 95
 limitations of 99
 of healthcare interventions 7
Systolic blood pressure 232

T

Techniques, comparisons of 26
Thoracolumbar, operative treatment of 18
Time lag bias 99
Treat analysis, intention to 42, 44, 50, 169, 173, 329

Treatment, alternative sources of 291

U

Undergo bypass surgery 9
Urine 136

V

Validated medical research 21
Verification bias 136, 147
Vitamin C, deficiency of 5
Voluntarily consent 276

W

Well-designed and poorly-designed data fields, comparing 301*t*
Willingness to pay 113, 115, 121, 128